Controversies in Vascular Neurosurgery

Erol Veznedaroglu
Editor

Controversies in Vascular Neurosurgery

Springer

Editor
Erol Veznedaroglu, MD, FACS, FAHA, FAANS
Chairman Department of Neurosurgery
Drexel University College of Medicine
Director Drexel Neuroscience Institute
Philadelphia, PA
USA

ISBN 978-3-319-27313-6 ISBN 978-3-319-27315-0 (eBook)
DOI 10.1007/978-3-319-27315-0

Library of Congress Control Number: 2016945033

Printed on acid-free paper

This Springer imprint is published by Springer Nature
The registered company is Springer International Publishing AG Switzerland

Preface

Vascular neurosurgery has seen an unprecedented level of advancement in the last decade. The progress of endovascular treatments has allowed safer, easier access to pathology untreatable in the past. With this advancement, controversy and diverging philosophies have left many practitioners confused as to what is best practice, or even appropriate. The genesis of *Controversies in Vascular Neurosurgery* was based on providing the practitioner a concise easy-to-use guide on current controversies with a practical approach. All too often, physicians leave didactic sessions that discuss controversies feeling that they have gained little more than an overview of a topic without any true guidance on how to manage a difficult disease entity. The philosophy of this book is to provide insight into the best *combined* approach with direction from those who are experts in the field and many of whom use all the tools available themselves. Clearly there is not nor will there ever be one uniform approach for difficult neurovascular pathology. Having access to a concise source of information that discusses what the different tools are and how best to use them is paramount to understanding the ever-evolving field of vascular neurosurgery.

Topics covered include some of the most challenging from a data and patient selection standpoint in modern medicine today. For the first time in modern medicine, devices and advancements in treatment have surpassed available data to support or challenge its use. In treatment of acute stroke, most of our current data is from a pre-perfusion imaging era. The ability to obtain complete revascularization safely is no longer the issue, but what patients do we select. A better understanding of AVM natural history has given pause to past treatment paradigms, despite having meaningful advancements in treatment. The authors have been carefully chosen to provide a true balanced vantage point of treatment paradigms that they themselves use, thus the ability to understand the thought process of the surgeons' approach to a specific challenging disease where there may be no one right path. The development of new technology lends itself not only to the expansion of treatment options, but also to the use of these treatment options that may not in fact lend itself to the best overall outcome or result. The use of flow diverters for cerebral aneurysms is covered with not only the most appropriate use but also avoidance of use that does not necessarily provide the best choice of treatment.

After over a decade of involvement in teaching controversy courses, hands-on sessions, and publications on the subject, it was evident that one reliable source to provide a practical and useful guide is sorely lacking. The basis of management of these complex diseases is looking at it from a treatment of disease standpoint using all available tools, not from what surgical option is best. The common coil versus clip is an antiquated and political notion. The modern surgeon looks at the disease and thinks of what tools he or she has that allows best outcome. The format of this book is based on this concept. Each chapter has a specific disease, and it is discussed by experienced surgeons who discuss their approach and thought process involved. The conclusion will be an evaluation by a third author who will provide best evidence and pearls in the treatment of that disease. The true benefactor of this book will be the patient; our biases as physicians should never become a patient's morbidity.

Philadelphia, PA, USA Erol Veznedaroglu

Contents

Paraclinoid Aneurysms: Who to Treat with Craniotomy?

1

Amit Singla, Kyle M. Fargen, and J. Mocco

Introduction

The term "paraclinoid aneurysms" was first used by S Nutik to identify the aneurysms arising from internal carotid artery (ICA) opposite to the origin of the ophthalmic artery (OA) [39]. Since that time, various anatomical landmarks have been used to define these aneurysms.

In the Bouthhillier classification of ICA into seven segments, the clinoidal segment (C5) begins at the proximal dural ring and ends at the distal dural ring where the ICA becomes intradural. The ophthalmic segment (C6) begins after the clinoidal segment (C5) of the ICA and ends proximal to the origin of posterior communicating artery [8]. The clinoidal segment of the ICA extends between the proximal and distal dural ring. These aneurysms arising from the clinoidal segment of the ICA may expand through the distal dural ring and project intradurally. Batjer et al. used the term "paraclinoid aneurysms" for aneurysms arising from the segments of the ICA (C5–C6) between the roof of the cavernous sinus and the origin of the posterior communicating artery. This definition is most commonly used in the current literature to describe paraclinoid aneurysms. These aneurysms have a common close relationship with the bone of the skull base and with the dural folds around the ICA, and they are frequently large and giant.

A. Singla, MD
Department of Neurosurgery, Covenant Medical Center, Waterloo, IA, USA

K.M. Fargen, MD, MPH
Department of Neurosurgery, Medical University of South Carolina, Charleston, SC, USA

J. Mocco, MD, MS (✉)
Department of Neurological Surgery, Cerebrovascular Center, Mount Sinai Health System, New York, NY, USA
e-mail: j.mocco@mountsinai.org

E. Veznedaroglu (ed.), *Controversies in Vascular Neurosurgery*,
DOI 10.1007/978-3-319-27315-0_1

Classification of Paraclinoid Aneurysms

Various classification systems have been proposed for paraclinoid aneurysms [3, 4, 13, 14]:

Day classified paraclinoid aneurysms into two broad categories with one group referred to as "OA aneurysms," which arise from the ICA just distal to the origin of the ophthalmic artery. The other group was referred to as "superior hypophyseal artery aneurysms" which was further classified into paraclinoid and suprasellar variants based on the direction of projection of the aneurysm. The paraclinoid variant projects inferiorly and the suprasellar variant projects medially or superomedially above the diaphragma sellae into the suprasellar space [13].

Batjer et al. further classified paraclinoid aneurysms into three groups: (i) carotid OA aneurysms arising just distal to the ophthalmic artery and projecting superiorly or superomedially, (ii) superior hypophyseal aneurysms arising from the medial or inferomedial wall of the carotid artery and projecting medially, and (iii) proximal posterior carotid aneurysms arising from the posterior or posterolateral wall of the carotid artery (a.k.a ventral ICA aneurysms) with no apparent vessel of origin [4].

De Jesus et al. proposed separate classifications for C6 and C5 ICA segment aneurysms. They classified ophthalmic segment (C6) aneurysms topographically into medial, posterior, and anterior varieties based on location of the aneurysm's neck on the ophthalmic segment of the ICA or into ophthalmic, superior hypophyseal artery, and posterior paraclinoid aneurysms, based on the arterial bifurcation point at which the aneurysms arise. Aneurysms of the C5 segment were classified into medial, lateral, or anterior, depending on the surface of the ICA from which they originate. They originate without an apparent branch site of the ICA [14].

Based on the cerebral angiographic findings, Barami et al. classified paraclinoid aneurysms in four different types [3]. We believe that this classification system is most descriptive and helpful in the treatment planning.

- Type I: Origin from the dorsal surface of the ICA
  - Type Ia: Aneurysms are closely related to the ophthalmic artery (OA) origin.
  - Type Ib: Aneurysms have no branch relation and are often sessile.
- Type II: Origin from the ventral surface of the C6 segment of the ICA, no branch relation.
- Type III: Origin from the medial surface of C5 and C6 segments, are closely related to the superior hypophyseal artery (SHA) origin (seen best on the antero-posterior view of the carotid arteries).
  - Type IIIa from C6 segment of the ICA, above the dural reflection.
  - Type IIIb from C5 segment of the ICA, below the dural reflection.
- Type IV: Origin from the ventral clinoidal and ophthalmic segment of the ICA. They had no branch relations and widened the distal dural ring.

Microsurgical Versus Endovascular Treatment

With the development of latest technological advancements in endovascular techniques, there is a significant paradigm shift toward endovascular treatment for paraclinoid aneurysms. However, obliteration of the large/giant paraclinoid aneurysms with endovascular treatment has a lower success rate for total occlusion [30, 35]. Even with the advent of the latest endovascular techniques such as flow diverter stents, paraclinoid aneurysms remain a formidable challenge for vascular neurosurgeons. Thence, microsurgery still has a significant role in their management for certain indications.

Some of the indications for which microsurgical management remains a strong consideration include:

- Multiple aneurysms with distal aneurysms unsuited for endovascular management
- Ruptured aneurysms with anatomy not amenable for stand-alone coiling
- Aneurysms associated with hematoma which needs evacuation
- Progressive visual compromise due to mass effect from the aneurysm

Patients with paraclinoid aneurysms with other distal aneurysms not well suited for endovascular treatment or with hematoma from ruptured paraclinoid aneurysms needing evacuation may best be managed with microsurgery. Ruptured paraclinoid aneurysms with complex morphology such as those with a lower dome/neck ratio, which are not suitable for stand-alone coiling, are often better managed with microsurgery. The use of a stent or flow-diverting stents in such patients necessitates the use of antiplatelet medications, such as aspirin and clopidogrel, which may be undesirable in the setting of subarachnoid hemorrhage due to the frequent need for surgical procedures.

The significant incidence of increased mass effect after coiling resulting in worsening of the visual symptoms favors surgical decompression in patients presenting with progressive visual compromise [47]. Conceptually flow-diverting stents such as the Pipeline™ or SILK™ stent have shown promise in such a group of patients as no coils are placed in the aneurysm cavity itself thereby limiting mass effect. However, the literature on visual outcomes with the use of flow-diverter stents remains limited at this time.

Some of the relative contraindications for the endovascular management of complex, broad-based paraclinoid aneurysms include:

1. Resistance or contraindication to antiplatelet medications
2. Size <10 mm (off-label use for flow-diverter device)
3. Tortuous anatomy with difficult access via endovascular techniques
4. Patient's desire for immediate aneurysm occlusion
5. Patient's reluctance or inability to have close angiographic follow-up
6. Large or giant aneurysms at hospitals with unavailability of flow-diverter technology or the personnel trained in using flow-diverter devices

Adequate platelet inhibition is important in the prevention of in-stent thrombosis and re-stenosis making it imperative to ensure that adequate antiplatelet effects are achieved in patients undergoing stent placement. This is especially important for flow-diverting stents due to the high percentage of wall coverage with metal. Platelet inhibition from aspirin and clopidogrel varies broadly, and some patients are classified as being "resistant" or low responders if their platelet inhibition is inadequate. In these patients who are "resistant" to the standard antiplatelet regimen, placement of the intracranial stents can significantly increase the incidence of thromboembolic complications [32, 42]. These patients may be better managed with microsurgical techniques. Likewise, patients with tortuous anatomy or atherosclerotic plaques along the ICA may have increased endovascular procedural risk, and therefore these patients may be better suited for microsurgery.

Some patients, especially those with a family history of ruptured brain aneurysms, may be anxious about aneurysmal rupture and may want to achieve aneurysm occlusion as soon as possible. In those patients, microsurgical techniques should be offered. Further, endovascular treatment mandates close follow-up with angiography to evaluate for recurrence. The patients who are reluctant to undergo follow-up or in whom follow-up angiography may be contraindicated may prefer to have the aneurysm microsurgically clipped. The availability of the resources and the personnel trained in the latest endovascular techniques such as flow-diverting stents may further influence decision making, as not all endovascular treatments may be available depending on treating center.

The efficacy of endovascular coiling for large or giant and partially thrombosed aneurysms is yet to be established because of their high recurrence rates. A retrospective series of large unruptured ophthalmic aneurysms associated with visual compromise treated with endovascular coiling reported only 50 % near complete occlusion and 37.5 % significant aneurysm residual. Only 50 % of patients had complete aneurysm occlusion at the final follow-up in 16 patients; 7 patients needed carotid sacrifice due to continued aneurysm filling [27]. Addition of a stent to the endovascular coiling for large/giant carotid aneurysms has not been shown to improve aneurysm occlusion rates. A series on 15 large and giant carotid aneurysms treated mostly with stent-assisted coiling reported only 47 % complete or nearly complete occlusion at last follow-up; 80 % of patients required retreatment [26].

Surgical Treatment

The surgical options available for aneurysms difficult to treat with endovascular techniques include:

- Surgical clipping
- Trapping with or without a bypass procedure

Balloon Test Occlusion

Although occlusion of an intracranial aneurysm with preservation of the parent artery is the desired outcome during aneurysm surgery, it may not always be feasible. Often the aneurysms are large or giant with broad necks, have a calcified wall, or the necks are ill defined which may make surgical reconstruction challenging. In such cases, endovascular or surgical carotid occlusion might be a more reasonable and definitive treatment option. Balloon test occlusion (BTO) should be performed in such instances to assess collateral circulation to prevent ischemic complications prior to performing carotid occlusion as a definitive treatment [28, 36]. Serbienko has been credited with the novel technique of temporary arterial balloon occlusion for assessing cerebrovascular reserve. Complete angiography with and without compression of the involved carotid artery to assess the collateral circulation is recommended when BTO is planned [28].

For BTO, patients undergo digital subtraction angiography (DSA) with a 30-min period of temporary ICA occlusion using a balloon, including a 10-min period of induced hypotension, during which mean arterial pressure is lowered by 20–30 % of baseline value. Intravenous heparin is administered during the procedure to maintain the activated clotting time of 250–300s to decrease the likelihood of thromboembolic complications. During BTO, the patients undergo serial clinical examinations to detect any neurological changes and the collateral circulation is assessed. In addition, many techniques have been described in the literature such as single-photon emission CT (SPECT) and xenon CT perfusion scans to further evaluate cerebrovascular reserve besides the clinical assessment [3]. Further management is dependent on the patient's ability to tolerate the test clinically and adequacy of collateral cerebral circulation without any perfusion defects on SPECT; permanent occlusion of the ICA and trapping of the aneurysm can be performed relatively safely in such cases. Sekhar et al. used a range of cerebral blood flow measurement with xenon-CT examination to determine the revascularization need. They recommended revascularization if patients develop neurological deficits or if CBF is 15–35 mL/100 g per minute or less even in the absence of neurological deficits. No revascularization was recommended for patients with cerebral blood flow (CBF) of >35 mL/100 g per minute [50]. Nevertheless, carotid occlusion even after a successful BTO with no intraoperative neurological changes and with a normal SPECT is not completely safe and carries a 15–20 % risk of development of ischemia/infarction [49]. If the patients have failed the BTO with clinical examination or through supplementary investigations, they require a revascularization procedure with a bypass graft [50].

Carotid Ligation

Historically, the treatment for intracranial aneurysms started with carotid ligation when Horsley ligated bilateral carotid arteries in a patient who was operated for a suspected tumor but was found to have an intracranial aneurysm. Thereafter, proximal surgical ligation became the primary treatment modality for intracranial aneurysms for decades [17]. A large series of 461 patients with carotid artery ligation was published by Sahs and Locksley with reported mortality of 20.7 % and a 30 % stroke rate [45]. The efficacy of carotid ligation in inducing thrombosis within an aneurysm is reported to be inversely proportional to the degree of collateral circulation and decreases with more distal aneurysm location along the ICA. Paraclinoid aneurysms may be treated effectively with carotid ligation; however, the likelihood of thrombosis is reported to be slightly less than the aneurysms located along more proximal ICA segments because of the potential for retrograde flow through the ophthalmic artery [19].

The ischemic complications following carotid ligation can arise from thromboembolism or hypoperfusion. The incidence of ischemic complications after ICA ligation is possible due to thrombus which forms in the lumen of ICA from the point of occlusion to first important branching point, usually the ophthalmic artery. Due to the turbulent retrograde flow through the ophthalmic artery, emboli may break off of the top of the intraluminal thrombus and can cause distal thromboembolism. Another potential complication with carotid ligation is de novo aneurysm formation with new aneurysms reported in 1–10 % of patients undergoing carotid ligation [9]. However, carotid ligation remains a viable option in a carefully selected patient when the other reconstructive options are deemed less safe.

Microsurgical Management

Preoperative Planning

The adjacent complex neurovascular and bony anatomy makes the microsurgical treatment of paraclinoid aneurysms technically challenging. The success of the microsurgical treatment correlates to a multitude of factors such as establishing control of the proximal artery, adequate exposure of the aneurysm neck with or without anterior clinoidectomy, and successful obliteration of the aneurysm with minimal manipulation of the surrounding nerves. Preoperative imaging studies are carefully assessed for size and position of the aneurysm neck and determine the relation of the aneurysm neck to the surrounding structures. The timing and extent of the surgical bony drilling and the technique of proximal control should be the part of the preoperative planning. The extent of the removal of anterior clinoid, extra- versus intradural resection of anterior clinoid, and removal of the optic strut are still the areas of debate without clear consensus. Many believe that removal of the anterior clinoid, roof of the bony optic canal, and the optic strut is important for satisfactory exposure and safe clipping [13, 14].

Intraoperative Neuromonitoring

Intraoperative neuromonitoring is performed with somatosensory evoked potentials (SSEP) with median nerve stimulation and electroencephalography (EEG). Cerebral protectants can be administered if intraoperative neuromonitoring demonstrates slowing or asymmetry. EEG is also used to demonstrate burst suppression and help optimize the cerebral protection with the use of cerebral protectants.

Intraoperative Angiography

Intraoperative angiography is important particularly with paraclinoid aneurysms because of the difficulty in visualizing the aneurysm neck and working around the optic nerve. Intraoperative angiography is planned prior to the craniotomy by either inserting the femoral sheath or prepping the groin for later insertion of femoral sheath depending on personal preference.

Surgical Exposure

The patient is positioned supine with the head rotated to the contralateral side 40° to improve the lateral view under the optic nerve and extended only about 15–20° (more extension can steepen the view to the aneurysm). The head is fixated with a three-point skeletal fixation device such as Mayfield clamp. A standard pterional craniotomy is sufficient for the majority of cases especially for small aneurysms. A curvilinear skin incision starts at the zygomatic arch 1 cm anterior to the tragus and curves to the midline, just behind the hairline. Frontotemporal pterional craniotomy is performed with two burr holes using 4 mm round cutting or the M8 drill bit; one in the squamous temporal bone and another in the "key hole" region. In the elderly patients due to thin and adherent dura three to four burr holes are drilled and dura is carefully separated from the undersurface of the bone using a combination of blunt dissection and elevators. The craniotomy is completed using the craniotome. The craniotomy extends from the temporal burr hole inferiorly and then arcing anteromedially lateral to the supraorbital notch and then connecting with the "key hole" burr hole. The drill is used to take off the lesser wing of the sphenoid medially to the superior orbital fissure, with a flat surface over the orbit connecting the anterior and middle cranial fossae. Cranial base modification with orbital and/or zygomatic osteotomy is generally performed in cases with large or giant aneurysms. We prefer to perform modification of orbitozygomatic (OZ) craniotomy in such cases, as generally for paraclinoid aneurysms, only orbital osteotomy is required for adequate exposure. When performing orbital osteotomy, the periorbita is separated from the superior and lateral orbital rim using blunt dissection. The superior orbital rim is cut perpendicularly using the saw and the cut is then extended to the inferior orbital fissure carefully protecting the dura on one side and the periorbita on the other. The lateral orbital rim is cut inferiorly close to its junction with the floor of the orbit directed toward the inferior orbital fissure to complete the orbital osteotomy.

Proximal Control

The timing and the technique of proximal control depends on the size, morphology of the aneurysm, its relationship to the surrounding structures, and experience of the operating surgeon. Proximal control of these aneurysms is difficult due to their intimate relationship with the skull base and anterior clinoid process. Various sites for proximal control include [31]:

(a) Exposure of the cervical ICA is recommended as a routine for proximal control in large and giant aneurysms. In small aneurysms in which the neck is visible on angiography, typically the neck is prepped only without surgical exposure of the ICA [11, 37].

(b) Exposure of the petrous ICA in the floor of middle cranial fossa extradurally after the craniotomy. The middle fossa floor is drilled along the course of the canal of petrosal nerve. Petrous bone over the ICA is unroofed up to where the carotid artery turns vertically to prevent injury to the cochlea. The temporary occlusion is then achieved using the surgical patties (Fukushima technique) or with the Fogarty catheter (Spetzler technique) [2].
(c) Exposure of the cavernous ICA can be achieved after opening the distal dural ring. However, as the aneurysm is encountered first with this technique with the potential for rupture, this technique is less favored.
(d) Endovascular techniques with placement of the balloon in the cervical ICA using the transfemoral approach. Simultaneous retrograde suction decompression can be performed for large/giant aneurysms. This is becoming more common now with the improvement in the endovascular techniques [20].

Techniques of Proximal Control/Methods to Reduce Aneurysm Size

Paraclinoid aneurysms are often large and have a tendency to compress the adjacent optic apparatus. The adequate visualization of the aneurysm neck and reconstructing the parent vessel without occluding important arteries are important for successful clip obliteration of the aneurysm. Even with extensive bone removal with anterior clinoidectomy and optic canal roof drilling, the neck of the aneurysm can still be difficult to define. This often requires decompressing aneurysm size for giant and large aneurysms so that the clipping can be performed safely. Various techniques have been described over the years for adequate decompression of the large/giant paraclinoid aneurysms.

Proximal control by clamping the carotid artery in the neck may not adequately decompress the dome due to collateral filling of the aneurysm through the ophthalmic artery and cavernous branches [4]. Direct puncture followed by "suction decompression" of large and giant aneurysms via a No. 21 butterfly-type scalp vein needle described by Flamm was reported to adequately decompress the aneurysm [23]. However, it is technically challenging and may lead to bleeding if the needle accidentally slips out of the aneurysm at the moment of clip application [4]. This technique is still practiced by some surgeons. Good results were recently reported with direct aneurysm puncture with or without aneurysmotomy to decompress the optic nerves during clipping of visually symptomatic aneurysms [15].

In 1990, Batjer and Samson described the alternative technique of retrograde suction decompression (RSD) of the aneurysm via surgical exposure and placement of the vascular clamp across the cervical ICA. For distal occlusion, the temporary clip was applied on the supraclinoid ICA proximal to the posterior communicating artery origin. Direct cannulation of the cervical ICA with an 18-gauge angiocatheter was then performed followed by gentle aspiration using a 20-ml syringe. They reported success in achieving aneurysmal collapse and clipping in more than 40 cases using retrograde suction decompression. One elderly patient with severe extracranial and intracranial atherosclerosis suffered an arterial dissection which necessitated emergency carotid endarterectomy [5]. Fan et al. suggested the revised technique where instead of direct clamping and cannulating of the ICA, the CCA and ECA were isolated, and suction decompression was carried out via the ECA [22].

A year later after the original open technique of RSD was described, Scott et al. suggested an endovascular way of RSD based on the similar principles [48]. The cervical ICA is reached via a transfemoral approach with a 5-Fr 100-cm double lumen occlusion balloon catheter. The balloon is inflated in the ICA proximal to the paraclinoid aneurysm. A temporary clip is placed across the ICA proximal to the posterior communicating artery. The aneurysm is then collapsed by gentle aspiration through the distal lumen of the balloon catheter. Since the initial description, several authors have utilized this technique with some variations [2, 38]. The endovascular technique of RSD obviates the need for exposure of the carotid artery in the neck, and the intraoperative angiogram can be performed simultaneously. However, the endovascular adjunct can potentially result in additional complications such as thromboembolic complications and vessel dissection [2, 21, 38]. One recent single-center series found no statistically significant difference in complications between ophthalmic artery aneurysms treated with and without endovascular suction decompression [24].

Anterior Clinoidectomy

The anterior clinoid process (ACP) is the continuation of the lesser sphenoid wing, which is bridged to the sphenoid body by the optic strut (forming the floor of the optic canal) and the roof of the optic canal. It is located on the superomedial aspect of the superior orbital fissure. Anterior clinoidectomy can be performed extra- or intradurally without a clear consensus for the superiority of one over the other. Both the intradural and the extradural clinoidectomies require elevating the dura to the orbitotemporal periosteal fold (OTPF) a.k.a meningo-orbital band, which is located at the lateral aspect of the superior orbital fissure.

Extradural Clinoidectomy

For extradural clinoidectomy, OTPF is cut sharply to develop the plane between the temporal dura and the connective tissue covering the superior orbital fissure. The dura is elevated further posteriorly with using microdissector to expose the superior and the lateral aspect of the ACP. Extradural clinoidectomy along with unroofing the optic canal and the resection of optic strut is performed using the high-speed 3 mm diamond drill. The advantages of extradural clinoidectomy include having the dura as a brain protectant while drilling and avoiding contamination of the subarachnoid space with the bone dust [6, 33]. The disadvantages include not having the control on the aneurysm in case of accidental rupture during drilling and limited exposure of the aneurysm [37].

Intradural Clinoidectomy

After the sphenoid wing is flattened and the OTPF is reached by elevating the dura, the dura is opened sharply using a no.15 scalpel in the C-shaped fashion and reflected with the base at the Sylvian fissure. The Sylvian fissure is opened with the Arachnoid knife to expose the aneurysm. The aneurysm neck is then inspected to determine the need for anterior clinoidectomy. Small aneurysms can often be clipped by sectioning the falciform ligament without the need for anterior clinoidectomy or optic strut resection. However, in most cases, the ACP will have to be resected along with the optic strut and deroofing the optic canal for proper visualization. A small flap of dura is created around the ACP and optic nerve canal, which is used to protect the aneurysm during drilling. The advantages with intradural clinoidectomy include direct visualization of the aneurysm dome and adjacent neurovascular structures; the need for and the extent of clinoidectomy can be determined [37], and it provides improved exposure of ophthalmic segment aneurysms [1].

Subsequent Bony Exposure and Distal Dural Ring Dissection

After the anterior clinoidectomy, the optic canal is unroofed with the high-speed drill with a 2 mm round diamond-tip drill bit. The thinned out bony roof is then elevated with a microdissector away from the optic nerve. This helps in the early decompression of the optic nerve. Copious irrigation during the drilling can decrease the chances of heat injury to the optic nerve. Similarly, the optic strut is drilled with the high-speed drill. The distal dural ring is then incised lateral to the optic sheath. The distal dural ring is anterior to the origin of the ophthalmic artery, and the artery should be elevated before the cut in the distal dural ring to prevent the injury to the artery. Opening the distal dural ring anchoring the ICA reveals the proximal portion of the aneurysm neck.

Aneurysm Dissection/Clipping

Ophthalmic artery aneurysms have their neck on the superior carotid wall with the dome projecting upward. The ophthalmic artery origin is defined and carefully separated from the aneurysm neck. Mostly, the incision along the upper half of the distal dural ring is sufficient to expose the aneurysmal neck in large aneurysms. Proximal control at this stage can help soften the aneurysm and can make the visualization of the aneurysm neck easier. Superior hypophyseal artery aneurysms are more complex because of their inferomedial orientation and require a more circumferential distal dural ring incision.

The side-angled clip is optimal for ophthalmic aneurysms so that the clip blades lay parallel to the ophthalmic segment of the ICA. For small ophthalmic artery aneurysms, the straight clip might be sufficient. Superior hypophyseal artery aneurysms are better clipped with the angled fenestrated clip due to their inferomedial orientation.

Indocyanine green (ICG) angiography is performed to confirm aneurysm occlusion and flow preservation in the surrounding vasculature. The intraoperative angiogram is also performed to confirm the aneurysm occlusion after clipping. The closure is performed in the standard fashion.

Surgical Outcomes

Due to their unique location with close proximity to neurovascular structures, complex morphology with often large/giant configuration, and difficult proximal control, paraclinoid aneurysms pose considerable challenge to the operating neurosurgeon. Historically, they have been associated with high morbidity and mortality [7, 14, 16]. Drake et al. reported good outcomes (GOS score of 4 or 5) in only 40 % of patients (with 14 paraclinoid aneurysms) following microsurgery, while 60 % of patients died [18]. However, the refinements in microsurgical techniques have greatly improved surgical safety with subsequent clinical series demonstrating better outcomes for paraclinoid aneurysms [10, 43]. Hoh et al. reported that combined surgical and endovascular treatment of paraclinoid aneurysms resulted in excellent or good outcomes in 90 % of the 145 surgically treated aneurysms [29].

Complications

Visual Outcomes

Large and giant paraclinoid aneurysms can be symptomatic with visual disturbances due to their close proximity to the anterior visual apparatus. Monocular blindness can result from the mobilization of the optic nerve, compromise of the perforators to the optic nerve, or the heat injury to the optic nerve. In the majority of cases, the visual symptoms can improve or remain stable following clipping [12, 13]; often they can get worse following surgery [37]. However, coiling does not appear to be superior than clipping with respect to visual outcomes. In fact, there are numerous case reports and series suggesting against the use of coils in visually symptomatic large to giant aneurysms [41, 46, 51, 52]. A recent meta-analysis showed improvement in visual outcomes in 70 % patients after surgical clipping and 43 % patients after coiling; worsening was seen in 9 % patients after clipping and 26 % patients after coiling [47]. Surgical clipping was the only variable that was significantly associated with improvement of visual symptoms[56]. Microsurgery carries an advantage of immediate optic nerve decompression, which is specifically effective in patients with acute hemorrhages. Endovascular coil embolization may not provide symptomatic relief due to chronic optic nerve compression in such symptomatic cases [27].

Recently, an article on the visual outcomes after flow-diverter stent covering the ophthalmic artery for ICA aneurysms reported a high rate (39.3 %) of new ophthalmic complications. The initial angiogram showed normal ophthalmic artery patency in 24/28 cases (85.7 %) [44]. Another concern with the use of flow diverting stent is the increase in aneurysm size further increasing the associated mass effect [25] which may cause ophthalmoplegia and visual loss due to cranial nerve compression.

Intraoperative Aneurysm Rupture

Intraoperative aneurysm rupture is reported to occur ranging from 0.8 % to 14.3 %; most frequently, this occurs during dissection of the aneurysm. In case of large/giant aneurysms, they can be adherent to the gyrus rectus, and inadvertent lifting of the frontal lobe can result in intraoperative aneurysmal rupture. Careful dissection of the aneurysm dome should be performed under proximal control with temporary clipping to manage this complication [11, 34, 36].

Cranial Nerve Palsies

Cranial nerve palsies are commonly reported in the range of 5–25 % following treatment of paraclinoid aneurysms both after clipping and coiling. They have been attributed to injury during clinoid removal, clip blade advancement, or overzealous sinus packing. Fortunately, most of them are transient [14, 29, 40].

ICA Occlusion and Ischemia

Dolenc et al. reported an unplanned ICA occlusion rate of 2.8 % with no neurological deficits [16], and later Hoh et al. reported 2 % morbidity related to unplanned ICA occlusion in 180 microsurgical treatments of paraclinoid aneurysms [29]. The incidence of ICA occlusions can be lowered with the use of a variety of clips, including angled fenestrated clips. The use of intraoperative neuromonitoring and angiography can help in early detection and in lowering the incidence of postoperative ICA thrombosis.

Cerebrospinal Fluid Rhinorrhea

Cerebrospinal fluid (CSF) rhinorrhea can occur when frontal or ethmoidal sinuses are opened during the craniotomy or drilling of the pterion or when the optic strut is pneumatized. The temporalis muscle can be folded and packed into the optic strut tightly to decrease the incidence of CSF rhinorrhea. Bone cement or temporalis muscle strip can be used to obliterate the sinuses if opened.

Mortality

Operative mortality (death during the first 30 days after surgery, related or not to surgical procedure) from surgical treatment in patients with paraclinoid aneurysms ranges from 0% to 17.6% [11, 20, 24, 29, 37]. ICA occlusion is most likely the cause for operative mortality [11].

Conclusions

The advancement in endovascular techniques has revolutionized the treatment of paraclinoid aneurysms. However, microsurgery remains an important treatment option for a subset of patients presenting with aneurysms in this location. Patients with multiple ipsilateral aneurysms, those with ruptured paraclinoid aneurysms associated with a hematoma, patients with visual loss secondary to optic apparatus compression, and those with subarachnoid hemorrhage and in which stand-alone coiling techniques are insufficient may be better suited to open surgical clipping. Further, additional relative contraindications toward endovascular treatment may favor microsurgical treatment. Careful surgical planning in regard to proximal control, understanding the adequacy of collaterals, need for bony drilling for neck exposure, and careful dissection around the important adjacent neurovascular structures are paramount to surgical success.

References

1. Andaluz N, Beretta F, Bernucci C, Keller JT, Zuccarello M. Evidence for the improved exposure of the ophthalmic segment of the internal carotid artery after anterior clinoidectomy: morphometric analysis. Acta Neurochir (Wien). 2006;148(9):971–5. doi:10.1007/s00701-006-0862-x; discussion 975–976.
2. Arnautovic KI, Al-Mefty O, Angtuaco E. A combined microsurgical skull-base and endovascular approach to giant and large paraclinoid aneurysms. Surg Neurol. 1998;50(6):504–18; discussion 518–520.
3. Barami K, Hernandez VS, Diaz FG, Guthikonda M. Paraclinoid carotid aneurysms: surgical management, complications, and outcome based on a new classification scheme. Skull Base. 2003;13(1):31–41. doi:10.1055/s-2003-820555.
4. Batjer HH, Kopitnik TA, Giller CA, Samson DS. Surgery for paraclinoidal carotid artery aneurysms. J Neurosurg. 1994;80(4):650–8. doi:10.3171/jns.1994.80.4.0650.
5. Batjer HH, Samson DS. Retrograde suction decompression of giant paraclinoidal aneurysms. Technical note. J Neurosurg. 1990;73(2):305–6. doi:10.3171/jns.1990.73.2.0305.
6. Beretta F, Andaluz N, Zuccarello M. Aneurysms of the ophthalmic (C6) segment of the internal carotid artery: treatment options and strategies based on a clinical series. J Neurosurg Sci. 2004;48(4):149–56.
7. Boet R, Wong GK, Poon WS, Lam JM, Yu SC. Aneurysm recurrence after treatment of paraclinoid/ophthalmic segment aneurysms – a treatment-modality assessment. Acta Neurochir (Wien). 2005;147(6):611–6. doi:10.1007/s00701-005-0524-4; discussion 616.
8. Bouthillier A, van Loveren HR, Keller JT. Segments of the internal carotid artery: a new classification. Neurosurgery. 1996;38(3):425–32; discussion 432–423.
9. Briganti F, Cirillo S, Caranci F, Esposito F, Maiuri F. Development of "de novo" aneurysms following endovascular procedures. Neuroradiology. 2002;44(7):604–9. doi:10.1007/s00234-001-0732-4.

10. Cawley CM, Zipfel GJ, Day AL. Surgical treatment of paraclinoid and ophthalmic aneurysms. Neurosurg Clin N Am. 1998;9(4):765–83.
11. Colli BO, Carlotti Jr CG, Assirati Jr JA, Abud DG, Amato MC, Dezena RA. Results of microsurgical treatment of paraclinoid carotid aneurysms. Neurosurg Rev. 2013;36(1):99–114. doi:10.1007/s10143-012-0415-0; discussion 114–115.
12. Date I, Asari S, Ohmoto T. Cerebral aneurysms causing visual symptoms: their features and surgical outcome. Clin Neurol Neurosurg. 1998;100(4):259–67.
13. Day AL. Aneurysms of the ophthalmic segment. A clinical and anatomical analysis. J Neurosurg. 1990;72(5):677–91. doi:10.3171/jns.1990.72.5.0677.
14. De Jesus O, Sekhar LN, Riedel CJ. Clinoid and paraclinoid aneurysms: surgical anatomy, operative techniques, and outcome. Surg Neurol. 1999;51(5):477–87; discussion 487–478.
15. de Oliveira JG, Borba LA, Rassi-Neto A, de Moura SM, Sanchez-Junior SL, Rassi MS, . . . Giudicissi-Filho M. Intracranial aneurysms presenting with mass effect over the anterior optic pathways: neurosurgical management and outcomes. Neurosurg Focus. 2009;26(5), E3. doi: 10.3171/2009.3.FOCUS0924.
16. Dolenc VV. A combined transorbital-transclinoid and transsylvian approach to carotid-ophthalmic aneurysms without retraction of the brain. Acta Neurochir Suppl. 1999;72:89–97.
17. Drake CG. Earlier times in aneurysm surgery. Clin Neurosurg. 1985;32:41–50.
18. Drake CG, Vanderlinden RG, Amacher AL. Carotid-ophthalmic aneurysms. J Neurosurg. 1968;29(1):24–31. doi:10.3171/jns.1968.29.1.0024.
19. Elhammady MS, Wolfe SQ, Farhat H, Ali Aziz-Sultan M, Heros RC. Carotid artery sacrifice for unclippable and uncoilable aneurysms: endovascular occlusion vs common carotid artery ligation. Neurosurgery. 2010;67(5):1431–6. doi:10.1227/NEU.0b013e3181f076ac; discussion 1437.
20. Eliava SS, Filatov YM, Yakovlev SB, Shekhtman OD, Kheireddin AS, Sazonov IA, . . . Okishev DN. Results of microsurgical treatment of large and giant ICA aneurysms using the retrograde suction decompression (RSD) technique: series of 92 patients. World Neurosurg. 2010;73(6), 683–87. doi: 10.1016/j.wneu.2010.03.017.
21. Fahlbusch R, Nimsky C, Huk W. Open surgery of giant paraclinoid aneurysms improved by intraoperative angiography and endovascular retrograde suction decompression. Acta Neurochir (Wien). 1997;139(11):1026–32.
22. Fan YW, Chan KH, Lui WM, Hung KN. Retrograde suction decompression of paraclinoid aneurysm – a revised technique. Surg Neurol. 1999;51(2):129–31.
23. Flamm ES. Suction decompression of aneurysms. Technical note. J Neurosurg. 1981;54(2):275–6. doi:10.3171/jns.1981.54.2.0275.
24. Fulkerson DH, Horner TG, Payner TD, Leipzig TJ, Scott JA, Denardo AJ, . . . Goodman JM. Endovascular retrograde suction decompression as an adjunct to surgical treatment of ophthalmic aneurysms: analysis of risks and clinical outcomes. Neurosurgery. 2009;64(3 Suppl), ons107–11; discussion ons111–102. doi: 10.1227/01.NEU.0000330391.20750.71.
25. Hammoud D, Gailloud P, Olivi A, Murphy KJ. Acute vasogenic edema induced by thrombosis of a giant intracranial aneurysm: a cause of pseudostroke after therapeutic occlusion of the parent vessel. AJNR Am J Neuroradiol. 2003;24(6):1237–9.
26. Hauck EF, Welch BG, White JA, Replogle RE, Purdy PD, Pride LG, Samson D. Stent/coil treatment of very large and giant unruptured ophthalmic and cavernous aneurysms. Surg Neurol. 2009;71(1):19–24. doi:10.1016/j.surneu.2008.01.025; discussion 24.
27. Heran NS, Song JK, Kupersmith MJ, Niimi Y, Namba K, Langer DJ, Berenstein A. Large ophthalmic segment aneurysms with anterior optic pathway compression: assessment of anatomical and visual outcomes after endosaccular coil therapy. J Neurosurg. 2007;106(6):968–75. doi:10.3171/jns.2007.106.6.968.
28. Heros RC, Nelson PB, Ojemann RG, Crowell RM, DeBrun G. Large and giant paraclinoid aneurysms: surgical techniques, complications, and results. Neurosurgery. 1983;12(2):153–63.
29. Hoh BL, Putman CM, Budzik RF, Carter BS, Ogilvy CS. Combined surgical and endovascular techniques of flow alteration to treat fusiform and complex wide-necked intracranial

aneurysms that are unsuitable for clipping or coil embolization. J Neurosurg. 2001;95(1):24–35. doi:10.3171/jns.2001.95.1.0024.

30. Hope JK, Byrne JV, Molyneux AJ. Factors influencing successful angiographic occlusion of aneurysms treated by coil embolization. AJNR Am J Neuroradiol. 1999;20(3):391–9.
31. Kattner KA, Bailes J, Fukushima T. Direct surgical management of large bulbous and giant aneurysms involving the paraclinoid segment of the internal carotid artery: report of 29 cases. Surg Neurol. 1998;49(5):471–80.
32. Kim B, Kim K, Jeon P, Kim S, Kim H, Byun H, . . . Jo K. Thromboembolic complications in patients with clopidogrel resistance after coil embolization for unruptured intracranial aneurysms. AJNR Am J Neuroradiol. 2014;35(9), 1786–92. doi: 10.3174/ajnr.A3955.
33. Kim JS, Lee SI, Jeon KD, Choi BS. The pterional approach and extradural anterior clinoidectomy to clip paraclinoid aneurysms. J Cerebrovasc Endovasc Neurosurg. 2013;15(3):260–6. doi:10.7461/jcen.2013.15.3.260.
34. Kumon Y, Sakaki S, Kohno K, Ohta S, Ohue S, Oka Y. Asymptomatic, unruptured carotid-ophthalmic artery aneurysms: angiographical differentiation of each type, operative results, and indications. Surg Neurol. 1997;48(5):465–72.
35. Lanzino G, Wakhloo AK, Fessler RD, Hartney ML, Guterman LR, Hopkins LN. Efficacy and current limitations of intravascular stents for intracranial internal carotid, vertebral, and basilar artery aneurysms. J Neurosurg. 1999;91(4):538–46. doi:10.3171/jns.1999.91.4.0538.
36. Liu Y, You C, He M, Cai BW. Microneurosurgical management of the clinoid and paraclinoid aneurysms. Neurol Res. 2008;30(6):552–6. doi:10.1179/174313208X298101.
37. Nanda A, Javalkar V. Microneurosurgical management of ophthalmic segment of the internal carotid artery aneurysms: single-surgeon operative experience from Louisiana State University, Shreveport. Neurosurgery. 2011;68(2):355–70. doi:10.1227/NEU.0b013e3182039819; discussion 370–351.
38. Ng PY, Huddle D, Gunel M, Awad IA. Intraoperative endovascular treatment as an adjunct to microsurgical clipping of paraclinoid aneurysms. J Neurosurg. 2000;93(4):554–60. doi:10.3171/jns.2000.93.4.0554.
39. Nutik S. Carotid paraclinoid aneurysms with intradural origin and intracavernous location. J Neurosurg. 1978;48(4):526–33. doi:10.3171/jns.1978.48.4.0526.
40. Nutik SL. Removal of the anterior clinoid process for exposure of the proximal intracranial carotid artery. J Neurosurg. 1988;69(4):529–34. doi:10.3171/jns.1988.69.4.0529.
41. Pickett GE, Laitt RD, Herwadkar A, Hughes DG. Visual pathway compromise after hydrocoil treatment of large ophthalmic aneurysms. Neurosurgery. 2007;61(4):E873–4. doi:10.1227/01.NEU.0000298918.55119.7C; discussion E874.
42. Prabhakaran S, Wells KR, Lee VH, Flaherty CA, Lopes DK. Prevalence and risk factors for aspirin and clopidogrel resistance in cerebrovascular stenting. AJNR Am J Neuroradiol. 2008;29(2):281–5. doi:10.3174/ajnr.A0818.
43. Raco A, Frati A, Santoro A, Vangelista T, Salvati M, Delfini R, Cantore G. Long-term surgical results with aneurysms involving the ophthalmic segment of the carotid artery. J Neurosurg. 2008;108(6):1200–10. doi:10.3171/JNS/2008/108/6/1200.
44. Rouchaud A, Leclerc O, Benayoun Y, Saleme S, Camilleri Y, D'Argento F, . . . Mounayer C. Visual outcomes with flow-diverter stents covering the ophthalmic artery for treatment of internal carotid artery aneurysms. AJNR Am J Neuroradiol. 2014 doi: 10.3174/ajnr.A4129.
45. Sahs AL. Cooperative study of intracranial aneurysms and subarachnoid hemorrhage. Report on a randomized treatment study. I. Introduction. Stroke. 1974;5(4):550–1.
46. Schmidt GW, Oster SF, Golnik KC, Tumialan LM, Biousse V, Turbin R, . . . Miller NR. Isolated progressive visual loss after coiling of paraclinoid aneurysms. AJNR Am J Neuroradiol. 2007;28(10), 1882–89. doi: 10.3174/ajnr.A0690.
47. Schuss P, Guresir E, Berkefeld J, Seifert V, Vatter H. Influence of surgical or endovascular treatment on visual symptoms caused by intracranial aneurysms: single-center series and systematic review. J Neurosurg. 2011;115(4):694–9. doi:10.3171/2011.5.JNS101983.

48. Scott JA, Horner TG, Leipzig TJ. Retrograde suction decompression of an ophthalmic artery aneurysm using balloon occlusion. Technical note. J Neurosurg. 1991;75(1):146–7. doi:10.3171/jns.1991.75.1.0146.
49. Segal DH, Sen C, Bederson JB, Catalano P, Sacher M, Stollman AL, Lorberboym M. Predictive value of balloon test occlusion of the internal carotid artery. Skull Base Surg. 1995;5(2):97–107.
50. Sekhar LN, Sen CN, Jho HD. Saphenous vein graft bypass of the cavernous internal carotid artery. J Neurosurg. 1990;72(1):35–41. doi:10.3171/jns.1990.72.1.0035.
51. Tawk RG, Villalobos HJ, Levy EI, Hopkins LN. Surgical decompression and coil removal for the recovery of vision after coiling and proximal occlusion of a clinoidal segment aneurysm: technical case report. Neurosurgery. 2006;58(6):E1217. doi:10.1227/01.NEU.0000215995.09860.0A; discussion E1217.
52. Turner RD, Byrne JV, Kelly ME, Mitsos AP, Gonugunta V, Lalloo S, . . . Fiorella D. Delayed visual deficits and monocular blindness after endovascular treatment of large and giant paraophthalmic aneurysms. Neurosurgery. 2008;63(3), 469–74; discussion 474–65. doi: 10.1227/01.NEU.0000324730.37144.4B.

Paraclinoid Aneurysms: Flow Diverters and Endovascular Treatment

2

Ashish Sonig, L. Nelson Hopkins, Kenneth V. Snyder, Elad I. Levy, and Adnan H. Siddiqui

A. Sonig, MD MS MCh
Department of Neurosurgery, Jacobs School of Medicine and Biomedical Sciences, University at Buffalo, State University of New York, Buffalo, NY, USA

Department of Neurosurgery, Gates Vascular Institute at Kaleida Health, Buffalo, NY, USA

L.N. Hopkins, MD FACS • A.H. Siddiqui, MD PhD FAHA FAANS (✉)
Department of Neurosurgery, Gates Vascular Institute at Kaleida Health, Buffalo, NY, USA

Departments of Neurosurgery and Radiology, Jacobs School of Medicine and Biomedical Sciences, University at Buffalo, State University of New York, Buffalo, NY, USA

Toshiba Stroke and Vascular Research Center, University at Buffalo, State University of New York, Buffalo, NY, USA

Jacobs Institute, Buffalo, NY, USA
e-mail: asiddiqui@ubns.com

K.V. Snyder, MD PhD
Department of Neurosurgery, Gates Vascular Institute at Kaleida Health, Buffalo, NY, USA

Toshiba Stroke and Vascular Research Center, University at Buffalo, State University of New York, Buffalo, NY, USA

Departments of Neurosurgery, Radiology, and Neurology, Jacobs School of Medicine and Biomedical Sciences, University at Buffalo, State University of New York, Buffalo, NY, USA

E.I. Levy, MD MBA FACS FAHA FAANS
Department of Neurosurgery, Gates Vascular Institute at Kaleida Health, Buffalo, NY, USA

Departments of Neurosurgery and Radiology, Jacobs School of Medicine and Biomedical Sciences, University at Buffalo, State University of New York, Buffalo, NY, USA

Toshiba Stroke and Vascular Research Center, University at Buffalo, State University of New York, Buffalo, NY, USA

E. Veznedaroglu (ed.), *Controversies in Vascular Neurosurgery*,
DOI 10.1007/978-3-319-27315-0_2

Abbreviations

ACT	activated coagulation time
AP	anteroposterior
BTO	balloon test occlusion
CBF	cerebral blood flow
CE	Conformité Européene
ECA	external carotid artery
F	French
FDA	Food and Drug Administration
FRED	Flow-Redirection Endoluminal Device
GDC	Guglielmi detachable coil
ICA	internal carotid artery
ISAT	International Subarachnoid Aneurysm Trial
ISUIA	International Study of Unruptured Intracranial Aneurysms
PComA	posterior communicating artery
PED	Pipeline embolization device
PUFS	Pipeline for Uncoilable or Failed Aneurysms
rSO_2	regional oxygen saturation
SAH	subarachnoid hemorrhage
SCENT	Safety and Effectiveness of an Intracranial Aneurysm Embolization System for Treating Large or Giant Wide Neck Aneurysms
SPECT	single photon emission computed tomography
SSEPs	somatosensory evoked potentials
TIA	transient ischemic attack

Introduction

Paraclinoid aneurysms arise from the internal carotid artery (ICA) located adjacent to the anterior clinoid process, between the distal dural ring at the end of the cavernous segment and the origin of the posterior communicating artery (PComA). The proximity of these aneurysms to the optic apparatus, multiple dural attachments, osseous anatomy, and the need for adequate exposure through anterior clinoid bone removal, prior to securing these aneurysms, make them more complex than distal ICA aneurysms for microsurgical management.

Microsurgical anatomical complexity is less of a concern relative to the endovascular management of paraclinoid aneurysms. The major endovascular challenge is tortuosity of the carotid siphon, which resides in the paraclinoid segment. Over the years, the treatment of these aneurysms has progressively shifted, from microneurosurgery [1–3] to endovascular neurosurgery [4–6]. This has paralleled the shift for most aneurysms in the intracranial circulation except those at the anterior communicating artery, the middle cerebral artery, and the PComA associated with a fetal type circulation. In the second part of the International Study of Unruptured

Intracranial Aneurysms (ISUIA), the mortality and morbidity of patients treated by endovascular means were less than those associated with open microsurgery [7]. The International Subarachnoid Aneurysm Trial (ISAT) had similar findings, concluding that independent survival is more common after endovascular treatment than microsurgery [8]. The long-term ISAT follow-up data showed that the microsurgical group carried a significantly higher probability of dependency and death than the endovascular cohort [9]. The probability of disability-free survival was significantly greater in the endovascular group at 10 years.

Endovascular management of most intracranial aneurysms has become the standard of care at most centers. If the dome-to-neck ratio is favorable (>2), these aneurysms can be managed by primary coiling alone. However, in cases of wide-necked aneurysms, balloon-assisted and stent-assisted coiling strategies have been effective. The introduction of flow diverters has resulted in a rapid shift in treatment from traditional endovascular strategies for most aneurysms of the paraclinoid region [10].

This chapter provides an overview of the clinical anatomy, demographics, and endovascular management options for paraclinoid aneurysms with a focus on flow diversion.

Anatomy and Classification Systems

The segment of the ICA between the distal dural ring and origin of the PComA is called the "paraclinoid" segment [11–14]. The paraclinoid segment is the anterior-most segment of the ICA. The ICA changes its direction from an anteriorly directed cavernous flow as initially medially directed around the proximal half and then laterally directed around the distal half of a semicircle hinging around the optic strut underneath the anterior clinoid process. The ICA ends up with flow directed posterolaterally as the segment merges with the communicating segment. The paraclinoid ICA is intradural in location and therefore ruptures in this location result in subarachnoid hemorrhage. Although the anatomical details of the paraclinoid region are fixed, they pose differing challenges for microneurosurgery and endovascular approaches. Open microsurgery involves working in close proximity with the anterior clinoid process, optic strut, and distal dural ring. Hence, earlier work on paraclinoid aneurysms focused on microsurgical anatomy, and various classification systems were developed to showcase the unique anatomical relationships, which bear importance during microsurgical approaches.

The first detailed classification was based on anatomic dissection and was proposed by Gibo et al. [15]. Those authors classified the ICA mainly into four portions: cervical (C1), petrous (C2), cavernous (C3), and supraclinoid (C4). Bouthillier et al. [16] later included two additional segments, lacerum and clinoid. They proposed the following classification: cervical (C1), petrous (C2), lacerum (C3), cavernous (C4), clinoid (C5), ophthalmic (C6), and communicating (C7). This gave recognition to the importance of the transition zone as the ICA moves from the cavernous to intradural space (Fig. 2.1). Day [1] classified ICA aneurysms on the

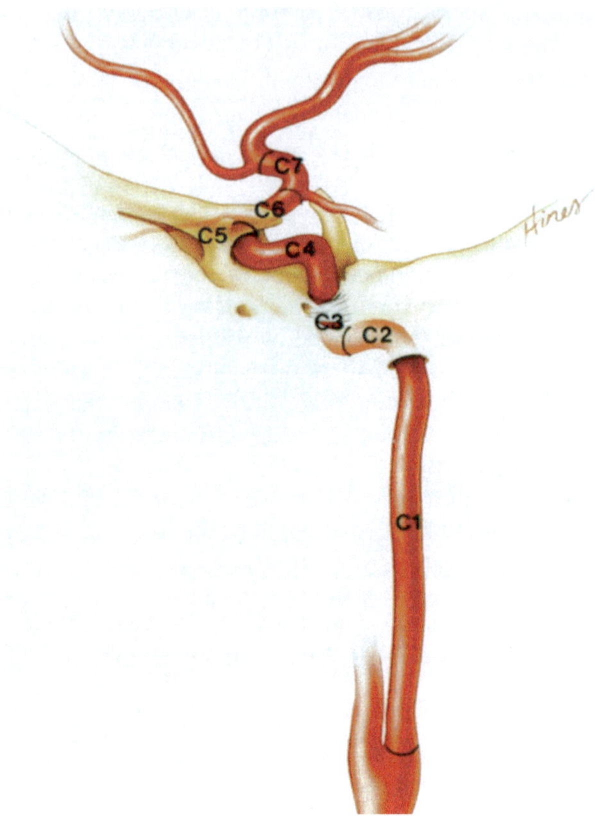

Fig. 2.1 According to the 1996 classification scheme [16], the seven segments of the internal carotid artery are as follows: *C1* cervical, *C2* petrous, *C3* lacerum, *C4* cavernous, *C5* clinoid, *C6* ophthalmic, and *C7* communicating (With permission from Bouthillier et al. [16])

basis of surgical considerations in two broad categories, ophthalmic artery and superior hypophyseal artery aneurysms. Later, Batjer et al. [17] added a third group to the classification, proximal posterior carotid aneurysms, which were those aneurysms arising from the posterior or posterolateral wall of the carotid artery.

Lasjaunias et al. [18] gave the first detailed embryological classification. Their classification was based on embryonic arteries: ventral pharyngeal hyoid, mandibular, primitive maxillary, trigeminal, dorsal ophthalmic, and ventral ophthalmic. On the basis of these arteries, the ICA was divided into the following segments: cervical, petrous, vertical cavernous, horizontal cavernous, clinoid, and cisternal segments.

Most recently, Shapiro et al. [19] produced a meticulous endovascular classification that simplifies the anatomy into cervical, petrous, cavernous, paraophthalmic, communicating, choroidal, and terminal segments. This classification bears importance to endovascular strategies because each segment has its own specific endovascular considerations. Cervical aneurysms tend to be healed dissections with pseudoaneurysms and pose no risk for rupture but act as a reservoir for embolic material. This is true for petrous aneurysms as well; however, the bony encasement of the artery has to be considered during intervention. Cavernous aneurysms can lead to cranial neuropathies either before or after treatment as well as rupture, which present as direct carotid cavernous fistulae. These fistulae allow for both arterial and venous approaches for management. Up to this segment, occlusion of side branches off the carotid artery is typically not consequential. The paraophthalmic segment is the transition intracranially and therefore aneurysmal rupture may present as a subarachnoid hemorrhage. Paraophthalmic aneurysms may also present as cranial neuropathies including visual field defects from direct optic nerve compression. This segment is also the most tortuous intracranial segment, and aneurysm catheterization and optimal wall apposition of intracranial stents, including flow diverters, can be challenging. Although the ophthalmic artery frequently has a dual supply from both internal and external carotid arteries, retinal artery occlusion is a well-recognized complication following treatment of paraophthalmic aneurysms. When associated with a large fetal posterior communicating artery, the communicating segment is a special challenge for which endovascular strategies remain suboptimal. The choroidal and terminal segments pose challenges for flow diversion when more than one flow diverter is used because of the risk for thrombosis of end vessel perforators in these locations.

Natural History, Treatment Indications, and Management Strategies

In one of the earliest studies on the natural history of unruptured intracranial aneurysms, the incidence of paraclinoid aneurysms was found to be 5.4 % [20]. In the first ISUIA (a retrospective study), ICA aneurysms comprised 28.5 % of all aneurysms [21]. The second ISUIA (a prospective study) suggested a possible 30 % incidence of ICA aneurysms [7]. In both studies, aneurysms arising from the cavernous ICA and PComA segment were not included in the cohort of ICA aneurysms, making paraclinoid aneurysms the commonest intracranial aneurysms. Like all intracranial aneurysms, paraclinoid aneurysms occur more frequently in women [7,21].

In the first ISUIA, the risk of first-time, de novo rupture of an aneurysm of <10 mm was 0.05 % per year [21]. The risk increased elevenfold when there was a previous history of rupture. For aneurysms >10 mm, the rupture risk was 1 % with or without previous history of rupture. In the second ISUIA, the 5-year cumulative rupture risk for ICA aneurysms (non-cavernous and non-PComA) ranged from 0 (<7 mm) to 40 % (>25 mm) [7].

When one considers studies from geographical locations with a higher incidence of aneurysms, the rupture risk is even greater. In a Finnish population study, the annual rupture rate for aneurysms <7 mm was 0.9 % [22]. Similarly, a high risk of rupture was seen in a Japanese population [23] with aneurysms <5 mm; the annual rupture rate was 0.34 % and 0.95 % per year for single and multiple aneurysm cases, respectively.

The decision to treat an unruptured aneurysm is often complicated. Among patients treated in the United States between 2001 and 2008, the overall risk of complications and mortality was higher following microsurgery than endovascular

Table 2.1 Predictors comprising the PHASES aneurysm rupture risk score

	Points
(P) Population	
North American, European (other than Finnish)	0
Japanese	3
Finnish	5
(H) Hypertension	
No	0
Yes	1
(A) Age	
<70 years	0
≥70 years	1
(S) Size of aneurysm	
<7.0 mm	0
7.0–9.9 mm	3
10.0–19.9 mm	6
≥20 mm	10
(E) Earlier SAH from another aneurysm	
No	0
Yes	1
(S) Site of aneurysm	
ICA	0
MCA	2
ACA/Pcom/posterior	4

With permission from Greving et al. [26]

To calculate the PHASES risk score for an individual, the number of points associated with each indicator can be added up to obtain the total risk score. For example, a 55-year-old North American man with no hypertension, no previous SAH, and a medium-sized (8 mm) posterior circulation aneurysm will have a risk score of 0+0+0+3+0+4=7 points. This score corresponds to a 5-year risk of rupture of 2.4 %

Abbreviations: *SAH* subarachnoid hemorrhage, *ICA* internal carotid artery, *MCA* middle cerebral artery, *ACA* anterior cerebral arteries (including the anterior cerebral artery, anterior communicating artery, and pericallosal artery), *Pcom* posterior communicating artery, *Posterior* posterior circulation (including the vertebral artery, basilar artery, cerebellar arteries, and posterior cerebral artery)

intervention [24]. In one meta-analysis, the periprocedural risk of adverse outcome, including mortality, was 4.8 % for aneurysms treated endovascularly [25]. Based on aneurysm size and patient demographics and comorbidities, the annual risk of rupture can range from 0 to 15 % [26]. A simple management algorithm is that the complication rate of the treatment should be less than the rupture risk of the aneurysm. In a pooled analysis of individual patient data from 6 prospective cohort studies with subarachnoid hemorrhage (SAH) as the outcome, the variables of aneurysm size, aneurysm site, patient age, previous history of rupture, hypertension, and geographical location of population were found to be significant predictors of rupture risk (Table 2.1) [26].

Similarly, an understanding of the relation of the aneurysm and associated branch vessels is equally important. In a study by Tanaka et al. [27], paraclinoid aneurysms were associated with the ophthalmic artery in 32.9 % of cases and with the superior hypophyseal artery in 47.1 %. In 20 % of cases, no branch vessel was associated with these aneurysms. Although superior hypophyseal artery occlusion is rarely symptomatic, retinal ischemia following ophthalmic artery occlusion is well recognized.

Treatment of Symptomatic Paraclinoid Aneurysms

Most paraclinoid aneurysms are asymptomatic and discovered incidentally during workup for unrelated pathologies (frequently headaches). SAH is the commonest presentation of symptomatic paraclinoid aneurysms. Anterior optic pathway compression is the next commonest clinical manifestation of these aneurysms. The incidence of visual impairment ranges from 25 % [28] to 33 % [29,30] in some series. Visual outcome following treatment is a key consideration in the selection of microsurgery or endovascular management. If there is significant mass effect on the optic nerve with a concurrent visual field loss, microsurgery remains a superior option to rapidly decompress the optic apparatus and maximize potential for visual function recovery. However, some studies have suggested equal efficacy of endovascular or surgical clipping with respect to improved visual outcomes [31] whereas others have shown improved outcomes following clipping [32]. In a systematic review, it was shown that surgical clipping resulted in better visual outcomes [33]. That being said, it is important to appreciate that there is risk of visual loss following microsurgery as well. In one surgical series, new-onset optic nerve dysfunction was observed in 27 % of patients [34]. Acute visual loss after open surgery may be caused by occlusion of the ophthalmic artery, ischemia to the optic nerve secondary to perforator injury or manipulation of the nerve, or retinal ischemia [35,36].

In an endovascular series, the use of platinum coils alone to embolize paraclinoid aneurysms in patients presenting with visual field defects did not result in significant improvement of vision [37]. Inflammation following coiling and new thrombus formation post-coiling were suspected as the commonest reasons for non-improvement or deterioration in vision. However, one study demonstrated improvement in vision following coiling [38]. In this analysis of 12 patients with mass effect on the anterior optic pathway who were treated by coiling, 5 patients (42 %) had complete resolution of symptoms, 4 (33 %) had significant improvement of symptoms, and 3 (25 %) were unchanged.

Endovascular management of paraclinoid aneurysms has become the preferred management option. One of the reasons is the increased morbidity of open surgery, secondary to complex surgical anatomy of the region. The amount of exposure needed can vary from a proximal cervical carotid exposure to resection of the anterior clinoid process and optic strut. In cases of carotid cave and superior hypophyseal artery aneurysms, mobilization of the optic nerve, optic nerve sheath incision, and exposure of the distal dural ring are often needed. This adds to the morbidity and to new visual deficits.

On the contrary, the anatomical location of the paraclinoid aneurysm does not add to the difficulty of the procedure when endovascular management is considered. Instead, it is the tortuosity of the ICA, the angle the long axis of the aneurysm forms with the ICA, aspect ratio, absolute neck dimensions, relation of branch vessel, and, for giant aneurysms, the inflow and outflow accessibility that decides the choice of treatment. Endovascular management has evolved from primary coiling, then balloon-assisted and subsequently stent-assisted coiling, to most recently the use of flow diverters.

Endovascular Considerations: Techniques, Results, and Outcomes

Historical Perspective

Endovascular techniques to treat cavernous and paraclinoid aneurysm are similar. It is important to note that it was the treatment of carotid-cavernous fistula that accelerated the development of endovascular options. Brooks [39] can be credited for laying the foundation of endovascular surgery. In 1930, he used a piece of muscle in the ICA to treat a carotid cavernous fistula. For the next 4 decades, this procedure was used and refined by others. In one of the first and largest series on temporary occlusion of the intracranial and cervical carotid arteries, Serbinenko [40] described temporary arterial occlusions in 304 cases, with complications occurring in just two cases.

The safety of temporary occlusion of the ICA formed the premise for the use of detachable balloons to treat cavernous carotid artery aneurysms. Higashida et al. [41] applied this technique for treatment of such aneurysms in 87 patients. In 68 (78.2 %) patients, therapeutic occlusion (or endovascular sacrifice or deconstruction) of the ICA across or just proximal to the aneurysm neck was performed. In 1985, these authors modified the technique by filling the balloon with hydroxyethyl methacrylate, a permanent solidifying agent, after which the balloon was guided into the aneurysm to preserve the parent artery. This technique was successfully used in 19 (22 %) of the 87 patients. The results were equally impressive, with 68 % of the 19 patients achieving complete occlusion at follow-up.

Therapeutic ICA Occlusion

In one of the first systematic reviews of the literature on ICA occlusion in conjunction with partial aneurysm coiling, it was found that the technique of therapeutic ICA occlusion was reasonably safe and resulted in occlusion of the aneurysm in most patients [42].

Current Status

Endovascular sacrifice of the carotid artery for the treatment of paraclinoid aneurysm is considered as the last option when conventional options of coiling, clipping, or flow diversion are not feasible or aneurysmal recurrence is observed despite the above treatments. In such cases, carotid occlusion without a bypass is a reasonable option, provided adequate collateral circulation has been demonstrated by balloon test occlusion (BTO).

Compared with surgical ligation, endovascular vessel sacrifice is preferred, because occlusion of the ICA can be achieved in a minimally invasive fashion with the same effect. Another advantage is the ability to achieve parent vessel occlusion close to or within the aneurysm segment with partial occlusion of the aneurysm with coils. This is advantageous as only a short segment of the vessel is available for thrombus formation compared to the entire cervical segment during open ligation, thus reducing thromboembolic phenomena. However, vessel sacrifice has its own perils. Thromboembolic complications and delayed ischemia have been well characterized following successful BTO and ICA deconstruction [43]. In addition, increased compensatory flow around the circle of Willis is suspected to lead to de novo aneurysm formation in up to 20 % of cases following carotid sacrifice [44].

One prerequisite for vessel sacrifice is the documentation of adequate collateral flow by performing a BTO. Once a hypotensive challenge is added to the assessment, the accuracy of the test reaches 100 % to predict a major stroke following sacrifice. In one study, none of the patients developed major stroke following vessel sacrifice once they had passed hypotensive challenge; one patient developed minor symptoms following treatment but recovered completely [45].

Some authors have used BTO to assess retrograde filling of the ophthalmic artery from the external carotid artery during the treatment of ophthalmic artery aneurysms [46]. Retrograde filling of the ophthalmic artery from the external carotid artery and the appearance of a choroidal blush help in devising a strategy for safe and efficacious occlusion of ophthalmic artery aneurysms, especially those incorporating the ophthalmic artery [46].

BTO Technique

BTO is performed with the patient under conscious sedation. A 6-French (F) sheath is placed, and diagnostic angiography is performed to assess the cerebrovascular anatomy. However, if a recent cerebral angiogram is available, one can proceed directly with the BTO. After the sheath has been placed, sufficient heparin is administered to achieve an activated coagulation time (ACT) of approximately 250–300 s. The choice of balloon catheter can vary. We prefer to use a 6 F Cello™ balloon guide catheter (Covidien). This catheter has the advantage of a double lumen. The central lumen can be used to continuously irrigate the occluded vessel with heparinized saline, thus preventing thrombotic complications. Once the balloon tip is delivered over a 0.035-inch wire to the desired location, the ACT is confirmed and a baseline neurological examination is performed. The balloon is inflated until anterograde flow is confirmed through stasis of contrast material in the distal ICA. This strategy prevents overinflation of the balloon and complications such as vessel dissection.

Under normotensive conditions, the patient's neurological status and occlusion of the balloon are assessed every 3 min, for a period of 15–20 min. If the patient tolerates normotensive occlusion, the hypotensive challenge is initiated. The mean arterial pressure is reduced by 30 % and even further to 60 mmHg; periodic neurological examinations are performed. Generally, hypotensive challenge is carried out for 10–15 min. The test is aborted if there is a change in mental status or neurological examination.

Neurological Evaluation During BTO

Clinical neurological evaluation is the commonest method; however, other options are as follows:

1. Cerebral blood flow (CBF) testing: In one study, cerebral blood flow (CBF) of <30 ml/g/min was associated with deterioration in sustained attention during temporary balloon occlusion [47]. CBF was measured simultaneously using the intracarotid 133Xe washout method.
2. Cerebral oximetry: regional oxygen saturation (rSO_2) of the brain can be used to assess the outcome of BTO. In one study, rSO_2 of the brain was measured and compared simultaneously with near infrared spectroscopy [48]. Asymmetric single photon emission computed tomography (SPECT) patterns always accompanied a profound decrease in rSO_2 that coincided with a reduction in stump pressure.
3. Neurophysiologic monitoring: electroencephalography and short latency somatosensory evoked potentials (SSEPs) are important adjuncts in the assessment of BTO. These methods are important in the setting of general anesthesia or preexisting poor neurological examination. A CBF of <15 ml/100 g/min coincides with >50 % loss of SSEP amplitude [49].

Complications are uncommon with BTO. In one of the largest series of 500 consecutive BTO patients, carotid dissection was seen in 1.2 % cases [50]. The incidence of pseudoaneurysm or embolism was 0.2 % each with 0 % mortality.

Primary and Balloon-Assisted Coiling

Guglielmi detachable coils (GDCs) were introduced in 1990 for the treatment of cerebral aneurysms and approved by the FDA in September of 1995. One important aspect in primary aneurysm coiling is the fundus to neck ratio. A ratio of >2 is considered favorable. In one of the largest series of primary coiling of paraclinoid aneurysms in 73 patients, 63 % of aneurysms had unfavorable anatomy and 66.7 % aneurysms that needed retreatment had unfavorable anatomy [51]. In another series of 71 aneurysms in which GDCs were used primarily, near-total aneurysm occlusion was seen in 85 % of patients at 6 months [6]. For the treatment of wide-necked and large aneurysms, the use of balloon-assisted coiling [4,52] and dual [53] or multiple [54] catheters preceded the advent of stent-assisted coiling.

Navigation of Microcatheters

Paraclinoid aneurysms pose a challenge for microcatheter navigation due to their close proximity to the carotid siphon with its tortuosity and the angles these aneurysms make with the parent vessel, which make the task sometimes quite difficult. Appropriately shaped microcatheters can be of tremendous help to the interventionist. The tip of the microcatheter can be shaped with steam and a mandrill [55]; however, pre-shaped catheters are now readily available. The commonest shapes that are used are straight, 45-degree J, C, and S (Fig. 2.2) [55–57].

Steering of the microcatheter without the use of a microwire has been described [56,57]. This can be antegrade, where the microcatheter is pushed into the aneurysm directly or retrograde when it goes distal to the aneurysm and it snaps into the aneurysm after being pulled. This maneuver can be very dangerous, particularly in small aneurysms. Once in the aneurysm, coils can be delivered typically using viewing angles, which allow clear visualization of the neck so as to prevent inadvertent herniation of coils into the parent vessel.

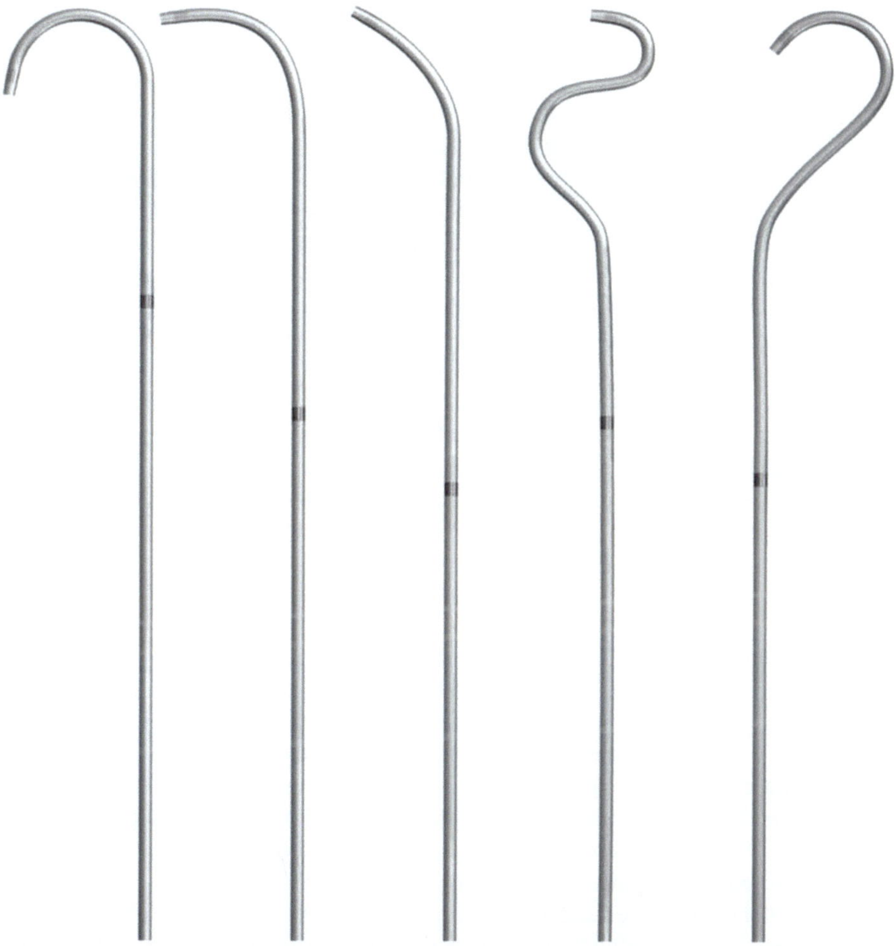

Fig. 2.2 Various shapes of SL-10 catheters (Stryker Neurovascular). From *left* to *right*: J-shaped, 90-degree, 45 angled, S-shaped, and C-shaped (With permission from Stryker Neurovascular)

Stent-Assisted Coiling

Stent-assisted coiling came to the fore to aid the treatment of aneurysms with wide necks and a <2 fundus-to-dome ratio. In most paraclinoid aneurysm series, stent-assisted coiling was predominantly used for wide-necked aneurysms (Table 2.2) [58–60]. The commonest stents used are Neuroform 2TM, Neuroform 3TM, Neuroform EZ (Stryker Neurovascular), and Enterprise TM (Cordis).

Compared to the Neuroform 2TM, the Neuroform 3TM has more interconnects between the cells to prevent the prolapse of the stent into the aneurysm. All Neuroform stents need a 0.027 inner diameter catheter for delivery. The Neuroform EZ is a modification of the 2TM and 3TM and has an easier deployment mechanism, like that of the Enterprise Vascular Reconstruction Device System (VRDS; Cordis). One advantage of the Enterprise stent is that it is delivered through a 0.021-inch inner diameter catheter for deployment. The closed-cell design of the Enterprise has an inherent ability for recapture after partial deployment and easy redeployment. However, the closed-cell, laser-cut design also has the propensity to kink around tight bends as can frequently be the case with paraclinoid aneurysms.

In one prospective registry, a higher rate of thromboembolic events was associated with Enterprise stent-assisted coiling when compared to Neuroform stents [61]. However, in one of the largest comparative analyses between the Enterprise and Neuroform stents, it was found that the rates of mortality, recanalization, and intracranial hemorrhage were higher in conjunction with Neuroform stent-assisted coiling [62]. In our opinion, Enterprise and Neuroform stents are equally safe and efficacious. Table 2.2 shows the results of primary and stent-assisted coiling of paraclinoid aneurysms [4,6,51,52,58–60,63–65]. More recently, newer stents have been employed in the paraclinoid location but long-term results are not available; these include the Liberty stent (Penumbra, Alameda, CA), Low-profile Visualized Intraluminal Support (LVIS) stent (MicroVention), Leo stent (Balt, Montmorency, France), Atlas stent (Stryker), and Solitaire (Covidien, Irvine, CA). They most importantly differ in their strut designs, construction materials, and delivery catheters.

Flow Diversion

Large, wide-necked, and fusiform aneurysms are the most challenging for endovascular treatment, with higher rates of retreatment. When compared to the recanalization rates for small aneurysms, those for large and giant aneurysms may be as high as 17 % [66]. To address these challenges, "flow diverters" became available as an option. The earliest flow diverters that were used were the Silk (Balt) and the Pipeline embolization device (PED; Covidien). The PED was approved by the FDA in April 2011 and is currently the only approved flow diverter in the USA. Flow diverters are self-expanding stents with low porosity and higher metal coverage than the earlier stents that were used to aid coiling. They work by inducing thrombosis in the aneurysm but preserving flow in adjacent vessels. Another advantage of the flow diverter is that multiple aneurysms located along the same or an adjacent vessel segment can be treated with a single device (Fig. 2.3).

Table 2.2 Series of >50 patients with paraclinoid aneurysm treated by primary or stent-assisted coiling

Authors, year	Title	No. patients	Number of paraclinoid aneurysm treated endovascularly	Primary coiling (with or without balloon)	Stent coiled	Available follow-up (number of patients unless otherwise noted)	Mean follow-up	Radiographic follow-up
Kwon et al. 2014 [52]	Angiographic and clinical result of endovascular treatment in paraclinoid aneurysms	113	116	74	36 (stent coiled +2 (only stent)	80	20.4 months	Complete occlusion in 56 aneurysms (70 %)
Ogilvy et al. 2011 [59]	Stent-assisted coiling of paraclinoid aneurysms: risks and effectiveness	91	94	24	70	80	[a]>2 years	Complete occlusion in 15/20 coiling and 40/60 stent coiling
D'Urso et al. 2012 [4]	Coiling for paraclinoid aneurysms: time to make way for flow diverters?	118	126	108	18	106	31.9 months	Complete occlusion in 66 aneurysms (62 %)
Wang et al. 2013 [60]	Endovascular treatment of paraclinoid aneurysms: 142 aneurysms in one center	126	142	24	118	112	16.6 months	Complete occlusion in 71 aneurysms (63.4 %)

(continued)

Table 2.2 (continued)

Authors, year	Title	No. patients	Number of paraclinoid aneurysm treated endovascularly	Primary coiling (with or without balloon)	Stent coiled	Available follow-up (number of patients unless otherwise noted)	Mean follow-up	Radiographic follow-up
Park et al. 2003 [51]	Endovascular treatment of paraclinoid aneurysms: experience with 73 patients	70	73	73	0	49	13.9 months	Complete occlusion in 43 (87.8 %)
Sorimachi et al. 2012 [64]	Long-term follow-up of intra-aneurysmal coil embolization for unruptured paraclinoid aneurysms	138	140	140		111	65.6 months	[b]
Chalouhi et al. 2013 [58]	Stent-Assisted Coiling of Intracranial Aneurysms Predictors of Complications, Recanalization, and Outcome in 508 Cases	508	122	0	122	87 %	26 months	Recanalization, 12 % (51/424); retreatment, 6.4 % (27/424)
Thornton et al. 2000 [6]	Endovascular treatment of paraclinoid aneurysms	66	71	71	0	61	16 months	Complete occlusion in 33 (54 %)

Yadla et al. 2011 [65]	Open and endovascular treatment of unruptured carotid-ophthalmic aneurysms: clinical and radiographic outcomes	161	147	75	72	118	10.9 months	81 aneurysms (68.6 %) had angiographic evidence of 100 % occlusion at last follow-up
Chen et al. 2013 [63]	Experiences and complications in endovascular treatment of paraclinoid aneurysms	47	50	30 (1 stenting alone)	19	50	18.6 months	Complete occlusions in 36 patients; incomplete occlusions in 11 patients; partial occlusion in 3

[a]Exact mean duration not available
[b]Complete occlusion rate not provided

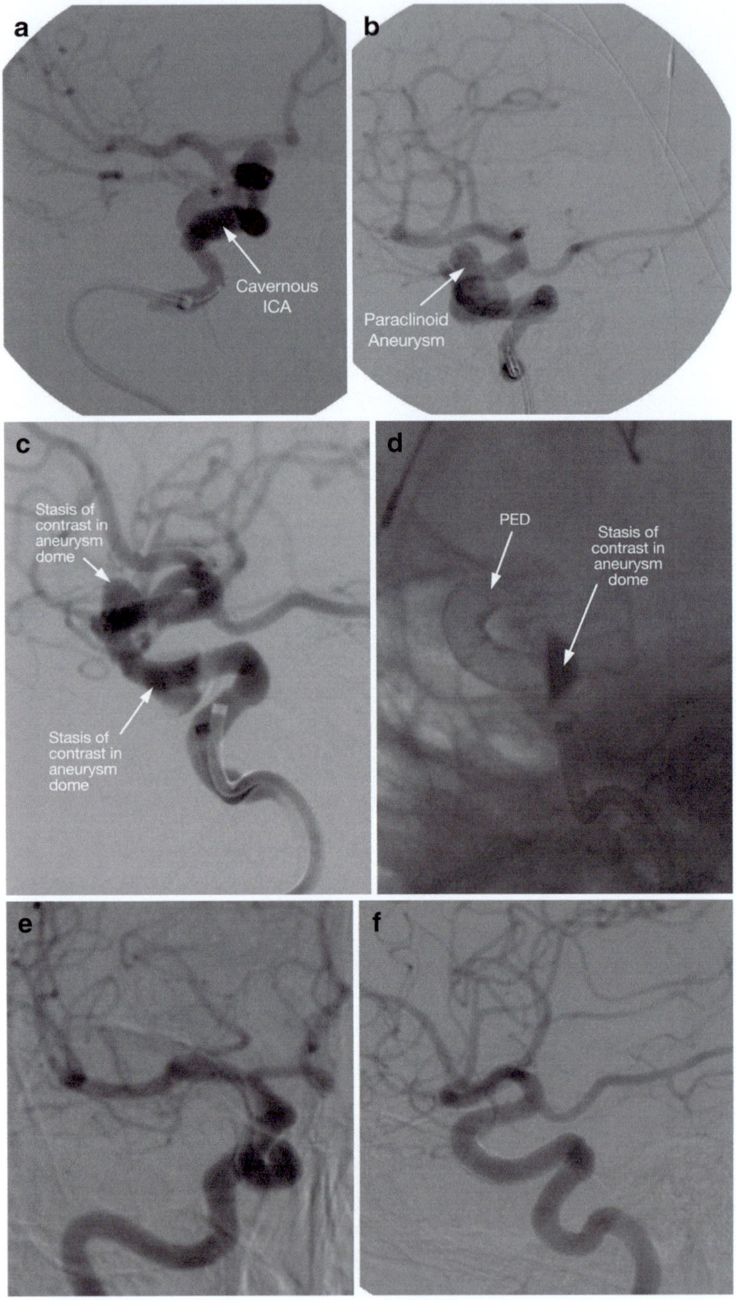

Fig. 2.3 This patient is a 62-year-old woman who was found to have sudden onset of left-hand weakness and a facial droop. Evaluation revealed a giant right internal carotid artery (ICA) aneurysm involving cavernous and paraclinoid locations. Digital subtraction angiogram: right ICA injection shows the guide catheter in the right ICA with a multilobulated giant ICA aneurysm located at the cavernous (**a**) and paraclinoid (**b**) portions. A significant change in flow was noticed after the deployment of three Pipeline embolization devices (PED; Covidien) (**c** and **d**). Two-month follow-up angiography, anteroposterior (AP) (**e**) and lateral (**f**) views, shows complete aneurysm obliteration

Strategies for Improving Results with the PED

Dual Antiplatelet Therapy

The rationale for antiplatelet usage is central to a lower incidence of thromboembolic complications. In the Pipeline for Uncoilable or Failed Aneurysms (PUFS) trial, patients received aspirin (325 mg daily for 2 days) and clopidogrel (75 mg daily for 7 days) prior to PED placement or a 600-mg loading dose of clopidogrel 1 day before the procedure [10]. Following the procedure, they were placed on 325 mg of aspirin daily for at least 6 months and 75 mg of clopidogrel daily for at least 3 months. We follow a similar protocol. Additionally, preprocedure aspirin and clopidogrel response testing [67] and aspirin therapy are considered vital by many experts, whereas others consider this testing to be unreliable. Studies have shown that a suboptimal response (>240) to clopidogrel is associated with increased thromboembolic complications [68–70]. If the clopidogrel response is nontherapeutic, we discontinue that agent and consider alternative antiplatelet agent, such as prasugrel (loading dose of 60 mg; maintenance dose of 5 mg once daily) if no history of stroke or transient ischemic attack (TIA) or ticagrelor (180 mg loading dose, then 90 mg twice daily for maintenance). Maintenance doses of aspirin above 100 mg reduce the effectiveness of ticagrelor and should be avoided. If a patient is started on ticagrelor, aspirin (75–100 mg daily) should be used instead.

Correct Sizing

Undersizing or oversizing of the stent (based on the size of the ICA) can alter the metal coverage over the neck of the aneurysm, causing incomplete occlusion and endoleaks [71]. Even modest oversizing can significantly increase the porosity. The calibration of the angiographic system can be inaccurate. We recommend measuring the size of the guide tip in both anteroposterior (AP) and lateral planes (as the actual size of the guide tip is always known). This yields the ratio of actual size and the measured size and helps in greater accuracy during calculation of the ICA diameters.

Metal coverage can also be altered by the method of deployment [72] and the number of devices deployed [73]. By controlling the push on the PED and the pull on the microcatheter, 50 % metal coverage at the aneurysmal neck can be achieved, causing flow reduction by 62 %.

Optimal Deployment and Judicious Overlapping

Optimal deployment of the devices that takes into consideration the location of perforators and branch vessels is equally important. Generally for a paraclinoid aneurysm, the distal margin of the stent should be just proximal to the origin of the PComA; and invariably in most cases, the origin of the ophthalmic artery is covered. In up to 25 % of cases, the ophthalmic artery may occlude in a delayed fashion [74]. However, because there is additional ophthalmic supply from the external carotid artery and this is a chronic process, visual disturbances and loss are reported but remain rare events.

As a rule, overlapping of devices should be avoided, as adequate metal coverage over the neck of the aneurysm can be achieved by dynamic push-pull on a single device. However, when more than two devices are needed, such as for giant aneurysms, and overlap occurs, judicious sizing of the devices can alter the metal coverage to maximum. When two devices of the same diameter are used, the variation in metal coverage is highest. However, when two devices of different size are used, more uniform coverage is produced [73].

Use of Coils

Flow diverters afford endoluminal treatment in contrast to the endosaccular treatment offered by coils. Endosaccular treatment has the advantage of immediate dome protection. By allowing a combination of flow diversion and coiling, benefits of both endoluminal (lesser recurrence) and endovascular (dome protection) treatment can be achieved. This is particularly important in the setting of large (Fig. 2.4) or giant wide-necked aneurysms, where the risks of PED prolapse into the dome of the aneurysm and delayed aneurysmal rupture are higher. Additionally, coils promote earlier thrombosis in the aneurysm as compared to the flow diverter alone [75].

Indications

The PED is currently approved for use in the USA by the FDA for >10 mm aneurysms in the proximal ICA from the petrous to the paraclinoid segment. In Europe, where many more flow diverters are approved, any aneurysm can be treated; however, the Silk stent is approved only with adjunctive use of coils. Currently there are multiple ongoing FDA-regulated trials, which are attempting to expand indications, such as those involving the Surpass stent (Stryker Neurovascular, Fremont, California) for >10 mm aneurysms up to the ICA terminus and the Flow-Redirection Endoluminal Device (FRED (MicroVention, Tustin, California)) for aneurysms >7 mm up to the ICA terminus as well as proximal vertebral artery aneurysms. The PED is currently being evaluated for aneurysms smaller than 7 mm up to the ICA terminus. Despite these restrictions, flow diverters have been utilized and reported in essentially all intracranial territories as well as some extracranial locations.

Fig. 2.4 This patient is a 44-year-old woman in whom a right paraclinoid aneurysm was discovered during evaluation subsequent to a transient ischemic attack. She underwent simultaneous coiling and PED placement. Digital subtraction angiogram shows a large saccular right paraclinoid unruptured aneurysm in AP (**a**) and lateral (**b**) projections. (**c**) A Triaxial system (consisting of a Cook shuttle, Flexor® Shuttle® guiding sheath [all Cook Medical], Navien™ 058 Intracranial Support Catheter [Covidien], and Marksman microcatheter [Covidien]) was used for better stability. A Prowler LPES microcatheter (Codman Neurovascular) was used to deliver Axium coils (Covidien). (**d**) PED deployed with coils in situ. (**e**) Three-month follow-up angiogram shows no residual aneurysm

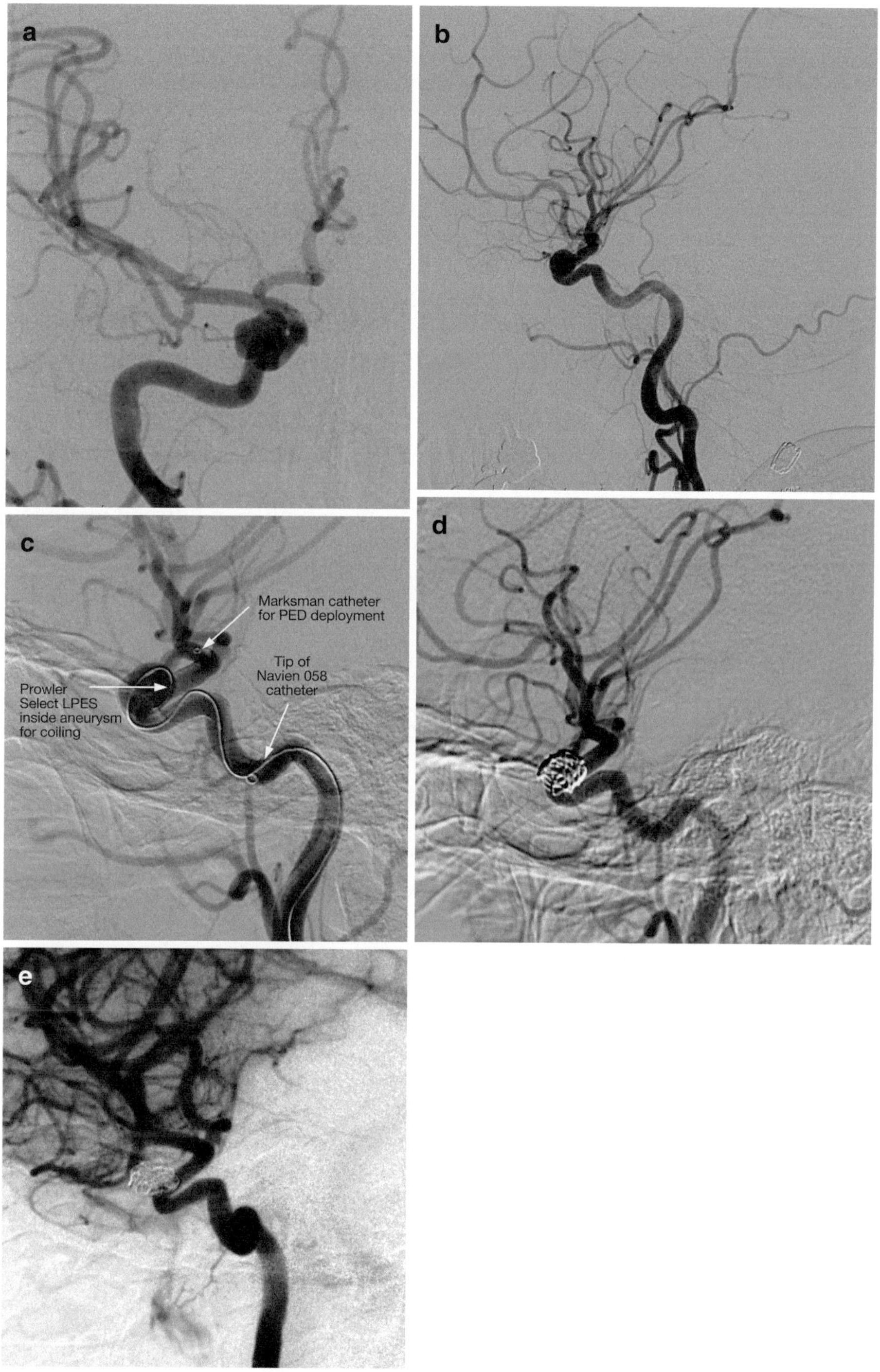
a
b
c
Marksman catheter for PED deployment
Tip of Navien 058 catheter
Prowler Select LPES inside aneurysm for coiling
d
e

Complications

Complications following Pipeline embolization may be related to the device, thromboembolism, perforator or branch vessel occlusion, hemorrhage in the territory of treated artery or remote, as well as delayed aneurysm rupture. Also, as with all interventions, access site-related complications, such as groin/retroperitoneal hematoma and nephropathy, do occur.

In a systemic review of ten studies, 448 intracranial aneurysms were treated with the PED, of which 83.5 % (374) were in the anterior circulation [76]. The overall symptomatic complication rate (IA ruptures, ischemic events, non-aneurysm-related intracranial hemorrhages, worsening of mass effect, and femoral or retroperitoneal hematomas) was 10.3 % (n = 46). The intracranial complication rate (hemorrhage and ischemia) was 6.3 % (n = 28). Procedure-related death occurred in 9 (2.2 %) of the 413 patients.

In one of the largest multicenter series to date involving 17 centers worldwide, peri- and postprocedure complications of PED in 906 aneurysms were analyzed of which 660 had anterior location [77]. A total of 311 (47.12 %) anterior circulation aneurysms were large (>10 mm). In this study, the overall mortality and morbidity of anterior circulation aneurysms were 3.4 % in small aneurysms and 7.9 % in large aneurysms. Tables 2.3 and 2.4 give the details of complications on the basis of aneurysm location and time frame, respectively.

Radiological Outcomes

In one of the first prospective single-center registries, 53 patients with 63 aneurysms underwent treatment with PED (33 small, 22 large, and 8 giant, wide-necked aneurysms) [78]. Complete angiographic occlusion of the aneurysm was achieved in 56 % (n = 42) of aneurysms at 3 months, 92.8 % (n = 28) at 6 months, and 95 % (n = 18) at 12 months.

Similar impressive results were seen in the PUFS trial [10]. PUFS was a multicenter, prospective, interventional single-arm trial of PED for the treatment of uncoilable or failed aneurysms of the ICA. A total of 108 patients with unruptured large or giant wide-necked ICA aneurysms were enrolled in the study. At 6 months, complete occlusion was achieved in 73.6 %. At 1 year of follow-up, 79 of 91 (86.8 %) patients had complete aneurysm occlusion. The FDA approved the use of the PED based on the results of this trial.

Most studies have shown impressive complete occlusion rates when aneurysms were treated by flow diverters. Table 2.5 provides a summary of studies in which more than 20 aneurysms were treated by flow diverters [5,77,79–86]. The rates of complete occlusion of paraclinoid aneurysms treated with PED at the end of 6 months varied from 76.2 % [5] to 91.6 % [84]; more importantly, the recanalization rate after achieving complete occlusion was 0 % [86].

PED in Ruptured Aneurysms

Paraclinoid aneurysms, which represent 1.5–9 % of all ruptured aneurysms, are an uncommon cause of SAH when compared to other aneurysms [87]. The argument against the use of PED in ruptured aneurysms is mainly due to the need for dual

Table 2.3 Complications by aneurysm location and size

Complications	Anterior ICA ≥10 mm (n=275)	Anterior ICA <10 mm (n=294)	95 % CI; P Value
Mean aneurysm size (mm)	16.8±6.2	5.2±2.2	(10.2–11.2); <.001
Spontaneous rupture	4 (0.7 %)	0 (0.0 %)	(0.2–1.5 %); .17
Intraparenchymal hemorrhage	6 (2.2 %)	6 (2.0 %)	(1.3–3.4 %); .73
Ischemic stroke	15 (5.5 %)	8 (2.7 %)	(3.2–6.2 %); .16
Parent artery stenosis	1 (0.4 %)	1 (0.4 %)	(0–0.7 %); 1.0
Cranial neuropathy	2 (0.7 %)	0 (0.0 %)	(0–0.7 %); .30
Neurologic morbidity	24 (8.7 %)	14 (4.5 %)	(5.6–9.2 %); .16
Neurologic mortality	11 (4.0 %)	4 (1.4 %)	(2.5–5.1 %); <.01
Neurologic morbidity and mortality (all patients)	26 (9.5 %)	14 (4.8 %)	(6.5–10.3 %); .01
Neurologic morbidity and mortality (patients with unruptured aneurysms)	24/263 (9.2 %)	11/270 (4.1 %)	(5.5–9.3 %); .03
Neurologic morbidity and mortality (patients with ruptured aneurysms)	2/12 (16.7 %)	3/24(12.5 %)	(10.0–27.1 %); .35
Neurologic morbidity and mortality (excluding ruptured, dissecting, or fusiform aneurysms)	15 (7.0 %)	9 (3.6 %)	(4.1–7.3 %); .19

Reproduced with permission from Kallmes et al. [77]
Note: n indicates the number of patients

Table 2.4 Occurrence of complications by time

Complications	<72 h	72 h–30 days	>30 Days
Spontaneous rupture	1 (0.1 %)	3 (0.4 %)	1 (0.1 %)
Intraparenchymal hemorrhage	3 (0.4 %)	11 (1.5 %)	4 (0.5 %)
Ischemic stroke	17 (2.3 %)	7 (0.9 %)	9 (1.2 %)
Parent artery stenosis	0 (0 %)	1 (0.1 %)	1 (0.1 %)
Cranial neuropathy	0 (0 %)	2 (0.3 %)	0 (0 %)
Neurologic morbidity	20 (2.7 %)	21 (2.8 %)	13 (1.8 %)
Neurologic mortality	4 (0.5 %)	13 (1.8 %)	7 (0.9 %)
Neurologic morbidity and mortality (all patients)	23 (3.1 %)	22 (3.0 %)	13 (1.8 %)
Neurologic morbidity and mortality (patients with unruptured aneurysms)	19/664 (2.9 %)	16/664 (2.4 %)	11/664 (1.7 %)
Neurologic morbidity and mortality (patients with ruptured aneurysms)	4/70 (5.7 %)	6/70 (8.6 %)	2/70 (2.9 %)
Neurologic morbidity and mortality (excluding ruptured, dissecting, or fusiform aneurysms)	13/549 (2.4 %)	12/549 (2.2 %)	5/549 (0.9 %)

Reproduced with permission from Kallmes et al. [77]
Note: n indicates the number of patients

antiplatelet agents and the inability to provide immediate dome protection. The authors of one multicenter series analyzed data for 26 patients with PED-treated ruptured aneurysms, of which 15 were ruptured paraclinoid aneurysms [88]. All patients received a loading dose of 650 mg of aspirin and 600 mg of clopidogrel before intervention. Following intervention, aspirin (325 mg) and clopidogrel (75 mg) were continued. Despite the use of dual antiplatelet agents, hemorrhagic complications were seen in only 2 of 26 patients, and complete occlusion was seen in 18 of 26 (74 %) patients at last follow-up. Among the 15 paraclinoid aneurysms that were treated, 7 were blister-type aneurysms. PED in the setting of a ruptured aneurysm is a viable option, especially when traditional endovascular methods and clipping are higher risk. Use of adjunctive coiling gives much needed dome protection [75,89]. Primary treatment of ruptured blister paraclinoid aneurysm with PED can be the preferred option [90].

Silk Stent

The Silk stent has CE marking and was the first flow diverter introduced for neurointervention. The indications for use are similar to those for the PED. However, there are a few differences in handling this device, when compared with the PED. The initial Silk stent had a difficult deployment mechanism and was replaced by a newer device, the Silk +, which has a 15 % increased radial force, flared ends, and improved radiopacity [91]. Additionally, the incidence of thromboembolic complication has been less with the newer device. Compared to the PED, shortening is seen more often in Silk stents, up to 50–60 % can occur, and they are difficult to negotiate along the curves. Table 2.5 summarizes the studies in which the Silk device was used to treat paraclinoid aneurysms.

Treatment with the Silk device is safe and efficacious. In some studies, similar occlusion rates to those with the PED were achieved [79,83,85], with up to 93 % occlusion rates [83] in paraclinoid aneurysms. There are very few studies that have directly compared the Silk device with the PED. In a multicenter study (Table 2.5) at 25 Italian centers, 295 IAs were treated with the Silk or PED [80]. The difference in hemorrhagic and ischemic stroke between the two cohorts was not significant. Ischemic or thromboembolic events occurred in 13 patients (4.8 %), 8 treated with the Silk and 5 with the PED. Technical complications such as failure to deploy, incorrect positioning, and in-stent stenosis were also similar in proportion in the two cohorts and were nonsignificant.

Other Flow Diverters

PED Flex

The first-generation PED had issues with deployment and inability to resheath. This has been addressed in the next-generation device, the PED Flex [92–95]. The PED Flex received CE approval in March of 2014 and FDA approval in February of 2015. This device is easier to deploy and is more precise and has the ability to be resheathed. However, during an initial experience, a few instances of difficult deployment of the distal end of the device have been encountered [94] (Fig. 2.5). The device comes with distal flaps that sometimes prevent the opening of the distal end. Resheathing within the microcatheter and redeployment provide one solution in this instance.

Table 2.5 Series of >20 paraclinoid aneurysm treated by flow diverters

Author(s), year	Title	No. aneurysms treated	No. of paraclinoid aneurysms treated	Type of flow diverter	Radiologic follow-up available (no. patients)	Complications	6-month angiography	12 months
Yu et al. 2012 [86]	Intracranial aneurysms: midterm outcome of Pipeline embolization device for intracranial aneurysms—prospective study in 143 patients with178 aneurysms	178	105	PED	140	30-day complications:143 patients Mortality: 1(1.4 %),ipsilateral ischemic stroke 1 (0.7 %), contralateral ICH 2 (1.4 %)	[a]78/140 (55.7 %) complete occlusion	61/75 (81 %) complete occlusion >12 months: [a]49/58 (84.5 %) complete occlusion; 0 recanalization
Saatci et al. 2012 [84]	Treatment of intracranial aneurysms using Pipeline flow-diverter embolization device: largest single-center experience with long-term follow-up results	251	134	PED	239	Worsening of mass effect 4 (0.16 %);SAH 1 (0.41 %); thromboembolic events 4 (0.14 %);in-stent stenosis needing treatment 3 (0.12 %)	[a]219/239; total occlusion rate 91.6 %.	7/20; results N/A

(continued)

Table 2.5 (continued)

Author(s), year	Title	No. aneurysms treated	No. of paraclinoid aneurysms treated	Type of flow diverter	Radiologic follow-up available (no. patients)	Complications	6-month angiography	12 months
Velioglu et al. 2012 [85]	Early and midterm results of complex cerebral aneurysms treated with Silk stent	87	63 (intradural ICA)	Silk	82	Minor thromboembolic event (TIA) (2.6 %); stroke due to embolic events (3.9 %); unexpected procedural technical events in 18 procedures (23.1 %)	[a]Specific time not available; overall control angiographic occlusion rates were as follows:87.8 % (72/82) total occlusion, 8.5 % residual aneurysm filling, and 3.7 % residual neck filling	N/A
Lanzino et al. 2012 [5]	Efficacy and safety of flow diversion for paraclinoid aneurysms: a matched-pair analysis compared with standard endovascular approaches	22	22	PED	22	Periprocedural technical complications: thrombus 1 (4.5 %),stent stenosis 1 (4.5 %),TIA 0, stroke 0, retroperitoneal hematoma 0	N/A	Class 1 16/22 (76.2 %);Class 3 7/22 (14.3 %);Class 2 5/22(9.5 %)

Kan et al. 2012 [82]	Early postmarket results after treatment of intracranial aneurysms with the Pipeline embolization device: a US multicenter experience	58	37	PED	19	Thromboembolic 1/19 (5.26 %); ICH: 2/19 (10.52 %); mortality 2/19 (10.52 %)	Among 19 patients with 3-month follow-up angiography, 68 % (13 patients) had complete aneurysm occlusion	N/A
Kallmes et al. 2015 [77]	International retrospective study of the Pipeline embolization device: a multicenter aneurysm treatment study	906	660	PED	Clinical follow-up (19.3 months, median)	ICH 12/569 (2.1 %); ischemic stroke 23/569 (4 %); parent artery stenosis 2/569 (0.35 %); mortality 15/569 (2.6 %)	Angiographic follow-up N/A	N/A
Berge et al. 2012 [79]	Flow-diverter Silk stent for the treatment of intracranial aneurysms: 1-year follow-up in a multicenter study	77	31 (intradural ICA)	Silk	77	[a]Periprocedural morbidity 5/65 (7.7 %),mortality 0 % Delayed: permanent morbidity 5/64 (7.8 %), mortality 2/64 (3 %).	[a]Complete occlusion 38 (68 %);[a]residual neck 3 (5 %); residual aneurysm 11 (20 %)	[a]Complete occlusion 59 (84 %) [a]Residual neck 1 year. 4 (6 %) [a]1 year. 3 (4 %)

(continued)

Table 2.5 (continued)

Author(s), year	Title	No. aneurysms treated	No. of paraclinoid aneurysms treated	Type of flow diverter	Radiologic follow-up available (no. patients)	Complications	6-month angiography	12 months
Piano et al. 2013 [83]	Midterm and long-term follow-up of cerebral aneurysms treated with flow-diverter devices: a single-center experience	104	83 ICA, 16 cavernous	Silk/ PED	91	Of 104 aneurysms, intra-/periprocedural 10,subarachnoid bleed (wire perforation) 3,parenchymal bleed delayed 10,parent vessel occlusion 4,TIA/ischemia 4,visual disturbances 1,intrastent thrombosis 1	78/91 (86 %) complete occlusion;11/91 (12 %) cases only a small remnant (<10 % of original aneurysmal sac)	0 % recanalization
Briganti et al. [80]	Italian multicenter experience with flow-diverter devices for intracranial unruptured aneurysm treatment with periprocedural complications—a retrospective data analysis	295	163 supraclinoid, 76 cavernous	Silk/ PED	[a]180	SILK cohort: 14/143 (5.1 %) ICH 5/143, ischemic: 8/143 PED cohort: 15/131(5.5 %) ICH 10/131, ischemic:5/131	At 3 months, 76 % of all aneurysms completely occluded	N/A

Fischer et al. 2012 [81]	Pipeline embolization device (PED) for neurovascular reconstruction: initial experience in the treatment of 101 intracranial aneurysms and dissections	101	79 (anterior circulation)	PED	[a]90	ICH 1/90;thromboembolic events 2/90;non-related ICH 2/90	At 3 months, complete occlusion in 47 (52 %)	74 % complete occlusion; 0 % recanalization

Abbreviations: *ICA* internal carotid artery, *ICH* intracranial hemorrhage, *N/A* data not available, *PED* Pipeline embolization device, *SAH* subarachnoid hemorrhage, *TIA* transient ischemic attack

[a]Not specific to paraclinoid data

Flow-Redirection Endoluminal Device (FRED)

The FRED is a new flow-diverting device [96–98]. It has a unique design of a "stent within a stent." The outer layer has 1 mm cell size and 16-wire weave design. The inner layer has a 48-wire braid design which is attached to the outer layer in a helical pattern with four flared ends, yielding full-length fluoroscopic visualization for good stent placement accuracy. The 48-wire inner stent layer provides a variable 22–44 % metal surface area plus a 16-wire outer stent layer combine for a significant reduction of blood flow into the aneurysm while providing a stable scaffold with excellent vessel apposition (Fig. 2.6).

Early results of this device are impressive. In a series of 24 patients with 34 aneurysms treated with the FRED, 1 disabling stroke and 2 minor strokes with complete recovery were seen [97]. At the 6-month follow-up evaluation, aneurysm occlusion was complete in 22 of 30 aneurysms. As mentioned, a trial of this device is under way in the USA (Pivotal Study of the FRED Stent System in the Treatment of Intracranial Aneurysms; https://clinicaltrials.gov/ct2/results?term=FRED&Search=Search).

Surpass

The Surpass flow diverter is a new-generation flow diverter. The device has high pore density that stays uniform across the aneurysm neck and is not affected by the diameter of the parent artery. As implants with various diameters and lengths are available, a single implant is sufficient to treat the target aneurysm(s) and parent artery (Fig. 2.7).

In one prospective series, 49 aneurysms were treated with the Surpass device [99]. A single device was used in 97 % of cases. There was no major periprocedural morbidity or mortality. During follow-up, four patients (10.4 %) experienced transient neurological deficit. At 6 months, 94 % showed complete occlusion. As mentioned, a trial of this device is under way in the USA (Safety and Effectiveness of an

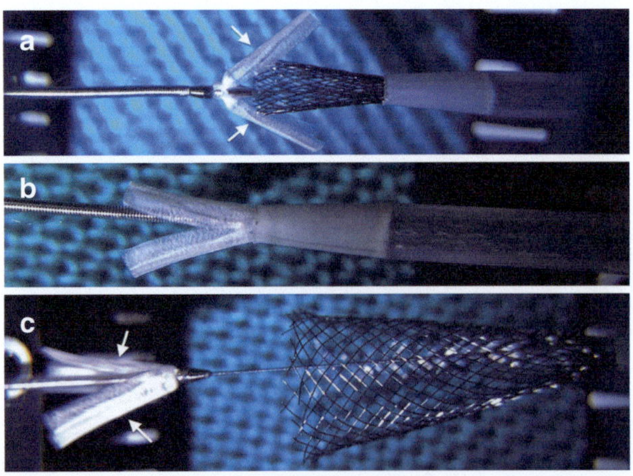

Fig. 2.5 In vitro distal end opening test explaining the "inverting flaps maneuver." (**a**) The implant opens instantly but sometimes the flaps (*white arrows*) do not open fully at the distal end of the device. (**b**) By resheathing the microcatheter, the flaps are displaced in an inverted fashion. (**c**) Unsheathing again allows full opening with perfect wall apposition (With permission from Martínez-Galdámez et al. [94])

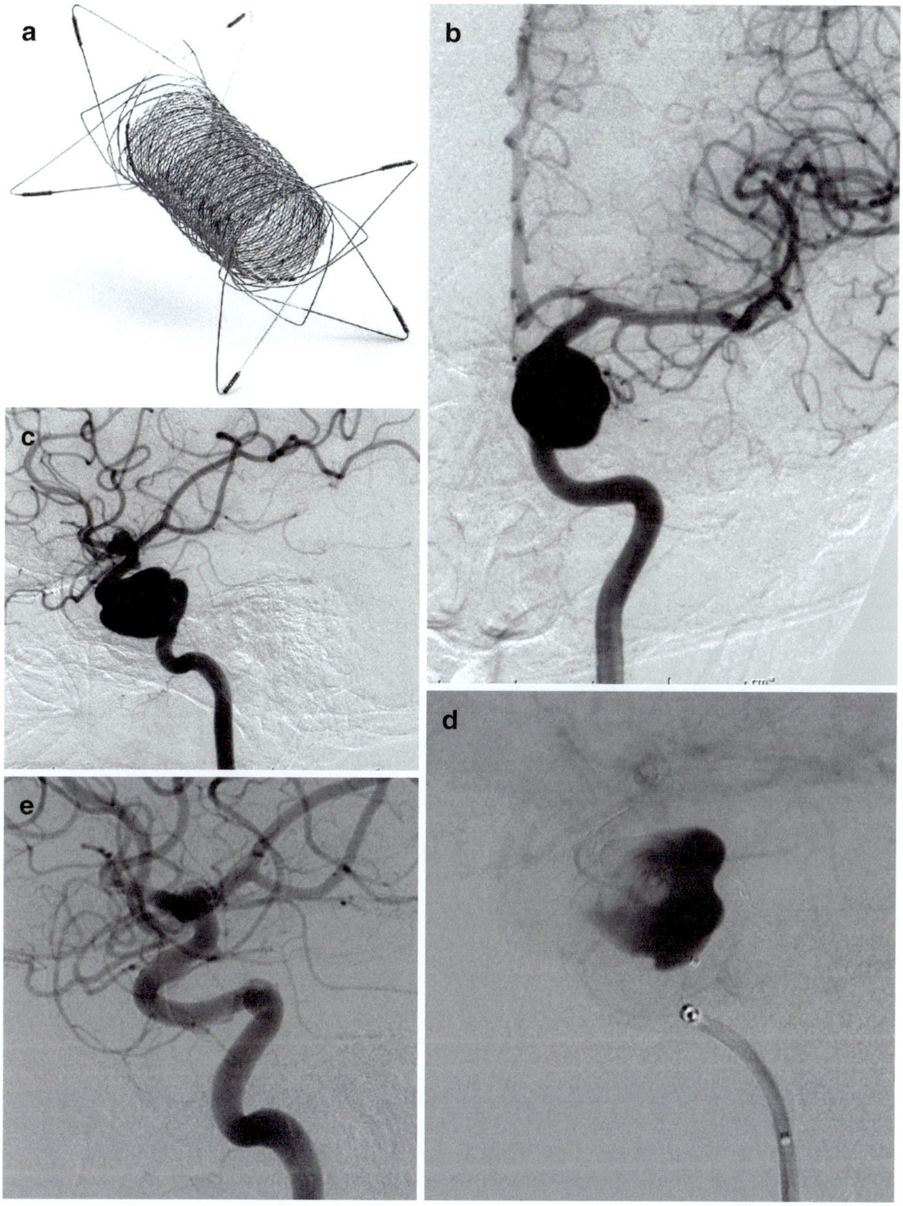

Fig. 2.6 (**a**) The Flow-Redirection Endoluminal Device (FRED, MicroVention) has an outer layer with 1 mm cell size and a 16-wire weave design. The inner layer has a 48-wire braid design and is attached to the outer layer in a helical pattern. The FRED is not approved by the FDA for commercial distribution; the device is investigational and is limited only for investigational use in the USA (Image obtained from Poncyljusz et al. [98]. http://www.ncbi.nlm.nih.gov/pmc/articles/PMC3796728/[This is an Open Access article distributed under the terms of the Creative Commons Attribution-Noncommercial 3.0 Unported License, permitting all non-commercial use, distribution, and reproduction in any medium, provided the original work is properly cited.]). This patient is 54-year-old woman who presented with diplopia. Workup showed a large left carotid-cavernous segment ICA aneurysm ((**b**) AP view and (**c**) lateral view) measuring 1.5 cm. (**d**) Stasis of contrast is seen following FRED deployment. (**e**) One-year follow-up angiogram showed complete occlusion of the aneurysm

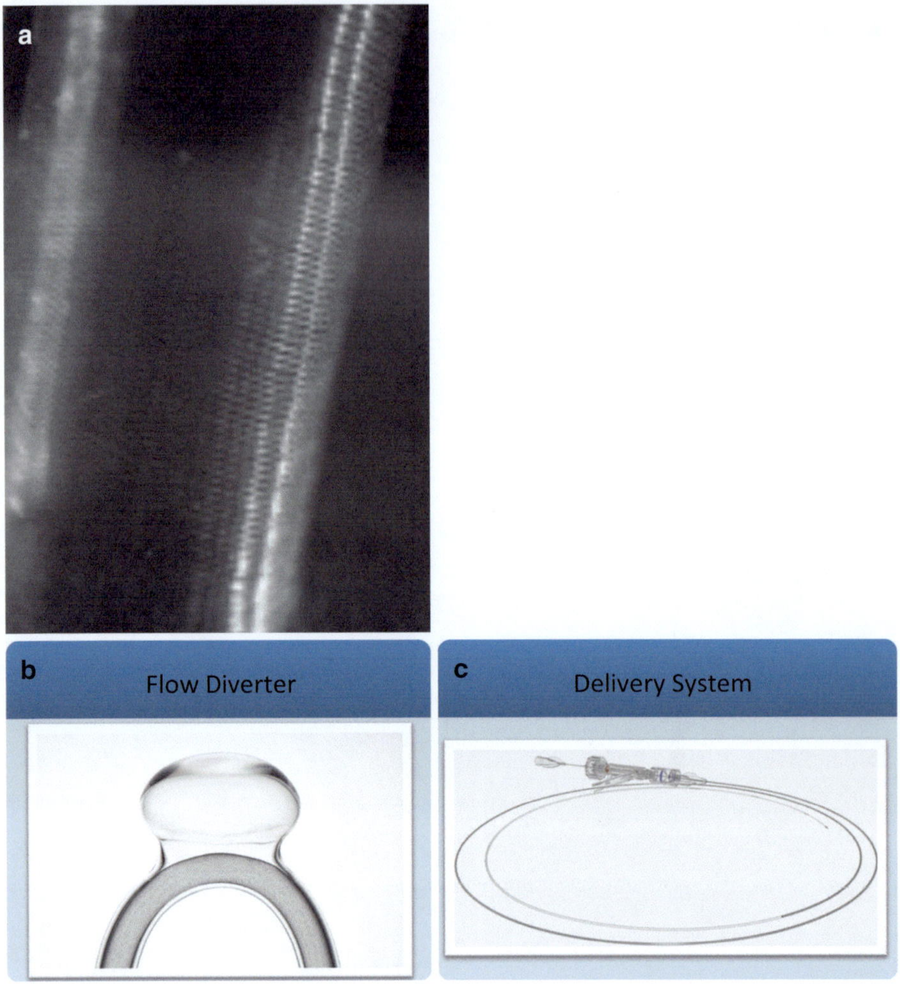

Fig. 2.7 The Surpass (Stryker Neurovascular) is a cobalt-chromium flow diverter (**a**) with low porosity (metal surface area coverage 30 %). This device has a self-expanding tubular-shaped mesh structure (**b**) with high pore density (21–32 pores/mm^2). It has a customized, preloaded, over-the-wire delivery system (**c**) (0.014-inch microwire). (With permission from Stryker Neurovascular). This patient is a 58-year-old woman who presented with headache and was found to have a left paraclinoid aneurysm ((**d**), AP projection; (**e**), lateral projection). She underwent treatment with a Surpass flow diverter. (**f**) and (**g**) Stasis of contrast is seen following device deployment. A 3-month follow-up angiogram is awaited

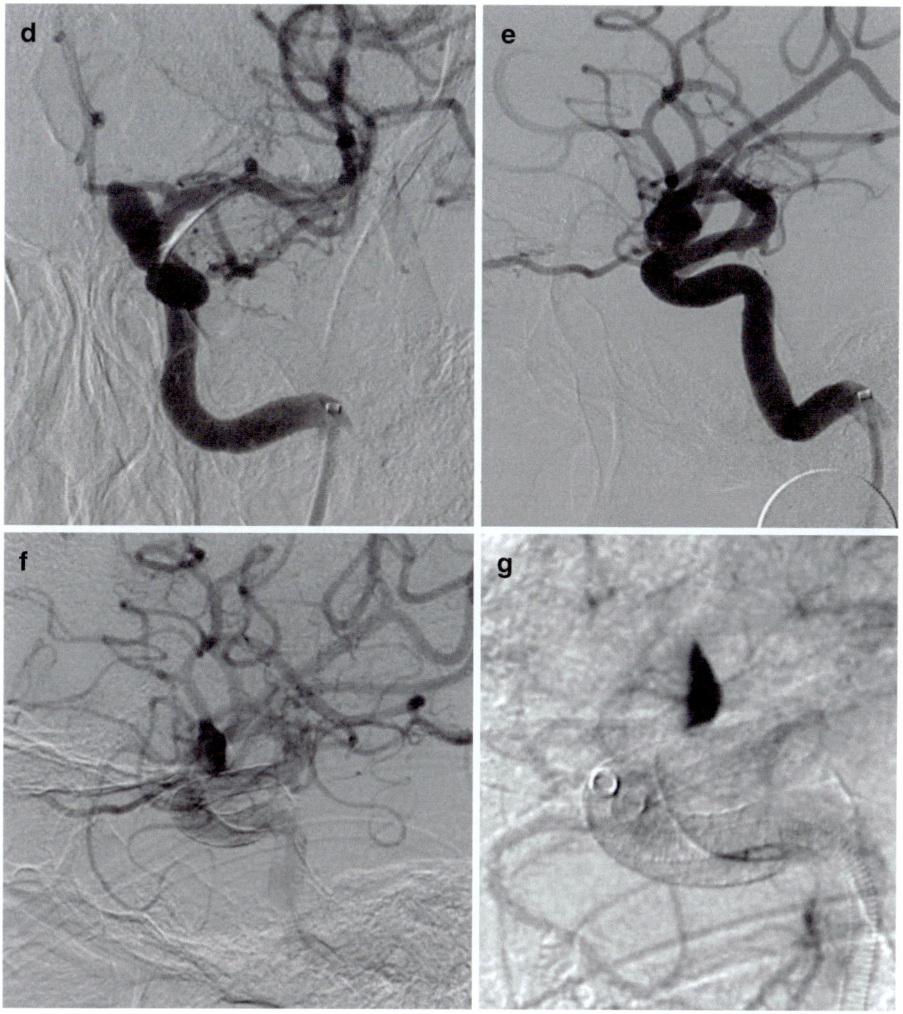

Fig. 2.7 (continued)

Intracranial Aneurysm Embolization System for Treating Large or Giant Wide Neck Aneurysms [SCENT]) [100].

Flow Diverters: The Future

A much higher rate of complete angiographic obliteration can be obtained with flow diversion when compared with other standard endovascular techniques. In a matched-pair analysis comparing PED flow diversion with standard endovascular options for the treatment of paraclinoid aneurysms, a significantly ($p = .03$) higher rate of complete occlusion was observed in the PED cohort with a similar complication rate [5].

In another study, 40 patients treated with the PED were matched with 120 patients treated with coiling. The rates of procedure-related complications did not differ. However, complete obliteration was achieved in a significantly higher proportion of aneurysms treated with Pipeline embolization (86 %) than with coiling (41 %; $P<0.001$) [101]. Flow diversion provides higher occlusion rates with similar complication rates compared with other conventional endovascular options.

Endovascular therapies suffered from perennial worse long-term occlusion rates as compared to microsurgery. Although those therapies had a better safety profile and were clearly less invasive, long-term occlusion rates – the goal of any endovascular intervention for aneurysms – did not even come close to those for microsurgical treatments. Flow diversion is beginning to change that, with long-term occlusion rates approaching microsurgical treatment occlusion rates with a safety profile similar to traditional endovascular therapies. We expect that as the manufacturers of second- and third-generation flow diverters begin addressing current issues of deliverability, reliability, thrombogenicity, and branch vessel management, we will likely see widespread adoption of this methodology in all intracranial locations.

References

1. Day AL. Aneurysms of the ophthalmic segment. A clinical and anatomical analysis. J Neurosurg. 1990;72:677–91.
2. Drake CG, Vanderlinden RG, Amacher AL. Carotid-ophthalmic aneurysms. J Neurosurg. 1968;29:24–31.
3. Seifert V, Guresir E, Vatter H. Exclusively intradural exposure and clip reconstruction in complex paraclinoid aneurysms. Acta Neurochir (Wien). 2011;153:2103–9.
4. D'Urso PI, Karadeli HH, Kallmes DF, et al. Coiling for paraclinoid aneurysms: time to make way for flow diverters? AJNR Am J Neuroradiol. 2012;33:1470–4.
5. Lanzino G, Crobeddu E, Cloft HJ, et al. Efficacy and safety of flow diversion for paraclinoid aneurysms: a matched-pair analysis compared with standard endovascular approaches. AJNR Am J Neuroradiol. 2012;33:2158–61.
6. Thornton J, Aletich VA, Debrun GM, et al. Endovascular treatment of paraclinoid aneurysms. Surg Neurol. 2000;54:288–99.
7. Wiebers DO, Whisnant JP, Huston 3rd J, et al. Unruptured intracranial aneurysms: natural history, clinical outcome, and risks of surgical and endovascular treatment. Lancet. 2003; 362:103–10.
8. Molyneux AJ, Kerr RS, Yu LM, et al. International subarachnoid aneurysm trial (ISAT) of neurosurgical clipping versus endovascular coiling in 2143 patients with ruptured intracranial aneurysms: a randomised comparison of effects on survival, dependency, seizures, rebleeding, subgroups, and aneurysm occlusion. Lancet. 2005;366:809–17.
9. Molyneux AJ, Birks J, Clarke A, et al. The durability of endovascular coiling versus neurosurgical clipping of ruptured cerebral aneurysms: 18 year follow-up of the UK cohort of the International Subarachnoid Aneurysm Trial (ISAT). Lancet. 2015;385:691–7.
10. Becske T, Kallmes DF, Saatci I, et al. Pipeline for uncoilable or failed aneurysms: results from a multicenter clinical trial. Radiology. 2013;267:858–68.
11. De Jesus O, Sekhar LN, Riedel CJ. Clinoid and paraclinoid aneurysms: surgical anatomy, operative techniques, and outcome. Surg Neurol. 1999;51:477–87. discussion 87–8.
12. Joo W, Funaki T, Yoshioka F, et al. Microsurgical anatomy of the carotid cave. Neurosurgery. 2012;70:300–11. discussion 11–2.

13. Kim JM, Romano A, Sanan A, et al. Microsurgical anatomic features and nomenclature of the paraclinoid region. Neurosurgery. 2000;46:670–80. discussion 80–2.
14. Nutik S. Carotid paraclinoid aneurysms with intradural origin and intracavernous location. J Neurosurg. 1978;48:526–33.
15. Gibo H, Lenkey C, Rhoton Jr AL. Microsurgical anatomy of the supraclinoid portion of the internal carotid artery. J Neurosurg. 1981;55:560–74.
16. Bouthillier A, van Loveren HR, Keller JT. Segments of the internal carotid artery: a new classification. Neurosurgery. 1996;38:425–32. discussion 32–3.
17. Batjer HH, Kopitnik TA, Giller CA, et al. Surgery for paraclinoidal carotid artery aneurysms. J Neurosurg. 1994;80:650–8.
18. Lasjaunias P, Santoyo-Vazquez A. Segmental agenesis of the internal carotid artery: angiographic aspects with embryological discussion. Anat Clin. 1984;6:133–41.
19. Shapiro M, Becske T, Riina HA, et al. Toward an endovascular internal carotid artery classification system. AJNR Am J Neuroradiol. 2014;35:230–6.
20. Locksley HB. Natural history of subarachnoid hemorrhage, intracranial aneurysms and arteriovenous malformations. Based on 6368 cases in the cooperative study. J Neurosurg. 1966;25:219–39.
21. International Study of Unruptured Intracranial Aneurysms Investigators. Unruptured intracranial aneurysms--risk of rupture and risks of surgical intervention. N Engl J Med. 1998;339:1725–33.
22. Juvela S, Poussa K, Lehto H, et al. Natural history of unruptured intracranial aneurysms: a long-term follow-up study. Stroke. 2013;44:2414–21.
23. Sonobe M, Yamazaki T, Yonekura M, et al. Small unruptured intracranial aneurysm verification study: SUAVe study, Japan. Stroke. 2010;41:1969–77.
24. Brinjikji W, Rabinstein AA, Nasr DM, et al. Better outcomes with treatment by coiling relative to clipping of unruptured intracranial aneurysms in the United States, 2001–2008. AJNR Am J Neuroradiol. 2011;32:1071–5.
25. Naggara ON, White PM, Guilbert F, et al. Endovascular treatment of intracranial unruptured aneurysms: systematic review and meta-analysis of the literature on safety and efficacy. Radiology. 2010;256:887–97.
26. Greving JP, Wermer MJ, Brown Jr RD, et al. Development of the PHASES score for prediction of risk of rupture of intracranial aneurysms: a pooled analysis of six prospective cohort studies. Lancet Neurol. 2014;13:59–66.
27. Tanaka Y, Hongo K, Tada T, et al. Radiometric analysis of paraclinoid carotid artery aneurysms. J Neurosurg. 2002;96:649–53.
28. Date I, Asari S, Ohmoto T. Cerebral aneurysms causing visual symptoms: their features and surgical outcome. Clin Neurol Neurosurg. 1998;100:259–67.
29. Ferguson GG, Drake CG. Carotid-ophthalmic aneurysms: visual abnormalities in 32 patients and the results of treatment. Surg Neurol. 1981;16:1–8.
30. Nonaka T, Haraguchi K, Baba T, et al. Clinical manifestations and surgical results for paraclinoid cerebral aneurysms presenting with visual symptoms. Surg Neurol. 2007;67:612–9. discussion 19.
31. Shimizu T, Naito I, Aihara M, et al. Visual outcomes of endovascular and microsurgical treatment for large or giant paraclinoid aneurysms. Acta Neurochir (Wien). 2015;157:13–20.
32. de Oliveira JG, Borba LA, Rassi-Neto A, et al. Intracranial aneurysms presenting with mass effect over the anterior optic pathways: neurosurgical management and outcomes. Neurosurg Focus. 2009;26, E3.
33. Schuss P, Guresir E, Berkefeld J, et al. Influence of surgical or endovascular treatment on visual symptoms caused by intracranial aneurysms: single-center series and systematic review. J Neurosurg. 2011;115:694–9.
34. Kumon Y, Sakaki S, Kohno K, et al. Asymptomatic, unruptured carotid-ophthalmic artery aneurysms: angiographical differentiation of each type, operative results, and indications. Surg Neurol. 1997;48:465–72.
35. Almeida GM, Shibata MK, Bianco E. Carotid-ophthalmic aneurysms. Surg Neurol. 1976;5:41–5.

36. Guidetti B, La Torre E. Carotid-ophthalmic aneurysms. A series of 16 cases treated by direct approach. Acta Neurochir (Wien). 1970;22:289–304.
37. Heran NS, Song JK, Kupersmith MJ, et al. Large ophthalmic segment aneurysms with anterior optic pathway compression: assessment of anatomical and visual outcomes after endosaccular coil therapy. J Neurosurg. 2007;106:968–75.
38. Kazekawa K, Tsutsumi M, Aikawa H, et al. Internal carotid aneurysms presenting with mass effect symptoms of cranial nerve dysfunction: efficacy and imitations of endosaccular embolization with GDC. Radiat Med. 2003;21:80–5.
39. Brooks B. The treatment of traumatic arteriovenous fistula. South Med J. 1930;23:00–1.
40. Serbinenko FA. Balloon catheterization and occlusion of major cerebral vessels. J Neurosurg. 1974;41:125–45.
41. Higashida RT, Halbach VV, Dowd C, et al. Endovascular detachable balloon embolization therapy of cavernous carotid artery aneurysms: results in 87 cases. J Neurosurg. 1990;72:857–63.
42. van der Schaaf IC, Brilstra EH, Buskens E, et al. Endovascular treatment of aneurysms in the cavernous sinus: a systematic review on balloon occlusion of the parent vessel and embolization with coils. Stroke. 2002;33:313–8.
43. Chen PR, Ortiz R, Page JH, et al. Spontaneous systolic blood pressure elevation during temporary balloon occlusion increases the risk of ischemic events after carotid artery occlusion. Neurosurgery. 2008;63:256–64. discussion 64–5.
44. Briganti F, Cirillo S, Caranci F, et al. Development of "de novo" aneurysms following endovascular procedures. Neuroradiology. 2002;44:604–9.
45. Standard SC, Ahuja A, Guterman LR, et al. Balloon test occlusion of the internal carotid artery with hypotensive challenge. AJNR Am J Neuroradiol. 1995;16:1453–8.
46. Ahn JH, Cho YD, Kang HS, et al. Endovascular treatment of ophthalmic artery aneurysms: assessing balloon test occlusion and preservation of vision in coil embolization. AJNR Am J Neuroradiol. 2014;35:2146–52.
47. Marshall RS, Lazar RM, Mohr JP, et al. Higher cerebral function and hemispheric blood flow during awake carotid artery balloon test occlusions. J Neurol Neurosurg Psychiatry. 1999;66:734–8.
48. Kaminogo M, Ochi M, Onizuka M, et al. An additional monitoring of regional cerebral oxygen saturation to HMPAO SPECT study during balloon test occlusion. Stroke. 1999;30: 407–13.
49. Liu AY, Lopez JR, Do HM, et al. Neurophysiological monitoring in the endovascular therapy of aneurysms. AJNR Am J Neuroradiol. 2003;24:1520–7.
50. Mathis JM, Barr JD, Jungreis CA, et al. Temporary balloon test occlusion of the internal carotid artery: experience in 500 cases. AJNR Am J Neuroradiol. 1995;16:749–54.
51. Park HK, Horowitz M, Jungreis C, et al. Endovascular treatment of paraclinoid aneurysms: experience with 73 patients. Neurosurgery. 2003;53:14–23. discussion 24.
52. Kwon WH, Jeong HW, Kim ST, et al. Angiographic and clinical result of endovascular treatment in paraclinoid aneurysms. Neurointervention. 2014;9:83–8.
53. Kwon OK, Kim SH, Kwon BJ, et al. Endovascular treatment of wide-necked aneurysms by using two microcatheters: techniques and outcomes in 25 patients. AJNR Am J Neuroradiol. 2005;26:894–900.
54. Kwon OK, Kim SH, Oh CW, et al. Embolization of wide-necked aneurysms with using three or more microcatheters. Acta Neurochir (Wien). 2006;148:1139–45. discussion 45.
55. Toyota S, Fujimoto Y, Iwamoto F, et al. Technique for shaping microcatheter tips in coil embolization of paraclinoid aneurysms using full-scale volume rendering images of 3D rotational angiography. Minim Invasive Neurosurg. 2009;52:201–3.
56. Cho YD, Rhim JK, Park JJ, et al. Microcatheter Looping to Facilitate Aneurysm Selection in Coil Embolization of Paraclinoid Aneurysms. Korean J Radiol. 2015;16:899–905.
57. Kwon BJ, Im SH, Park JC, et al. Shaping and navigating methods of microcatheters for endovascular treatment of paraclinoid aneurysms. Neurosurgery. 2010;67:34–40. discussion 40.

58. Chalouhi N, Jabbour P, Singhal S, et al. Stent-assisted coiling of intracranial aneurysms: predictors of complications, recanalization, and outcome in 508 cases. Stroke. 2013;44: 1348–53.
59. Ogilvy CS, Natarajan SK, Jahshan S, et al. Stent-assisted coiling of paraclinoid aneurysms: risks and effectiveness. J Neurointerv Surg. 2011;3:14–20.
60. Wang Y, Li Y, Jiang C, et al. Endovascular treatment of paraclinoid aneurysms: 142 aneurysms in one centre. J Neurointerv Surg. 2013;5:552–6.
61. Kadkhodayan Y, Rhodes N, Blackburn S, et al. Comparison of Enterprise with Neuroform stent-assisted coiling of intracranial aneurysms. AJR Am J Roentgenol. 2013;200:872–8.
62. King B, Vaziri S, Singla A, et al. Clinical and angiographic outcomes after stent-assisted coiling of cerebral aneurysms with Enterprise and Neuroform stents: a comparative analysis of the literature. J Neurointerv Surg. 2015;7(12):905–9.
63. Chen Z, Yang Y, Miao H, et al. Experiences and complications in endovascular treatment of paraclinoid aneurysms. J Clin Neurosci. 2013;20:1259–63.
64. Sorimachi T, Ito Y, Morita K, et al. Long-term follow-up of intra-aneurysmal coil embolization for unruptured paraclinoid aneurysms. Neurol Res. 2012;34:864–70.
65. Yadla S, Campbell PG, Grobelny B, et al. Open and endovascular treatment of unruptured carotid-ophthalmic aneurysms: clinical and radiographic outcomes. Neurosurgery. 2011;68: 1434–43. discussion 43.
66. Campi A, Ramzi N, Molyneux AJ, et al. Retreatment of ruptured cerebral aneurysms in patients randomized by coiling or clipping in the International Subarachnoid Aneurysm Trial (ISAT). Stroke. 2007;38:1538–44.
67. Gandhi CD, Bulsara KR, Fifi J, et al. Platelet function inhibitors and platelet function testing in neurointerventional procedures. J Neurointerv Surg. 2014;6:567–77.
68. Delgado Almandoz JE, Crandall BM, Scholz JM, et al. Pre-procedure P2Y12 reaction units value predicts perioperative thromboembolic and hemorrhagic complications in patients with cerebral aneurysms treated with the Pipeline Embolization Device. J Neurointerv Surg. 2013;5 Suppl 3:iii3–10.
69. Delgado Almandoz JE, Crandall BM, Scholz JM, et al. Last-recorded P2Y12 reaction units value is strongly associated with thromboembolic and hemorrhagic complications occurring up to 6 months after treatment in patients with cerebral aneurysms treated with the pipeline embolization device. AJNR Am J Neuroradiol. 2014;35:128–35.
70. Delgado Almandoz JE, Kadkhodayan Y, Crandall BM, et al. Variability in initial response to standard clopidogrel therapy, delayed conversion to clopidogrel hyper-response, and associated thromboembolic and hemorrhagic complications in patients undergoing endovascular treatment of unruptured cerebral aneurysms. J Neurointerv Surg. 2014;6:767–73.
71. Shapiro M, Raz E, Becske T, et al. Variable porosity of the Pipeline embolization device in straight and curved vessels: a guide for optimal deployment strategy. AJNR Am J Neuroradiol. 2014;35:727–33.
72. Ma D, Xiang J, Choi H, et al. Enhanced aneurysmal flow diversion using a dynamic push-pull technique: an experimental and modeling study. AJNR Am J Neuroradiol. 2014;35:1779–85.
73. Shapiro M, Raz E, Becske T, et al. Building multidevice Pipeline constructs of favorable metal coverage: a practical guide. AJNR Am J Neuroradiol. 2014;35:1556–61.
74. Puffer RC, Kallmes DF, Cloft HJ, et al. Patency of the ophthalmic artery after flow diversion treatment of paraclinoid aneurysms. J Neurosurg. 2012;116:892–6.
75. Lin N, Brouillard AM, Krishna C, et al. Use of coils in conjunction with the Pipeline embolization device for treatment of intracranial aneurysms. Neurosurgery. 2015;76:142–9.
76. Leung GK, Tsang AC, Lui WM. Pipeline embolization device for intracranial aneurysm: a systematic review. Clin Neuroradiol. 2012;22:295–303.
77. Kallmes DF, Hanel R, Lopes D, et al. International retrospective study of the Pipeline embolization device: a multicenter aneurysm treatment study. AJNR Am J Neuroradiol. 2015;36: 108–15.

78. Lylyk P, Miranda C, Ceratto R, et al. Curative endovascular reconstruction of cerebral aneurysms with the pipeline embolization device: the Buenos Aires experience. Neurosurgery. 2009;64:632–42; discussion 42–3; quiz N6.
79. Berge J, Biondi A, Machi P, et al. Flow-diverter Silk stent for the treatment of intracranial aneurysms: 1-year follow-up in a multicenter study. AJNR Am J Neuroradiol. 2012;33:1150–5.
80. Briganti F, Napoli M, Tortora F, et al. Italian multicenter experience with flow-diverter devices for intracranial unruptured aneurysm treatment with periprocedural complications--a retrospective data analysis. Neuroradiology. 2012;54:1145–52.
81. Fischer S, Vajda Z, Aguilar Perez M, et al. Pipeline embolization device (PED) for neurovascular reconstruction: initial experience in the treatment of 101 intracranial aneurysms and dissections. Neuroradiology. 2012;54:369–82.
82. Kan P, Siddiqui AH, Veznedaroglu E, et al. Early postmarket results after treatment of intracranial aneurysms with the Pipeline embolization device: a U.S. multicenter experience. Neurosurgery. 2012;71:1080–7; discussion 87–8.
83. Piano M, Valvassori L, Quilici L, et al. Midterm and long-term follow-up of cerebral aneurysms treated with flow diverter devices: a single-center experience. J Neurosurg. 2013;118: 408–16.
84. Saatci I, Yavuz K, Ozer C, et al. Treatment of intracranial aneurysms using the Pipeline flow-diverter embolization device: a single-center experience with long-term follow-up results. AJNR Am J Neuroradiol. 2012;33:1436–46.
85. Velioglu M, Kizilkilic O, Selcuk H, et al. Early and midterm results of complex cerebral aneurysms treated with Silk stent. Neuroradiology. 2012;54:1355–65.
86. Yu SC, Kwok CK, Cheng PW, et al. Intracranial aneurysms: midterm outcome of Pipeline embolization device--a prospective study in 143 patients with 178 aneurysms. Radiology. 2012;265:893–901.
87. Chan RS, Mak CH, Wong AK, et al. Use of the Pipeline embolization device to treat recently ruptured dissecting cerebral aneurysms. Interv Neuroradiol. 2014;20:436–41.
88. Lin N, Brouillard AM, Keigher KM, et al. Utilization of Pipeline embolization device for treatment of ruptured intracranial aneurysms: US multicenter experience. J Neurointerv Surg. 2015;7(11):808–15.
89. Chalouhi N, Zanaty M, Whiting A, et al. Treatment of ruptured intracranial aneurysms with the pipeline embolization device. Neurosurgery. 2015;76:165–72. discussion 72.
90. Yoon JW, Siddiqui AH, Dumont TM, et al. Feasibility and safety of Pipeline embolization device in patients with ruptured carotid blister aneurysms. Neurosurgery. 2014;75:419–29. discussion 29.
91. Lubicz B, Van der Elst O, Collignon L, et al. Silk flow-diverter stent for the treatment of intracranial aneurysms: a series of 58 patients with emphasis on long-term results. AJNR Am J Neuroradiol. 2015;36:542–6.
92. Colby GP, Lin LM, Caplan JM, et al. Immediate procedural outcomes in 44 consecutive Pipeline Flex cases: the first North American single-center series. J Neurointerv Surg 2015. Epub *July 1* 2015
93. Duckworth EA, Nickele C, Hoit D, et al. The first North American use of the Pipeline Flex flow diverter. BMJ Case Rep. 2015;30:2015.
94. Martinez-Galdamez M, Gil A, Caniego JL, et al. Preliminary experience with the Pipeline Flex Embolization Device: technical note. J Neurointerv Surg. 2015;7(10):748–51.
95. Martinez-Galdamez M, Perez S, Vega A, et al. Endovascular treatment of intracranial aneurysms using the Pipeline Flex embolization device: a case series of 30 consecutive patients. J Neurointerv Surg. 2016;8(4):396–401.
96. Diaz O, Gist TL, Manjarez G, et al. Treatment of 14 intracranial aneurysms with the FRED system. J Neurointerv Surg. 2014;6:614–7.

97. Mohlenbruch MA, Herweh C, Jestaedt L, et al. The FRED Flow-Diverter Stent for Intracranial Aneurysms: Clinical Study to Assess Safety and Efficacy. AJNR Am J Neuroradiol. 2015;36: 1155–61.
98. Poncyljusz W, Sagan L, Safranow K, et al. Initial experience with implantation of novel dual layer flow-diverter device FRED. Wideochir Inne Tech Maloinwazyjne. 2013;8:258–64.
99. De Vries J, Boogaarts J, Van Norden A, et al. New generation of flow diverter (Surpass) for unruptured intracranial aneurysms: a prospective single-center study in 37 patients. Stroke. 2013;44:1567–77.
100. Safety and Effectiveness of an Intracranial Aneurysm Embolization System for Treating Large or Giant Wide Neck Aneurysms (SCENT). NCT01716117. ClinicalTrials.gov [Internet]. [cited 2015 Jul 28]. Available from: https://clinicaltrials.gov/ct2/show/NCT01716117.
101. Chalouhi N, Tjoumakaris S, Starke RM, et al. Comparison of flow diversion and coiling in large unruptured intracranial saccular aneurysms. Stroke. 2013;44:2150–4.

Treatment Options for Paraclinoid Aneurysms: Discussion

3

Adam S. Arthur, Daniel A. Hoit, and Clarence B. Watridge

In the preceding two chapters, the authors have reviewed the literature and their experience with paraclinoid aneurysms. They pay particular attention to the indications and techniques used for treatment with open surgical clipping and flow diversion. Also mentioned were several other strategies for treating patients with these lesions including conservative management, carotid ligation, simple embolization, and balloon- or stent-assisted embolization.

With so many therapies available, it is difficult but important to organize a cohesive framework upon which to base treatment recommendations. In our view, patient presentation is the most important influence upon this decision. Paraclinoid aneurysms are generally brought to the attention of patients and their physicians as incidental findings, after subarachnoid hemorrhage, or as the culprits of symptoms from mass effect.

Open surgical outcomes and techniques have improved, and endovascular technology has advanced tremendously, but the bimodal distribution of patient presentation is both a historical and modern constant in the practice of cerebrovascular neurosurgery. Patients are generally either quite ill, or completely asymptomatic. Asymptomatic patients often fear that their aneurysm could, without warning, cause a devastating hemorrhage. It therefore becomes incumbent on the physician to provide sage counseling and to make treatment recommendations based on the available data for rupture risk and treatment risks.

The first option considered for incidentally discovered aneurysms should be conservative treatment. Small aneurysms generally have a low risk of hemorrhage distributed over the lifetime of the patient. Conversely, procedural risk is inherent to any open surgical or endovascular intervention and diminishes after treatment. For

A.S. Arthur, MD, MPH (✉) • D.A. Hoit, MD, MPH • C.B. Watridge, MD
Department of Neurosurgery, Semmes-Murphey Neurologic and Spine Clinic,
University of Tennessee, Memphis, TN, USA
e-mail: aarthur@semmes-murphey.com

E. Veznedaroglu (ed.), *Controversies in Vascular Neurosurgery*,
DOI 10.1007/978-3-319-27315-0_3

older patients and others with shorter life expectancies, the cumulative risk of hemorrhage is likely less than the procedural risk even for the most experienced operators. When no procedure is recommended, the physician must reassure the patient and explain the rationale for conservative therapy. Interval noninvasive imaging to monitor for any growth or change in the aneurysm may be performed, although scientific data for this recommendation are lacking. Despite these recommendations, some patients will remain ill at ease at the prospect of living with a potentially dangerous aneurysm. In our view, further clinical follow-up to facilitate discussion and understanding between physicians, patients, and caregivers is the basis of conservative management and should be considered a viable therapeutic option.

For those with larger aneurysms, younger patients or those with risk factors for subarachnoid hemorrhage, exclusion of the aneurysm from the circulation is warranted. In narrow-necked aneurysms, simple embolization is often effective and carries low periprocedural risk. Utilizing careful angiography, obliteration of the aneurysm can be achieved with coils alone and obviate the need for adjunctive technologies or surgical exposures. Coiled aneurysms should be followed for growth or recurrence, but published data indicate that shallow neck remnants pose little risk of hemorrhage. For wide-necked aneurysms, balloon-assisted coiling can result in aneurysm neck closure without placement of an intraluminal device. For many large wide-necked aneurysms, intraluminal stents or flow diversion offers the best chance for a complete angiographic treatment. Stent-assisted coiling and flow diversion both require the usage of dual antiplatelet medications, but both have been shown to have higher initial occlusion rates, higher likelihoods of improved or stable remnants, and lower recurrence rates for treated aneurysms.

Currently, flow-diverting devices are indicated by the FDA as "on label" in the USA only for the treatment of large cavernous segment and paraclinoid aneurysms but have been used extensively for smaller aneurysms, more distal anterior circulation aneurysms, and posterior circulation aneurysms with acceptable safety and efficacy margins both in the USA and abroad. For large lesions, and/or complex lesions encompassing both the paraclinoid and more proximal cavernous internal carotid artery, flow diversion has supplanted clip reconstruction, bypass, coiling, liquid embolics, and stent-assisted coiling. While access and device positioning can be challenging, flow diversion provides a gradual thrombosis of the aneurysm in many cases and allows for recovery of the native arterial endothelium, while preserving flow within the distal vascular territory. When access is possible, and there are no contraindications to antiplatelet therapy, we use flow diversion as a first option for treatment of these difficult cases. The use of coils in conjunction with flow diversion remains an area of investigation, and further definition of risk factors for complications of flow diversion including in-stent thrombosis, aneurysm rupture after flow diversion, and distal hemorrhagic or ischemic events is needed.

Open surgical clipping for asymptomatic paraclinoid aneurysms, once common, has become a much less common occurrence in our practice. We agree that this is an excellent option for younger patients or patients who harbor multiple accessible aneurysms that seem to merit treatment. This is a scenario that we encounter a few times a year in our current practice.

While there has been much discussion regarding the anatomical location of a paraclinoid aneurysm in regard to the cavernous sinus and dural rings, there has been less discussion about the extent of circumferential carotid arterial wall involvement. Many paraclinoid aneurysms involve much of the circumference of the carotid artery, and "reconstructing" an artery by clip application begs the question of how any unclipped arterial wall will behave in future years and just how much risk avoidance is achieved with open clipping. Any paraclinoid aneurysm with carotid artery wall involvement of 180° or more poses a significant risk of incomplete clipping and adjacent anatomical iatrogenic injury. It may well be that aneurysms with extensive circumferential arterial aneurysmal involvement are better candidates for either arterial sacrifice with or without bypass or flow diversion. The actual aneurysm anatomy as it relates to the extent of circumferential carotid artery wall involvement is an important factor in the consideration of the risk of surgical intervention.

In our practice, several factors deserve special attention when microneurosurgical clipping is required. Proximal control is of paramount importance. It is unusual to approach a paraclinoid aneurysm without exposure of the cervical internal carotid artery. In addition to proximal control, having access to the cervical carotid allows for needle aspiration of a large aneurysm to deflate the aneurysm for more facile clip application. Others have used endovascular balloon guide catheters for this purpose. Removal of the clinoid process is performed routinely by an extradural approach with an occasional completion of clinoid removal by a combined intradural and extradural exposure. Much care is given to protection of the optic nerve. This is accomplished by removal of the clinoid and opening the falciform ligament and dural investment for a generous length of the nerve. Temporary clipping proximal to the takeoff of the posterior communicating artery with cervical carotid occlusion isolates the paraclinoid segment for less dangerous clip application and optic nerve manipulation. Placement of the clip proximal to the posterior communicating artery allows for at least some continued perfusion of the carotid territory. Cerebral protection is accomplished by maintaining an adequate blood pressure as well as the use of cerebral protection agents. Once a clip reconstruction of the paraclinoid internal carotid artery has been accomplished, ensuring patency of the artery is accomplished by indocyanine green video angiography and, not infrequently, intraoperative arteriography. For aneurysms that involve more than 180° of the internal carotid, arterial sacrifice is considered if endovascular techniques are not feasible. In these cases, test balloon occlusion with SPECT imaging is performed. In the event the patient does not show adequate collateral flow and develops a neurologic impairment or decreased cerebral blood flow by SPECT, extracranial to intracranial arterial bypass is planned. High flow vein graft bypasses are used to replace the carotid blood flow if the patient develops a significant deficit, whereas, if the patient has no clinical deficit but abnormal SPECT imaging, superficial temporal artery to middle cerebral artery bypass is performed to augment the collateral circulation. Attention to every detail is required in the surgical approaches for these aneurysms and even then, a perfect result is not always obtained.

For symptomatic aneurysms, the most commonly encountered issue is how to deal with an aneurysm that threatens vision. For large paraclinoid aneurysms that present with visual deficits, every available option carries the risk of partial or even complete blindness. Conservative management carries a definitive risk of the progression of any visual deficit and aneurysm rupture. While open surgical treatment has been advocated for this situation, there are aneurysms that grow around or into the optic nerve or have thinned the nerve over time. It can be daunting to confront this situation in the operating room with the delicate nerve plastered against the dome of the aneurysm. Dissection of the aneurysm away from the nerve in these cases carries a significant risk of loss of vision. As has been often noted, endovascular treatment does not immediately remove the mass effect, and vision can worsen acutely as the aneurysm undergoes inflammatory changes after endovascular treatment. In such cases, the particulars of the patient's age, medical condition, and visual status should be taken into account in weighing which option might be the "least bad" choice. Occasionally, paraclinoid aneurysms will present with symptoms of headache or dysfunction of other cranial nerves as well. These symptoms can be very important when judging the risk of rupture and sudden death as they may be harbingers of aneurysm growth. At times, one has to accept that loss of vision in one eye or other cranial nerve deficits are preferable to a devastating subarachnoid bleed.

Ruptured paraclinoid aneurysms are usually thought to be best treated with some intervention, as the risk of rerupture is significant. Endovascular therapy is our first consideration. If the aneurysm is wide necked, we usually prefer to protect the patient against rerupture with a subtotal treatment, planning to treat definitively with stent assistance or flow diversion at a later date to avoid the need for antiplatelet medications in the acute setting. When the patient selection and aneurysm anatomy and morphology do not favor endovascular methods, an open surgical approach with either direct clipping or arterial sacrifice with or without bypass is chosen. Open surgical clipping for ruptured paraclinoid aneurysms has become an uncommon occurrence in our practice with this approach.

From this discussion, it is obvious that a "one-size-fits-all" management paradigm cannot apply to carotid paraclinoid aneurysms. Patient selection with a complete risk/reward analysis is necessary. A detailed knowledge of the aneurysm anatomy and morphology and an awareness of and expertise in which treatment methodologies are best suited for particular patients can provide the platform for the "experts" to be the best advocates for their patients.

Aneurysm Neck Remnants: A Strong Case Can Be Made for Re-treatment

4

Awais Vance and Babu G. Welch

Introduction

Endovascular treatment of intracranial aneurysms, both ruptured and unruptured, is now more prevalent than surgical methods. While the increased surveillance inherent to endovascular success has introduced the concept of "coil compaction," the neck remnant has been a topic of surgical discussion for generations. In 1965, McKissock classically reported the recurrence of a middle cerebral aneurysm following "excision and double clipping" [1]. While many such recurrences were historically found at autopsy, advanced imaging has not only improved detection but also increased consternation over the appropriate management of the aneurysm neck remnant (ANR).

For the purposes of debate, it is important to begin with an accurate definition of the aneurysm neck remnant (ANR). In the endovascular era, the definition provided by the Raymond-Roy classification, "the persistence of any portion of the original defect of the arterial wall as seen on any single projection but without opacification of the aneurysmal sac," serves our purpose [2]. Prior surgical definitions are well encapsulated by Feuerberg and colleagues who define "aneurysm rests" as "a remnant of the aneurysm proximal to the clip which still fills at angiography" [3].

In this publication that addresses common controversies in cerebrovascular surgery, we will argue that treatment of surgical or endovascular neck remnants is appropriate when one carefully evaluates the natural history of the ANR as it relates to the method of presentation, the lesion location, the size (or change in size) of the remnant, and the procedural tolerance of the patient.

Awais Vance, MD
Resident, Department of Neurosurgery, UT Southwestern Medical Center, Dallas, TX, USA

B.G. Welch, MD (✉)
Department of Neurosurgery, UT Southwestern Medical Center, Dallas, TX, USA
e-mail: Babu.Welch@UTSouthwestern.edu

E. Veznedaroglu (ed.), *Controversies in Vascular Neurosurgery*,
DOI 10.1007/978-3-319-27315-0_4

Incidence of the Aneurysm Neck Remnant (ANR)

When discussing the management endovascular and surgical neck remnants, it is crucial to understand the incidence. The true incidence of the surgical ANR is closely related to practice of intraoperative angiography, a former habit that is now sporadic, at best. As endovascular treatments have gained prominence, "delayed" postoperative studies have provided some useful data. In a treatise on the endovascular treatment of neck remnants, Lubicz and colleagues suggest a 4–19 % incidence of surgical neck remnants from their literature review [4]. Similar findings (15 % incomplete obliteration) were provided by the latest Barrow Ruptured Aneurysm Trial data reported 15 % incomplete aneurysm obliteration [3, 5]. Feuerberg et al reported an ANR incidence of 4.4 % (32 of 715, 2–9mm) during an observation period of 4–13 years. Thornton et al. suggested an incidence of 5.4 % in their review of 1,370 surgically clipped aneurysms [6]. Thus a minimum incidence of 4 % is a fair estimate for the surgical ANR.

A recent meta-analysis of coiled aneurysms showed immediate complete occlusion rates of 62 % [7]. Due to the likelihood of progressive thrombosis, the incidence of the ANR in endovascular treatment is better understood at follow-up. Using 12-month follow-up as a guide, our own evaluation of the literature suggests complete occlusion rates somewhere between 60 % and 80 % [8–10]. This is similar to the meta-analysis by Ferns et al. that cites a complete occlusion at follow-up of 61.5 %. The BRAT data also reports a similar initial endovascular complete occlusion rate of 58 % [5]. We would suggest that the reported incidence of endovascular ANR or residual aneurysm to be 20–40 %.

Natural History of ANR

For the sake of brevity, we will propose that many of the same factors that increase the risk of de novo aneurysm rupture (smoking, family history, uncontrolled hypertension) also affect the natural history of the ANR. Management of the ANR is encouraged when these positive risk factors are identified. A discussion of the effect of the method of presentation, the lesion location, and the size (or change in size) of the remnant is more important to the natural history.

The method of presentation appears to have an important influence on the natural history of the ANR. In the endovascular era, it is clear that the natural history of the ANR is aggressive when the remnant is associated a hemorrhagic presentation. In the previously mentioned paper by Feuerberg et al., a calculated risk of re-rupture for the surgical ANR was 3.7 % over a mean follow-up of 8 years [3].

In the CARAT study (2008), the overall risk of re-hemorrhage was 1.9 % and was similarly associated with degree of aneurysm occlusion (1.1 % for complete occlusion, 2.9 % for 91–99 % occlusion, 5.9 % for 70–90 %, 17.6 % for <70 %; $P<0.0001$) [11]. More recently, data from the ISAT study suggests a cumulative risk of delayed (>1 year after treatment) re-hemorrhage is 2.16 % and 0.64 % for coiled and clipped aneurysms, respectively. In this cohort there were 17 incidences of delayed re-hemorrhage, 13 out of 1,073 coiled and 4 out of 1,070 clipped aneurysms with three and two deaths, respectively [12]. Re-hemorrhage occurred up to 10 years after initial treatment. The re-hemorrhage risk varied with degree of occlusion, morphology, and location. Whether this variation is related to the concept of coil compaction or growth of the ANR is difficult to ascertain. Simply put the existence of the neck remnant is more likely with endovascular therapy, and endovascular therapy was directly related to the risk of re-hemorrhage in the largest trial on the topic of treatment of aneurysmal SAH to date.

While prior hemorrhagic presentation should prompt a discussion of re-treatment, new symptoms that can be attributed to an ANR should also raise concern. A classic example would be a posterior communicating artery aneurysm presenting with an acute oculomotor nerve palsy following treatment (Fig. 4.1). Neck remnants

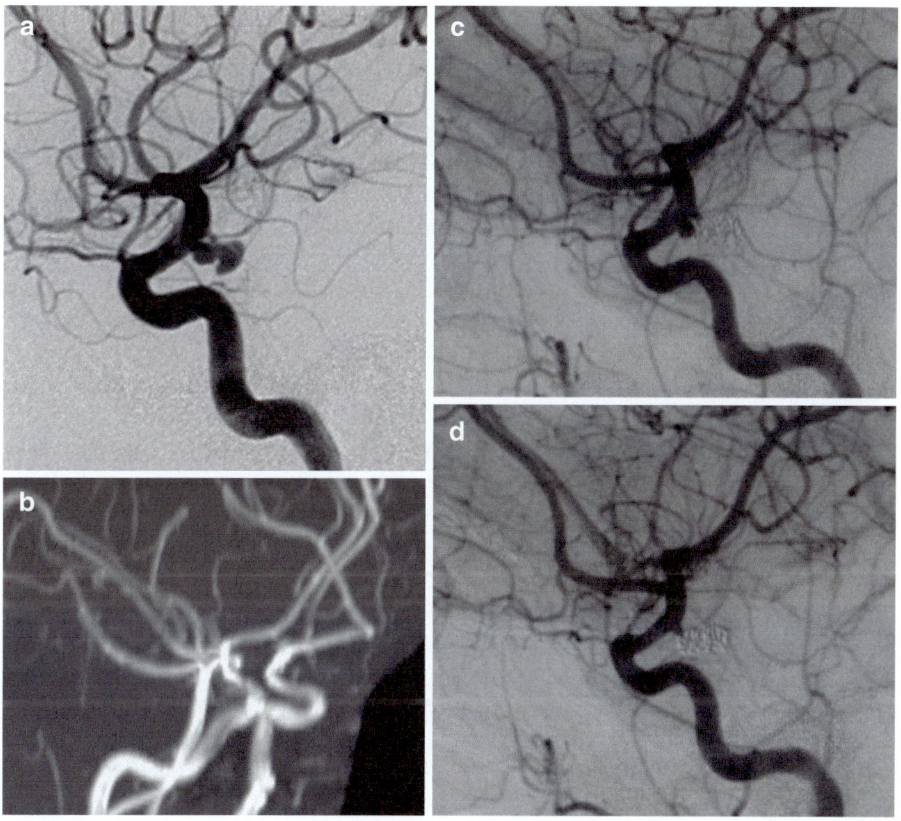

Fig. 4.1 45 year old female presented with new onset left oculomotor palsy and headache. She had a history of SAH from an aneurysm of the posterior communicating artery (**a**) 8 years prior to presentation. Despite a negative MRA (**b**), urgent angiography was performed that demonstrated a neck remnant (**c**). Surgical clipping was performed with a satisfactory result (**d**)

associated with aneurysms causing cranial nerve palsies, brainstem compression, or hydrocephalus warrant re-treatment especially if the neurologic symptoms are clearly associated with growth of the ANR.

Similar to the decision-making in unruptured aneurysms, location must also be considered in the assessment of the ANR. Following McKissock's initial report, Dr. Charles Drake and colleagues reported an evaluation of their own series detailing the management of symptomatic recurrences [13]. This review of 19 patients suggested it was more likely that the ANR would grow in the young patient. Expectedly, there were a disproportionate number (60 %) of posterior circulation lesions in this group. Feuerberg's own analysis of a larger cohort of surgical patients suggested a higher proportion of aneurysm rests in the anterior circulation and a single incidence of re-rupture in an MCA recurrence. Their review did not include any basilar apex aneurysm and had only one posterior circulation lesion. A more uniform evaluation of the effect of location on aneurysm "reopening" was performed by Ferns et al. [10]. In their evaluation of 46 studies (8,161 coiled aneurysms), the relative risk of aneurysm recurrence was 1.5 for posterior circulation lesions when compared with the anterior circulation.

The re-treatment of the cavernous aneurysm produces an interesting discussion in the era of flow diversion. Cavernous aneurysms have a much lower risk of rupture (0–1 %/year excluding giant aneurysms) [14], and the consequences of rupture are typically less than intradural aneurysms. We would advocate a less aggressive management scheme in the asymptomatic cavernous ANR.

Re-treatment Risk

An essential component of and essential, components of the discussion of management of the ANR should be the risk-to-benefit ratio of the treatment itself and the patient's tolerance of such a therapy. In the surgical era, patient tolerance was a much larger component of the re-treatment argument. Surgical morbidities range from 7 % to 15.7 % in earlier treatises on the topic [15, 16]. As endovascular treatments improve, the lower associated morbidity has resulted in a continued discussion concerning the management of the ANR. Ringer and colleagues reported a very low risk of death or permanent disability (1.28 %) in their series of 352 endovascular re-treatment procedures [17]. Other large retrospective series have reported similar low rates (<3 %) of complications from re-treatment [18, 19]. Given the risks associated with untreated ANR and the relatively low-risk endovascular re-treatment, we would argue in favor of treatment of the ANR that meets the more worrisome criteria above. Based on the morbidities above, endovascular and surgical benefits should be carefully weighed.

Advanced Imaging of ANR

Novel imaging techniques exist that may strengthen the argument for ANR management. These imaging techniques include aneurysm flow mapping and vessel wall characterization. Improved evaluation of the aneurysm wall will profoundly change the management of the ANR as well as the management of patients with multiple aneurysms.

Categorization of aneurysm flow (3D TOF MRA and 4D flow MRI) may be able improve the neurosurgeon's ability to predict the aggressive ANR. For example, water-hammer effects on the inflow zone may cause coil compaction, neck remnant growth, and rupture [20]. Computational fluid dynamic simulations have also been performed on post-processed catheter angiogram data to assess regional impact from inflow into the aneurysm. These findings have been associated with increased risk of aneurysm rupture [21, 22].

Similar to echocardiography, an evaluation of changes in or stress on the aneurysm wall secondary to tensile forces is directly related to aneurysm diameter and inversely proportional to wall thickness. High-resolution double inversion recovery black-blood MRI sequences can be used to directly measure wall thickness and thus give further information with regard to rupture risk of an aneurysm or ANR [23]. Similarly, T1-weighted black-blood imaging pre-/post-contrast can be used to assess aneurysm wall enhancement and intramural hemorrhage, both of which are associated with aneurysm rupture [24].

Conclusion

A strong case for re-treatment of the ANR can be made due to the aggressive behavior of select recurrent lesions and the improved morbidity provided by modern surgical and endovascular techniques. The ANR in a young patient with a previously ruptured lesion of the posterior circulation should raise the most concern. Similar trepidation should occur with the ANR that is associated with thromboembolic events, compressive symptoms causing neurologic deficits, or pain. As always the patient's age, current health, and SAH risk factors (e.g., hypertension, smoking) should be considered in the decision for re-treatment.

In the endovascular era, we have achieved the potential for lower treatment morbidity when compared with prior surgical approaches. Given the dire consequences of SAH and improved treatment modalities, a more aggressive approach to the management of the aneurysm neck remnant should be considered.

References

1. McKissock W. Recurrence of an intracranial aneurysm after excision. J Neurosurg. 1965;23:547–8.
2. Roy D, Milot G, Raymond J. Endovascular treatment of unruptured aneurysms. Stroke. 2001;32:1998–2004.
3. Natural history of postoperative aneurysm rests. 2009;66:30–4.
4. Lubicz B, Leclerc X, Gauvrit JY, Lejeune JP, Pruvo JP. Endovascular treatment of remnants of intracranial aneurysms following incomplete clipping. Neuroradiology. 2004;46:318–22.
5. Spetzler RF, et al. The barrow ruptured aneurysm trial: 3-year results. J Neurosurg. 2013;119:146–57.
6. Thornton J, et al. What percentage of surgically clipped intracranial aneurysms have residual necks? Neurosurgery. 2000;46:1294–8; discussion 1298–300.
7. Darflinger R, Thompson LA, Zhang Z, Chao K. Recurrence, retreatment, and rebleed rates of coiled aneurysms with respect to the Raymond-Roy scale: a meta-analysis. J NeuroInterventional Surg. 2015. doi:10.1136/neurintsurg-2015-011668.

8. Hayakawa M, et al. Natural history of the neck remnant of a cerebral aneurysm treated with the Guglielmi detachable coil system. J Neurosurg. 2000;93:561–8.
9. Raymond J, et al. Long-term angiographic recurrences after selective endovascular treatment of aneurysms with detachable coils. Stroke. 2003;34:1398–403.
10. Ferns SP, et al. Coiling of intracranial aneurysms: a systematic review on initial occlusion and reopening and retreatment rates. Stroke. 2009;40:e523–9.
11. Johnston SC, et al. Predictors of rehemorrhage after treatment of ruptured intracranial aneurysms: the Cerebral Aneurysm Rerupture After Treatment (CARAT) study. Stroke. 2008;39:120–5.
12. Molyneux AJ, Birks J, Clarke A, Sneade M, Kerr RSC. The durability of endovascular coiling versus neurosurgical clipping of ruptured cerebral aneurysms: 18 year follow-up of the UK cohort of the International Subarachnoid Aneurysm Trial (ISAT). Lancet. 2015;385:691–7.
13. Regrowth of aneurysm sacs from residual neck following aneurysm clipping. 2009; 70:556–60.
14. Wiebers DO, et al. Unruptured intracranial aneurysms: natural history, clinical outcome, and risks of surgical and endovascular treatment. Lancet. 2003;362:103–10.
15. Giannotta SL, Litofsky NS. Reoperative management of intracranial aneurysms. J Neurosurg. 1995;83:387–93.
16. Drake C, Friedman A, Peerless S. Failed aneurysm surgery: reoperation in 115 cases. J Neurosurg. 1984;61:848–56.
17. Defining the risk of retreatment for aneurysm recurrence or residual after initial treatment by endovascular coiling: a multicenter study. 2009;65:311–5; discussion 315.
18. Henkes H, et al. Repeated endovascular coil occlusion in 350 of 2759 intracranial aneurysms: safety and effectiveness aspects. Neurosurgery. 2006;58:224–32; discussion 224–32.
19. Teleb MS, et al. Safety and predictors of aneurysm retreatment for remnant intracranial aneurysm after initial endovascular embolization. J NeuroInterventional Surg. 2014;6:490–4.
20. Futami K, et al. Identification of the inflow zone of unruptured cerebral aneurysms: comparison of 4D flow MRI and 3D TOF MRA data. AJNR Am J Neuroradiol. 2014;35:1363–70.
21. Cebral JR, Mut F, Weir J, Putman CM. Association of hemodynamic characteristics and cerebral aneurysm rupture. AJNR Am J Neuroradiol. 2011;32:264–70.
22. Cebral JR, et al. Characterization of cerebral aneurysms for assessing risk of rupture by using patient-specific computational hemodynamics models. AJNR Am J Neuroradiol. 2005;26: 2550–9.
23. Park JK, Lee CS, Sim KB, Huh JS, Park JC. Imaging of the walls of saccular cerebral aneurysms with double inversion recovery black-blood sequence. J Magn Reson Imaging. 2009;30:1179–83.
24. Matouk CC, et al. Vessel wall magnetic resonance imaging identifies the site of rupture in patients with multiple intracranial aneurysms: proof of principle. Neurosurgery. 2013;72:492–6.

Remnant Intracranial Aneurysms: Safety and Feasibility of Observation Over Retreatment

5

Gerald W. Eckardt, Akinwunmi Oni-Orisan, Brian-Fred Fitzsimmons, and Glen Pollock

Introduction

The treatment of intracranial aneurysms has seen significant changes over the past 20 years with the advent of detachable coils and other endovascular techniques. With multiple modalities available to the surgeon and interventionalist, the decision of which treatment algorithm to recommend to patients can be challenging. Even more challenging can be the discussion following treatment of a patient's aneurysm, as not every procedure ends with complete occlusion of the index aneurysm. Protocols for follow-up imaging after aneurysm treatment are not readily available, and despite much research on this subject, evidence is still lacking. Once the treatment choice has been determined, a follow-up plan must be presented to each patient in such a manner that the risk of rupture or rerupture in the future is as low as feasibly possible. In this chapter, we will briefly overview the natural history of ruptured and unruptured intracranial aneurysms and the treatment modalities currently employed. Additionally, we will present research supporting the observation of remnant intracranial aneurysms found following treatment with open surgical clipping and endovascular techniques. Lastly, we will demonstrate the safety and practicality of close clinical and imaging observation for these patients in lieu of further immediate treatment as repeat craniotomy or endovascular procedures are not without risk (Figs. 5.1, 5.2, and 5.3).

G.W. Eckardt, MD • A. Oni-Orisan, MD • G. Pollock, MD, DVM (✉)
Department of Neurosurgery, Medical College of Wisconsin, Milwaukee, WI, USA
e-mail: gpolloc1@hotmail.com

B.-F. Fitzsimmons, MD
Department of Neurology, Medical College of Wisconsin, Milwaukee, WI, USA

E. Veznedaroglu (ed.), *Controversies in Vascular Neurosurgery*,
DOI 10.1007/978-3-319-27315-0_5

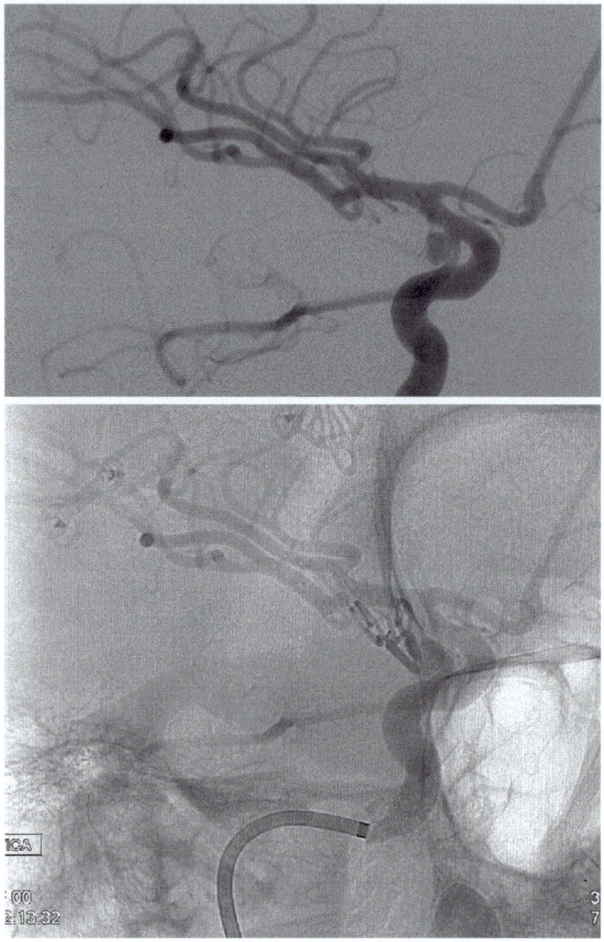

Fig. 5.1 Residual posterior communicating artery aneurysm discovered on follow-up angiogram for patient treated several years prior at an outside institution

Natural History of Intracranial Aneurysms

Aneurysmal subarachnoid hemorrhage (SAH) affects 9–15 persons per 100,000 people per year. The incidence does vary between different populations, but overall life risk is approximately 0.5 % per person [1, 2]. With progressive improvement in noninvasive imaging modalities, the diagnosis of incidentally discovered unruptured aneurysms is increasing. Clinical decision-making for the timing of treatment of these unruptured aneurysms is complex and dependent on multiple factors. Patient history that is positive for current smoking, a positive family or personal history of aneurysmal associated SAH, and hypertension are noted to increase the

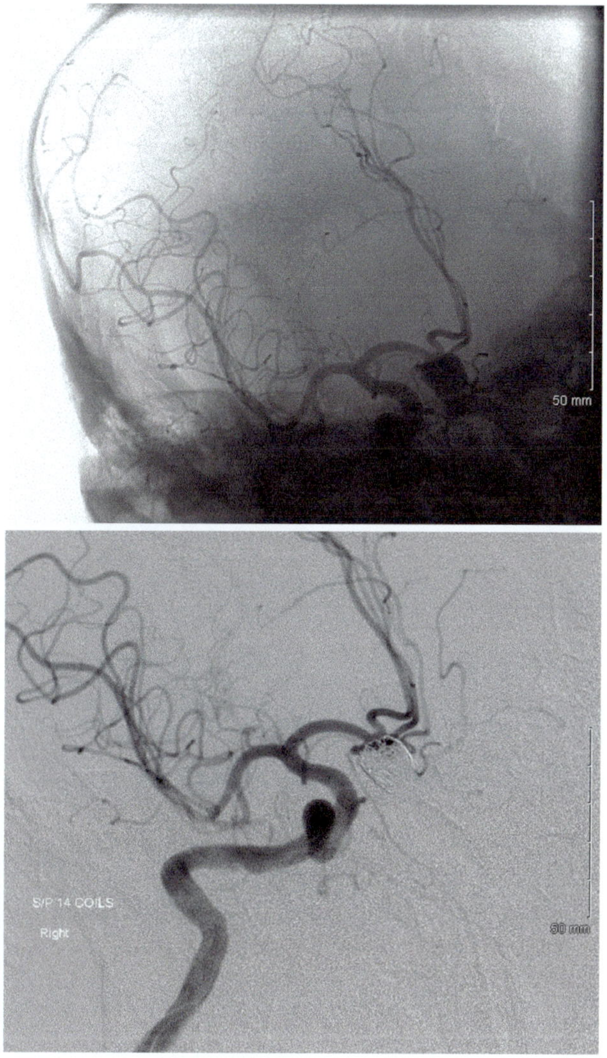

Fig. 5.2 Large anterior communicating artery aneurysm treated electively with endovascular coil embolization. Images demonstrate pre- and post-coil embolization frontal projections of a right internal carotid artery injection

overall lifetime risk for patients with known aneurysms and play an important role in the decision of how aggressive to be when it comes to treating unruptured aneurysms. Size, anatomic location, and individual aneurysm morphology must also be taken into account. Based on the data collected in the International Study of Unruptured Intracranial Aneurysms (ISUIA), aneurysms of less than 10 mm in diameter carried an annual rupture risk of 0.05 % in those patients without a personal history of SAH and 0.5 % in those with a history of SAH [3]. Similarly, posterior circulation aneurysms including the posterior communicating artery increased

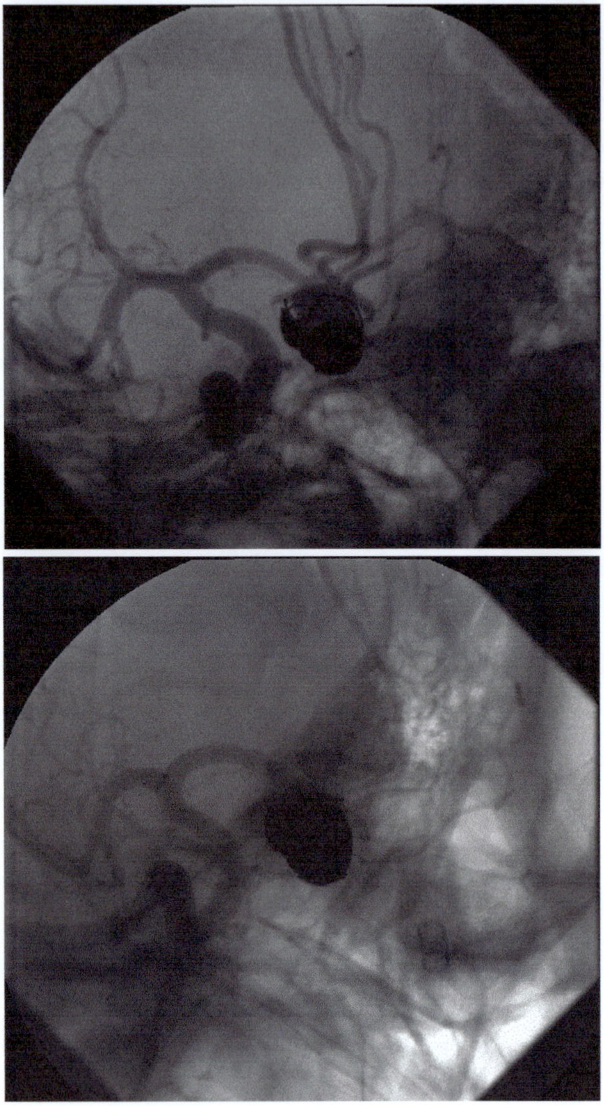

Fig. 5.3 The same patient returned for routine follow-up and was noted to have coil compaction and recanalization. He was successfully retreated with repeat coil embolization. *Note*: All of the images presented in this chapter were taken from de-identified patients from the Medical College of Wisconsin teaching hospital Froedtert Memorial Lutheran Hospital Radiology PACs system who presented for initial treatment or follow-up angiography

the relative risk of rupture by a factor of 2.3. Despite the lack of randomization in this study, it remains to be one of the key studies used to guide therapy for unruptured aneurysms.

Once the decision has been made to pursue treatment, deciding which treatment modality is paramount. Previous research has demonstrated improved outcomes of ruptured aneurysms with endovascular therapy. The 10-year data from the International Subarachnoid Aneurysm Trial (ISAT) demonstrated greater independence (82 % vs. 79 %, modified Rankin scale 0–2) and greater average survivability (82 % vs. 78 %) in those patients treated by endovascular embolization [4]. In the Barrow Ruptured Aneurysm Trial (BRAT), similar findings were noted for 3-year post-bleed modified Rankin scale (mRS) between endovascular treatment and surgical clipping, 35.8 % for clipping and 30 % for endovascular therapy with mRS >2 [5]. Also found in this study was surgical clipping provided higher degree of aneurysm obliteration (85 % vs. 52 %, respectively), decreased aneurysm recurrence, and decreased rate of retreatment for the index aneurysm (13 % retreatment for endovascular embolization at 3 years compared to 5 % for clipping).

These studies briefly emphasize the problem that the vascular neurosurgeons and interventionalists frequently encounter, that aneurysm remnants are common and require continued observation at a minimum. More importantly, which of these patients are at higher risk of rebleeding from their index aneurysm? How do we determine who should be retreated and who can be observed? Rerupture rates in the recent literature following treatment are low. In a study of over 1,000 patients treated at multiple centers over a 2-year period, rerupture rate was found to be 1.8 % which was similar to the 1-year rerupture risk (1.8 %) published in the ISAT trial [6]. That being said, there is a persistent risk to the patient with remnant aneurysm and at what point should retreatment be employed.

Remnant Aneurysms Following Surgical Clipping

Open surgical clipping of intracranial aneurysms has long been deemed one of the most technically demanding operations faced by neurosurgeons. Following the advent of the detachable GDC coils first utilized in 1991 by Guglielmi and colleagues, the treatment paradigm for intracranial aneurysms changed dramatically [7]. Currently, surgical clipping is thought, by some, to be the more definitive treatment for aneurysms. However, index aneurysm regrowth or aneurysm remnant (Fig. 5.1) after clipping has been described in the literature.

Despite routine scheduled follow-up imaging, there are sparse publications discussing angiographic follow-up after clipping in the literature compared to endovascular treatment. At one large-volume center, routine 1 and 3-year follow-up angiograms are ordered for all patients after clipping. Despite this schedule, as was previously stated, the actual percentage that obtained these repeat angiograms is small. In one study, late follow-up angiograms were performed on 102 patients who previously underwent surgical treatment of their aneurysm. The mean follow-up angiography period ranged from 2.6 to 9.7 years. Of the 167 aneurysms treated in this study population, 91.8 % were clipped and the remaining were treated by wrapping, bypass with trapping, or parent vessel occlusion. Ninety-two percent of the clipped aneurysms demonstrated no evidence of residua. The remaining aneurysms demonstrated residual necks in 8.2 % (12 patients). Of these incompletely clipped aneurysms, five aneurysms demonstrated regrowth with one diagnosed after subarachnoid hemorrhage [8]. There were no reported cases of SAH from those aneurysms without residua.

Similar studies demonstrate comparable results as it pertains to residua following clip placement on long-term angiographic follow-up. Akyüz et al. followed 166 surgically clipped ruptured aneurysms angiographically over a 3–7-year period. The results again demonstrated long-term aneurysm obliteration for those that demonstrated no residua following initial clip placement. Of those with known residua, five remained stable, one spontaneously thrombosed, and one demonstrated growth. Again despite known residua, no recurrent SAH was noted during the study period. Along with this finding, it was noted that two de novo aneurysms were detected and later treated [9]. Based on these results, despite the overall poor percentage of those patients that presented for late follow-up studies (approximately 10 % in this study), it is evident that clipping is a durable treatment modality but not without the potential for regrowth and SAH despite treatment.

There are several other studies that have looked at long-term durability of surgical clipping. Edner et al. described their experience of just over 100 SAH patients who were clipped at their institution. This study followed patients treated for aneurysmal SAH with surgical clipping for 20 years. One hundred and two patients who were 1- and 2-year survivors following SAH who were surgically treated between 1983 and 1985 were followed for 20 years. Forty-nine patients were alive at time of the study. Of these patients, none had experienced a repeat SAH. Aneurysm remnant was noted in eight patients and de novo aneurysms were found in seven patients. Of those deceased, one patient died secondary to SAH from a separate known untreated aneurysm [10]. The authors concluded that extreme long-term follow-up for successfully clipped aneurysm is not necessary, but this stance was a point of disagreement in the comment section of this publication.

Further studies with long-term results have attempted to identify risk factors for recurrence as well as a mean time from initial treatment to rerupture. Wermer et al. published a series of patients treated for SAH with surgical clipping with long-term outcomes (mean follow-up 8 years) and of 752 patients, only 18 had recurrent SAH. Risk factors for those recurrences were smoking, young age, and multiple aneurysms at the time of initial presentation. Of those that recurred, the vast majority (72 %) had bled from de novo aneurysms, and the mean interval from initial bleed and recurrence was 6.5 years with a range from 0.2 to 17 years [11].

These studies demonstrate several important points with respect to surgical clipped aneurysms. The likelihood of recurrence or remnant formation after aneurysm clipping is low but not absent. Repeat aneurysmal SAH from a surgically treated aneurysm, with or without remnant, is also low. The durability of surgical clipping cannot be denied, and in the age of increasingly popularity and technological advancements of endovascular therapy, neurosurgeons and interventionalists must keep this evidence in mind when discussing all available treatment options to their patients. Most importantly, this demonstrates the need for continued long-term observation of known aneurysms, particularly those that are not completely obliterated during initial treatment.

Remnant Aneurysms Following Endovascular Coil Embolization

Endovascular techniques for aneurysm treatment have continued to evolve since their initial use in the 1990s. Due to multiple studies [4, 5], particularly in the SAH population, the usage of endovascular techniques for the treatment of intracranial aneurysms has seen a significant increase around the globe. While the outcome data has been reassuring, the technique has also come under scrutiny for its durability and the potential for future rebleeding from treated aneurysms. In order to respond to this question of durability, there have been a number of studies published in the last 20 years concerning results and outcomes following endovascular treatment. As previously stated, techniques and outcomes have improved over the last 20 years, but no definitive evidence-based follow-up schedule is available. Further long-term data is still needed to address this.

Two early studies looked only at anterior communicating artery (Acomm) aneurysms treated with endovascular coiling (Figs. 5.2 and 5.3). Elias et al. followed 30 patients treated for ruptured Acomm aneurysms over a 2-year period with diagnostic angiograms at 6 months and 2 years of posttreatment. No further follow-up studies were performed past the 2-year angiogram if the treated aneurysm was fully obliterated. Residual neck remnants after treatment were noticed on 13 aneurysms and were persistently followed for up to 6 years. Only one was retreated and there were no rebleeds during the study time frame. A direct quote from this early paper accurately emphasized a lack of data concerning the subject in question when the authors stated, "The lack of information regarding both the frequency of residual filling or regrowth and long-term angiographic follow-up of patients with surgically treated aneurysms makes meaningful comparison between surgical treatments and endovascular treatment impossible" [12].

A second study examined both elective treated and anterior communicating artery aneurysms treated for rupture over a 9-year period at a single center. The ruptured group made up the vast majority of cases (85 %) and was found to have a higher likelihood of recurrence vs. those of the electively treated patients, 51 vs. 8, respectively. Also noted was the increase in rebleeding rate associated with ruptured aneurysms in this study. Although only 3.4 % of the patients presented with rebleeding, it was associated with a high mortality rate (88 %). This group retreated 27 of these recurrences endovascularly and two with surgical clipping. Of note, the majority of recurrences were noted within the first 6 months of treatment but were found as late as 3 years of posttreatment, and a de novo aneurysm was found to be the source of a distant rebleed in one patient 10 years after their initial treatment. The authors stated that long-term follow-up is recommended to assess for these recurrences, but no recommendation as to duration of follow-up was given [13]. Another group studied 466 patients with 501 aneurysms retrospectively to look for incidence of recurrence and risk factors for such. Their population was approximately 54 % ruptured patients, and they termed early follow-up less than 1 year and late follow-up after 1 year. They found a recurrence rate of 33 % at a mean time of 12.31

+/– 11.33 months. Of these recurrences, those that were deemed "major" actually presented later than the smaller recurrences (16.49 +/– 15.93 months). Approximately 50 % of the major recurrences were retreated, and they experienced only three rebleed events during their study period. They agreed that short-term follow-up was insufficient for these patients, but again no recommendations on follow-up imaging for remnants were offered [14].

Multiple other studies over the past 30 years have looked at similar populations of endovascular-treated patients. Follow-up periods have varied from months to years, and unlike the previous studies mentioned, the vast majority of the studies did not limit the patients by aneurysm location. Several of these studies are summarized in Table 5.1. As can be seen, percentage of remnant and residual aneurysms following treatment varied from 20 % to 50 %. These numbers clearly appear concerning, but in comparison, the number of rebleed events in each of these studies is significantly lower with some studies reporting zero rebleeds with follow-up period as long as 14 years [6, 12–26]. In a separate meta-analysis of 71 studies over a 5-year period, recurrent aneurysms were found in 24.4 % (321/1,316 patients) after an initial complete occlusion rate of 86 %. Retreatment was performed in 9.1 %, and rupture after endovascular therapy was found in only nine patients. The authors calculated the annual risk of rupture after endovascular therapy to be 0.2 % in their analysis of previously unruptured aneurysms [27].

As was stated before, the goal of aneurysm treatment is prevention of rupture or rerupture in the future. Follow-up imaging is directed toward monitoring those aneurysms that are not completely isolated from the parent circulation and present a possible future rebleed risk. There are three distinct possibilities for each treated aneurysm in terms of findings on follow-up imaging: stability, recanalization, or progression of thrombosis. Le Feuvre demonstrated complete occlusion immediately following embolization to be 52 %, with 32 % being >95 % occluded and 16 % of 90–95 %. Despite significant loss of follow-up in this study, there was a trend toward progressive thrombosis with 65 % demonstrating occlusion at 3 months and 82 % at 1 year [22]. Another study demonstrated a similar trend with aneurysms found to have remnant or residual aneurysms following initial therapy to further thrombose in 46 % or remain stable in 26 % [15]. Conversely, there are examples that demonstrate the opposite with those aneurysms exhibiting a change in their obliteration pattern toward recanalization on long-term follow-up in lieu of obliteration. Recanalization was found to be more common in the first 6 months, but late recanalization up to 2 years after therapy was also noted. Taking all this into consideration when considering options, it is important to note that the incidence of rebleed in this study was zero.

In addition to this, the supplement of coiling adjuncts such as balloon- or stent-assisted coiling methods must be considered as they also play an important role in the management of wide-necked and larger aneurysms. Evidence from current research demonstrates similar procedural risk profiles along with less recurrence noted on follow-up imaging. Yang et al. recently published their experience over a year period of stent-assisted coiling vs. coiling alone. Fifty-three percent of 512 patients were treated with stent-assisted coiling due to large neck size, low dome to

Table 5.1 Endovascular therapy for intracranial aneurysms

Clinical series	Dates	Number of patients	% Ruptured	Location of aneurysms	Duration of follow-up	Type of follow-up study	% Aneurysm remnants/ residuals
Elias et al.	Jan 1990–Dec 1998	30	100 %	Acomm	1–53 months	DSA	43 %
Finitsis et al.	Oct 1992–Oct 2001	280	85 %	Acomm	0–11 years, mean 3.09	DSA or MRA	21 %
Raymond et al.	Aug 1992–May 2002	466	54.00 %	All	1->37 months	DSA	33.60 %
Johnston et al.	1996–1998	1,001 (Clip 706)	100 %	All	0–9.6 years	Variable	24.1 %[a]
Thornton et al.	Jan 1995–Aug 1999	130	44 %	All	6–62 months	DSA	61 % initial, 39 % for late
Friedman et al.	1991–2000	83	100 %	All	0.2–70 months	DSA	64 %[b]
Sluzewski et al.	Jan 1995–Jan 2003	393	100 %	All	2–84 months	DSA	19 % at 6 months
Lindvall et al.	1996–2002	44	90 %	All	6–14 years	MRA	47–51 %
Gauvrit et al.	Jan 1998–Aug 2001	92	85 %	All	32–78 months[c]	DSA and MRA	38 % on long-term MRA
Hayashi et al.	Apr 1999–Dec 2005	58	12 %	All	Mean 32.1 months	MRA	28 %
Consoli et al.	Jan 2000–Dec 2005	241	100 %	All	2 years	DSA	27.40 %
Le Feuvre et al.	Feb 2002–Feb 2003	75	Not specified	All	1 year (DSA) 4 years[d]	DSA	35 % at 3 months and 18 % at 1 year
Ries et al.	Nov 1992–Dec 2005	323	63 %	All	6–132 months	DSA and MRA	21 %
Shankar et al.	Sep 2003–Dec 2006	124	60 %	All	0–53 months	MRA	48.4 % on initial MRA
Ansari et al.	Mar 2006–Oct 2007	84	63 %	All	13–42 months	DSA	51 % initial
Raslan et al.	Jan 2003–Jun 209	33	3 %	Acomm	0–48 months	DSA	24 %

Acomm anterior communicating artery aneurysm, *DSA* digital subtraction angiogram, *MRA* magnetic resonance angiogram
[a]Both endovascular and clip patients based on post-procedure angiogram or operative report
[b]Reported 26 % dog-ear remnant, 35 % residual neck, and 3 % aneurysm filling
[c]MRA long-term follow-up, study also provided short-term DSA and MRA at an interval of 5–25 months after embolization
[d]DSA performed on 34/75 patients at 1 year. 30/75 patients interviewed up to 4 years after embolization

neck ratio, or morphologic characteristics that prevented adequate treatment with coiling alone. In the setting of subarachnoid hemorrhage, coiling alone was preferred. They demonstrated a lower recurrence rate with the stent-assisted group, 5.2 % vs. 16.5 % in the coiling alone, at a mean follow-up period of 11.2 months (range 6–18 months). Also of interest was the initial complete occlusion rate after treatment in these patients. After coiling alone, 64.1 % of the patients demonstrated complete occlusion compared to 54.5 % of the stent-assisted group. Given that these aneurysms were selected due to their complex anatomy, this nonstatistically significant difference is not surprising. What was noted to be significant was the percentage of patients with remnant aneurysms that demonstrated progressive thrombosis on follow-up imaging. Patients with stent-assisted treatment demonstrated progressive thrombosis in 32.7 % compared to 15.1 % of those treated with coiling alone [28]. Despite several limitations to the study, particularly the significant loss of follow-up data in both groups, the trend toward progressive thrombosis in the stent-assisted patients again is supportive of the notion that remnant aneurysms can and often do thrombose with time.

A second similar study looked at stent-assisted treatment of anterior communicating artery aneurysms only. Over 6-year period, 44 patients harboring Acomm aneurysms were treated with stent-assisted coiling. Seventy-five percent of the patients in this study presented for follow-up imaging of at least 3 months (mean 65 weeks). Complete occlusion was found in 24 patients, residual neck in five, and residual aneurysm in four patients. Only one patient underwent retreatment due to persistent enlargement, and no patients experienced a bleed after treatment despite only 73 % initial complete occlusion [26].

As can be seen, there is a propensity of studies that demonstrate low rebleed risk despite the presence of remnant neck or aneurysms after endovascular therapy. Based on this published data, certain anatomical factors and other risk factors can guide the treating physician as to which aneurysms require a more stringent follow-up schedule. Initial angiographic result, aneurysm size, neck size, and history of rupture are factors that have demonstrated correlation with higher likelihood for recurrence and rebleed [14, 17, 19, 25]. Initial angiographic occlusion comes from patience, diligence, and experience in the angiography suite in attempt to obtain this goal of 100 % occlusion whenever possible and safe. Placing those patients with large aneurysms, large aneurysm necks, and subarachnoid hemorrhage in a separate class with a more frequent and intensive imaging follow-up schedule is recommended.

Although the vast majority of studies utilized repeat angiography as seen in Table 5.1, noninvasive imaging with magnetic resonance angiography (MRA) also can play an important role in posttreatment observation. Many surgeons and patients favor MRA for long-term and repeat imaging due to its noninvasive nature. Each of the studies demonstrates that MRA does have several advantages: noninvasive, no associated risks of a procedure, and may demonstrate more filling than formal angiography [19, 20, 24]. One particular study utilized time-of-flight MRA to assess long-term follow-up in 44 patients previously treated by endovascular coiling over a 6-year period and compared results of a DSA performed 3 years after treatment.

These patients then underwent MRA at a mean of 9.68 years (range 6–14 years) after their last endovascular treatment. Independent assessment by neuroradiologists demonstrated stable findings in 94 % of treated aneurysms once again demonstrating the high propensity for stability in previously treated aneurysms [18]. Certain centers have questioned whether MRA can replace DSA for follow-up imaging for reasons discussed above. One study compared MRA and DSA of similar time frames for follow-up after endovascular therapy of 80 aneurysms. They found 97 % correlation for diagnosis of recurrence of aneurysms when the modalities were examined by separate radiologists. Of the three that did not correlate, MRA identified a recurrence that was not visualized on DSA in one case and the opposite in the second two [34]. This demonstrates the accuracy and feasibility of transitioning long-term follow-up of aneurysms to noninvasive imaging.

Retreatment Risks

As discussed previously, the incidence and prevalence of aneurysm remnant following open surgery and endovascular therapy can be quite high, greater than 50 % in some reported studies [15, 16, 18, 25]. Patients with remnant aneurysms following treatment require counseling on the retreatment options and the potential risks this may pose.

Morbidity and mortality for endovascular therapy of unruptured aneurysms were presented by Oishi et al. in their recent publication concerning informed consent for patients undergoing endovascular therapy for unruptured aneurysms. They quote an overall morbidity of 4.4 % and mortality of 0.7 % [29]. Of those morbid events, thromboembolic events, groin hematomas, arterial dissections, aneurysm perforation, contrast-induced nephropathy, and radiation effects are most common in the literature. Groin hematomas are reported to be the most common overall complication involved in angiography [32, 33]. Data specific to intracranial aneurysm procedures are limited, but cardiac literature demonstrates groin hematoma rates of 9–32 % [31]. Reports of thromboembolic events range widely among studies from 2 % to 40 %. Of the thromboembolic events reported, all were diagnosed on post-procedure imaging, but the vast majority of these were not clinically relevant [30].

Similar to follow-up for previously clipped aneurysms, the evidence for risks of repeat craniotomy for aneurysm clipping is sparse. As can be said for other operations, the first operation is cleaner than the second and usually less complicated. Johnstone et al. showed that retreatment for aneurysm remnants was certainly not without risk when they reported life-threatening or disabling complication is 11 % of those aneurysms treated endovascularly and 17 % for those initially clipped [35].

Despite limited data specifically on repeat craniotomy for aneurysms, comparable data can be educational on this subject as it applies to other complex cranial cases. Arteriovenous malformations (AVMs) are complex and high-risk procedures faced by surgeons and interventionalists. One study demonstrated relatively low complication risk for initial surgery at a high-volume center (7.2 % with 1.9 % resulting in permanent neurologic deficit). Increasing complication rates were noted in larger AVMs, high number of preoperative embolizations, and unruptured AVMs [36]. Another study retrospectively examined epilepsy resections over a 30-year period in three separate types of operation: temporal lobectomy with or without amygdalohippocampectomy, extratemporal lobar or multilobar resections, or invasive electrode placement. The complication rates were divided into early period vs. more recent years, and overall the complication rates decreased dramatically, with the exception of a small increase in wound infections/meningitis and hemorrhage/hematoma in the invasive electrode placement group. These results were explained due to the addition of a second operation for removal of the electrodes or resection [37]. Despite the absence of data specifically outlying the risks of repeat craniotomy for remnant aneurysm surgery, the risk for repeat surgery is necessary to consider when discussing options with patients concerning their aneurysm.

Conclusion

Intracranial aneurysm rupture is the most common cause of spontaneous subarachnoid hemorrhage. SAH, even with treatment, can carry a significant risk of morbidity and mortality. The treatment of intracranial aneurysm typically consists of either surgical clipping or endovascular obliteration. However, even with significant advancements in the treatment of aneurysms, remnant aneurysm or aneurysm regrowth after treatment has been described. Surgical clipping of intracranial aneurysm has been established as a durable treatment option, although not without potential operative risks. Endovascular treatment is a less invasive way to achieve similar results of aneurysm occlusion. Despite this, however, the risk of remnant aneurysm after treatment may be higher. Given the lack of long-term randomized trials that compare the two treatment options, no specific guidelines can be established about the indications for surgical clipping and endovascular coiling of intracranial aneurysm. Angiographic follow-up is recommended after aneurysm treatment; however, if recurrence of the index aneurysm is found, continued observation vs. retreatment should be considered. Retreatment of remnant aneurysm is achievable, although these treatment paradigms may pose greater risk than the overall risk of observation as we have demonstrated here. Therefore, treatment decisions, including observation, should be carefully discussed with each patient, and they should be made aware that just because a remnant aneurysm exists, the right choice may be to continue with long-term clinical and radiographic follow-up as the current authors recommend.

References

1. Vlak M, Rinkel GJ, et al. Lifetime risks for aneurysmal subarachnoid haemorrhage: multivariable risk stratification. J Neurol Neurosurg Psychiatry. 2013;84:619–23.
2. Lawton MT, Gress DR, editors. Controversies in neurological surgery: neurovascular diseases. New York: Thieme; 2006.
3. Wiebers DO, Whisnant JP, et al. Unruptured intracranial aneurysms: natural history, clinical outcome, and risks of surgical and endovascular treatment. Lancet. 2003;362:103–10.

4. Molyneux A, Birks J, et al. The durability of endovascular coiling versus neurosurgical clipping of ruptured cerebral aneurysms: 18 year follow-up of the UK cohort of the International Subarachnoid Aneurysm Trial (ISAT). Lancet. 2015;385:691–7.
5. Spetzler RF, McDougall CG, et al. The Barrow Ruptured Aneurysm Trial: 3 year results. J Neurosurg. 2013;119:146–57.
6. Johnston SC, Dowd CF, et al. Predictors of rehemorrhage after treatment of ruptured intracranial aneurysms: the Cerebral Aneurysm Rerupture After Treatment (CARAT) Study. Stroke. 2008;39:120–5.
7. Hayakawa M, Murayama Y, et al. Natural history of the neck remnant of a cerebral aneurysm treated with the Guglielmi detachable coil system. J Neurosurg. 2000;93:561–8.
8. David C, Vishteh AG, et al. Late angiographic follow-up review of surgically treated aneurysms. J Neurosurg. 1999;91:396–401.
9. Akyüz M, Tuncer R, et al. Clinical article: angiographic follow-up after surgical treatment of intracranial aneurysms. Acta Neurochir. 2004;146:245–50.
10. Edner G, Almqvist H, et al. The Stockholm 20-year follow-up of aneurysmal subarachnoid hemorrhage outcome. Neurosurgery. 2007;60(6):1017–24.
11. Wermer MJ, Greebe P, et al. Incidence of recurrent subarachnoid hemorrhage after clipping for ruptured intracranial aneurysms. Stroke. 2005;36:2394–9.
12. Elias T, Ogungbo B, et al. Endovascular treatment of anterior communicating artery aneurysms: results of clinical and radiological outcome in Newcastle. Br J Neurosurg. 2003;17(3):278–86.
13. Finitsis S, Anxionnat R, et al. Endovascular treatment of ACom intracranial aneurysms: report on series of 280 patients. Interv Radiol. 2009;16:7–16.
14. Raymond J, Guilbert F, et al. Long-term angiographic recurrences after selective endovascular treatment of aneurysms with detachable coils. Stroke. 2003;34:1398–403.
15. Thornton J, Debrun G, et al. Follow-up angiography of intracranial aneurysms treated with endovascular placement of Guglielmi detachable coils. Neurosurgery. 2002;50(2):239–50.
16. Friedman J, Nichols D, et al. Guglielmi detachable coil treatment of ruptured saccular cerebral aneurysms: retrospective review of a 10-year single-center experience. Am J Neuroradiol. 2003;24:526–33.
17. Sluzewski M, van Rooij W, et al. Late rebleeding of ruptured intracranial aneurysms treated with detachable coils. Am J Neuroradiol. 2005;26:2542–9.
18. Lindvall P, Borota L, et al. Long-term follow-up of intracranial aneurysms treated with endovascular coiling: experience from one institution. Vasc Endovascular Surg. 2012;46(4):325–8.
19. Gauvrit J, Caron S, et al. Intracranial aneurysms treated with Guglielmi detachable coils: long-term imaging follow-up with contrast-enhanced magnetic resonance angiography. J Neurosurg. 2008;108:443–9.
20. Hayashi K, Kitagawa N, et al. Long-term follow-up of endovascular coil embolization for cerebral aneurysms using three-dimensional time-of-flight magnetic resonance angiography. Neurol Res. 2009;31:674–80.
21. Consoli A, Renieri L, et al. Five to ten years follow-up after coiling of 241 patients with acutely ruptured aneurysms: a single centre experience. Interv Neuroradiol. 2012;18:5–13.
22. Le Feuvre D, Taylor A. Endovascular cerebral aneurysm treatment: long-term outcomes. S Afr Med J. 2008;98(12):954–7.
23. Ries T, Siemonsen S, et al. Long-term follow-up of cerebral aneurysms after endovascular therapy – prediction and outcome of retreatment. Am J Neuroradiol. 2007;28:1755–61.
24. Shankar J, Lum C, et al. Long-term prospective follow-up of intracranial aneurysms treated with endovascular coiling using contrast-enhanced MR angiography. Am J Neuroradiol. 2010;31:1211–5.
25. Ansari S, Dueweke E, et al. Embolization of intracranial aneurysms with second-generation Matrix-2 detachable coils: mid-term and long-term results. J NeuroIntervent Surg. 2011;3:324–30.
26. Raslan A, Oztaskin M, et al. Neuroform stent-assisted embolization of incidental anterior communicating artery aneurysms: long-term clinical and angiographic follow-up. Neurosurgery. 2011;69(1):27–37.

27. Naggara O, White P, et al. Endovascular treatment of intracranial unruptured aneurysms: systematic review and meta-analysis of the literature on safety and efficacy. Radiology. 2010;256(3):887–97.
28. Yang H, Sun Y, et al. Comparison of stent-assisted coiling vs. coiling alone in 563 intracranial aneurysms: safety and efficacy at a high-volume center. Neurosurgery. 2015;77(2):241–7.
29. Oishi H, Yamamoto M, et al. Systematic review of complications for proper informed consent: endovascular therapy for unruptured intracranial aneurysms. No Shinkei Geka. 2013;41(10):907–16.
30. Chen M. A checklist for cerebral aneurysm embolization complications. J NeuroIntervent Surg. 2013;5:20–7.
31. Wong J, Ziewacz J, et al. Patterns in neurosurgical adverse events: endovascular neurosurgery. Neurosurg Focus. 2012;33(5), E14.
32. Samaniego E, Dabus G, et al. Avoiding complications in neurosurgical interventional procedures. J Neurosurg Sci. 2011;55(1):71–80.
33. Lawson M, Velat G, et al. Interventional neurovascular disease: avoidance and management of complications and review of the current literature. J Neurosurg Sci. 2011;55(3):233–42.
34. Lane A, Vivian P, et al. Magnetic resonance angiography or digital subtraction catheter angiography for follow-up of coiled aneurysms: do we need both? J Med Imaging Radiat Oncol. 2015;59(2):163–9.
35. CARAT Investigators. Rates of delayed rebleeding from intracranial aneurysms are low after surgical and endovascular treatment. Stroke. 2006;37(6):1437–42.
36. Theofanis T, Chalouhi N, et al. Microsurgery for cerebral arteriovenous malformations: postoperative outcomes and predictors of complications in 264 cases. Neurosurg Focus. 2014;37(3), E10.
37. Tebo C, Evins A, et al. Evolution of cranial epilepsy surgery complication rates: a 32-year systematic review and meta-analysis. J Neurosurg. 2014;120:1415–27.

Controversies in Vascular Neurosurgery: Aneurysm Remnants

6

David R. Santiago-Dieppa, Tianzan Zhou, Jeffrey S. Pannell, and Alexander A. Khalessi

The low prevalence but serious disability caused by hemorrhage of an incompletely occluded aneurysm understandably creates dispute regarding the proper management of these aneurysms. As mentioned in the previous sections, both aggressive and conservative management are feasible. The risks of retreatment and the risk of repeat hemorrhage both have to be carefully evaluated when deciding between aggressive treatment strategies and observation.

Incidence

The incidence of aneurysm neck remnants varies greatly depending on the procedure utilized for aneurysm repair. Clipped aneurysms are reported to have an 8 % rate of residual aneurysm [1]. As demonstrated in the international subarachnoid aneurysm trial (ISAT), the rate of residual aneurysms is higher for coiled aneurysms than microsurgical clipping: An 85 % obliteration for clipped and 53 % obliteration for coiled aneurysms was reported in the ISAT [2].

Natural History

Given the relatively low rate of residual aneurysms following microsurgical clipping, data on the evolution of aneurysm remnants following clipping is understandably sparse. In one study, out of 12 remaining residual necks after clipping, 5 demonstrated regrowth and 1 presented as a subarachnoid hemorrhage [1]. Another

D.R. Santiago-Dieppa, MD • T. Zhou, BS • J.S. Pannell, MD • A.A. Khalessi, MD, MS (✉)
Division of Neurosurgery, University of California – San Diego,
200 West Arbor Drive, San Diego, CA 92103, USA
e-mail: akhalessi@ucsd.edu

E. Veznedaroglu (ed.), *Controversies in Vascular Neurosurgery*,
DOI 10.1007/978-3-319-27315-0_6

study described seven residual clipped aneurysms, of which five remained stable, one thrombosed, and one demonstrated growth [3].

More data is available for residual coiled aneurysms. As demonstrated in Table 1 of the conservative management section, the percentage of patients with aneurysm remnants following coiling is higher than following microsurgical clipping. However, the percentage of repeat hemorrhage is comparatively low even after many years of follow-up. This is supported by studies demonstrating the tendency of aneurysmal remnants after coiling to either further thrombose or remains stable [4, 5].

Management

Given the risks of retreatment of aneurysmal remnants, it is important to stratify patients according to their risk of expansion and hemorrhage of the remnant. Certain risk factors have been shown to increase the risk of repeat hemorrhage in residual aneurysms. These risk factors are similar to the risk factors for naïve aneurysm rupture and include current smoking, family history of ruptured aneurysms, and hypertension. Furthermore, in remnants of aneurysms that had previously ruptured, aneurysms in the posterior circulation and aneurysms in young patients are more likely to exhibit growth and possible repeat hemorrhage [6].

As noted in both previous sections, retreatment of aneurysmal remnants may pose significant risks of morbidity and mortality. This is particularly true for surgical retreatment, where morbidity has been shown to range from 7 to 15.7 % [7, 8]. However, endovascular retreatment carries a significantly lower rate of morbidity and mortality. One study investigating endovascular treatment of repeat aneurysms showed that only 1.28 % of patients either died or had a permanent disability [9]. The relatively lower morbidity and mortality of endovascular management also lowers the clinical threshold for aggressive treatment strategies in the management of aneurysmal remnants.

Aggressive management should be considered for high-risk cases. In addition to family history, aneurysm characteristics, and symptoms suggestive of hemorrhage, new neurologic symptoms should also prompt immediate evaluation for intervention. These include cranial nerve palsy, brainstem compression, or hydrocephalus that can be attributed to the growth of an aneurysmal remnant.

Observation may be appropriate for uncomplicated cases such as remnants of unruptured aneurysms. Although angiography is commonly utilized to monitor these aneurysmal remnants, magnetic resonance angiography (MRA) is favored by many practitioners for their noninvasive nature. Furthermore, MRA has been found to have a 97 % correlation for diagnosis of recurrent aneurysm compared to DSA [10].

Advanced imaging techniques aimed at aneurysm flow mapping and vessel wall characterization may further identify high-risk aneurysmal remnants that would benefit an aggressive treatment strategy. 3D TOF MRA and 4D flow MRI may identify water hammer effects that may cause coil compaction, remnant growth, and rupture [11]. High-resolution double inversion recovery black-blood MRI can be used to measure wall thickness of the aneurysmal remnant [12]. Flow patterns and wall thickness are both correlated with the risk of aneurysm rupture and enable targeted selection of high-risk aneurysmal remnants for invasive management.

Conclusion

Unfortunately, current literature is too sparse to offer definitive risk stratification for optimal management of aneurysmal remnants. Patient and aneurysm characteristics that increase the risk of growth and hemorrhage of the aneurysmal remnants must be considered when choosing an approach as either approach may be appropriate depending on the clinical scenario. Aneurysm flow mapping and vessel wall characterization show promise at identifying high-risk remnants. Further studies are needed to quantify the risk factors of aneurysmal remnant hemorrhage and allow for more objective management guidelines.

References

1. David C, Vishteh AG, et al. Late angiographic follow-up review of surgically treated aneurysms. J Neurosurg. 1999;91:396–401.
2. Molyneux A, Birks J, et al. The durability of endovascular coiling vs neurosurgical clipping of ruptured cerebral aneurysms: 18 year follow-up of the UK cohort of the International Subarachnoid Aneurysm Trial (ISAT). Lancet. 2015;385:691–7.
3. Akyüz M, Tuncer R, et al. Clinical article: angiographic follow-up after surgical treatment of intracranial aneurysms. Acta Neurochir. 2004;146:245–50.
4. Thornton J, Debrun G, et al. Follow-up angiography of intracranial aneurysms treated with endovascular placement of Guglielmi detachable coils. Neurosurgery. 2002;50(2):239–50.
5. Le Feuvre D, Taylor A. Endovascular cerebral aneurysm treatment: long-term outcomes. S Afr Med J. 2008;98(12):954–7.
6. Lin T, Fox AJ, Drake CG. Regrowth of aneurysm sacs from residual neck following aneurysm clipping. J Neurosurg. 2009;70:556–60.
7. Giannotta SL, Litofsky NS. Reoperative management of intracranial aneurysms. J Neurosurg. 1995;83:387–93.
8. Drake C, Friedman A, Peerless S. Failed aneurysm surgery: reoperation in 115 cases. J Neurosurg. 1984;61:848–56.
9. Ringer AJ, et al. Defining the risk of retreatment for aneurysm recurrence or residual after initial treatment by endovascular coiling: a multicenter study. Neurosurgery. 2009;65:311–5. discussion 315.
10. Lane A, Vivian P, et al. Magnetic resonance angiography or digital subtraction catheter angiography for follow-up of coiled aneurysms: do we need both? J Med Imaging Radiat Oncol. 2015;59(2):163–9.
11. Futami K, Sano H, Misaki K, Nakada M, Ueda F, Hamada J. Identification of the inflow zone of unruptured cerebral aneurysms: comparison of 4D flow MRI and 3D TOF MRA data. Am J Neuroradiol. 2014;35(7):1363–70.
12. Park JK, Lee CS, Sim KB, Huh JS, Park JC. Imaging of the walls of saccular cerebral aneurysms with double inversion recovery black-blood sequence. J Magn Reson Imaging. 2009;30(5):1179–83.

Basilar Artery Aneurysm: Role for Open Surgery

7

W. Caleb Rutledge and Michael T. Lawton

Introduction

The relationship of the basilar artery to the brainstem and skull base makes basilar artery aneurysms among the most technically challenging aneurysms to treat microsurgically. Preservation of perforators supplying the brainstem, cerebellum, and cranial nerves, while operating in narrow and deep surgical corridors, is critical. Despite advances in microsurgical techniques, neuroanesthesia, and cerebral protection since Drake [5–9, 29], microsurgical clipping of these aneurysms still results in excess morbidity and mortality when compared to anterior circulation aneurysms.

Since publication of the landmark aneurysm trials, including the International Study of Unruptured Intracranial Aneurysms (ISUIA), which demonstrated worse outcomes with microsurgical clipping, and the International Subarachnoid Aneurysm Trial (ISAT), which showed better outcomes with coiling compared to clipping, endovascular treatments have largely replaced microsurgery as the primary treatment modality in management of both ruptured and unruptured aneurysms [1, 20, 24, 28, 32, 40, 41]. The benefits of coiling are more apparent for posterior circulation aneurysms. In the 3-year follow-up of the Barrow Ruptured Aneurysm Trial (BRAT), while there were no significant differences in outcomes among patients with anterior circulation aneurysms coiled or clipped, patients who underwent coil embolization of posterior circulation aneurysms continued to have significantly better outcomes than clipped patients [39].

Despite the shift toward endovascular treatment in management of aneurysms of the posterior circulation, particularly for P2 posterior cerebral artery (PCA), basilar trunk, vertebrobasilar junction, and vertebral artery aneurysms, there remains an

W.C. Rutledge • M.T. Lawton (✉)
Department of Neurological Surgery, University of California, San Francisco, 505 Parnassus Avenue, M780, San Francisco, CA 94143, USA
e-mail: Michael.Lawton@ucsf.edu

E. Veznedaroglu (ed.), *Controversies in Vascular Neurosurgery*,
DOI 10.1007/978-3-319-27315-0_7

important role for microsurgical clipping. While it is increasingly safe and effective, endovascular treatments, including coiling, balloon- and stent-assisted coiling, and flow diversion, are still more likely to result in residual aneurysm, aneurysm recurrence requiring re-treatment, and rarely aneurysmal rebleeding [3, 10–12, 14, 15, 17, 22, 25, 27, 31, 33, 34, 38]. Aneurysms of the distal anterior inferior cerebellar artery (AICA), superior cerebellar artery (SCA), P1 PCA, and basilar bifurcation are amenable to microsurgical clipping [36]. Wide-necked, thrombosed, large, or giant aneurysms prone to endovascular failure [2, 12, 27, 30] are also candidates for microsurgical clipping [13, 26, 37]. Microsurgical clipping of appropriately selected basilar artery aneurysms by well-trained and experienced cerebrovascular neurosurgeons is safe and effective and offers a durable cure.

At our center, microsurgery is considered a competitive alternative to endovascular therapy for P1 PCA, SCA, distal AICA, PICA, and some basilar bifurcation aneurysms. Conversely, endovascular treatment is preferred for P2 PCA, proximal AICA, basilar trunk, vertebrobasilar junction, and vertebral artery aneurysms, as these often require extensive cranial base approaches and carry a high risk of perforator infraction and cranial neuropathy.

The orbitozygomatic-pterional approach is used routinely because it provides the greatest exposure with flexibility to shift exposures from transsylvian to subtemporal. The subarachnoid dissection requires wide splitting of the Sylvian fissure to separate the frontal and temporal lobes and freeing the temporal lobe from granulations infratemporally or veins pretemporally. Dissection into the carotid and crural cisterns further mobilizes the temporal lobe to open the operative corridors. Three operative corridors to these aneurysms are established, including the optic-carotid triangle, supracarotid triangle, and carotid-oculomotor triangle, with the latter providing the widest and most useful window to the interpeduncular fossa (Fig. 7.1). The dissection down to the basilar aneurysm can be systematized to a series of steps with clear anatomical landmarks designed to gain early proximal control of the basilar trunk and clear identification of the quadrifurcation arteries and vital perforators. Dissection hazards vary with aneurysm projection, with the most common superior projecting aneurysms hiding perforators on the contralateral P1 PCA, anteriorly projecting aneurysms positioning the dome between the surgeon and the neck and posteriorly projecting aneurysms hiding the perforators originating from the distal basilar artery. The aneurysm's position above or below the posterior clinoid process can also complicate clipping. High-riding aneurysms require a steeper upward view that is more subtemporal in its trajectory. Low-riding aneurysms require a posterior clinoidectomy or even a transcavernous exposure.

Illustrative Case

Patient DS is a 59-year-old woman with a family history of aneurysmal subarachnoid history who presented with an incidentally discovered large basilar tip aneurysm (Fig. 7.2). The aneurysm was deemed a favorable candidate for microsurgical clipping given its size, projection, and relationship to the clinoid process. She

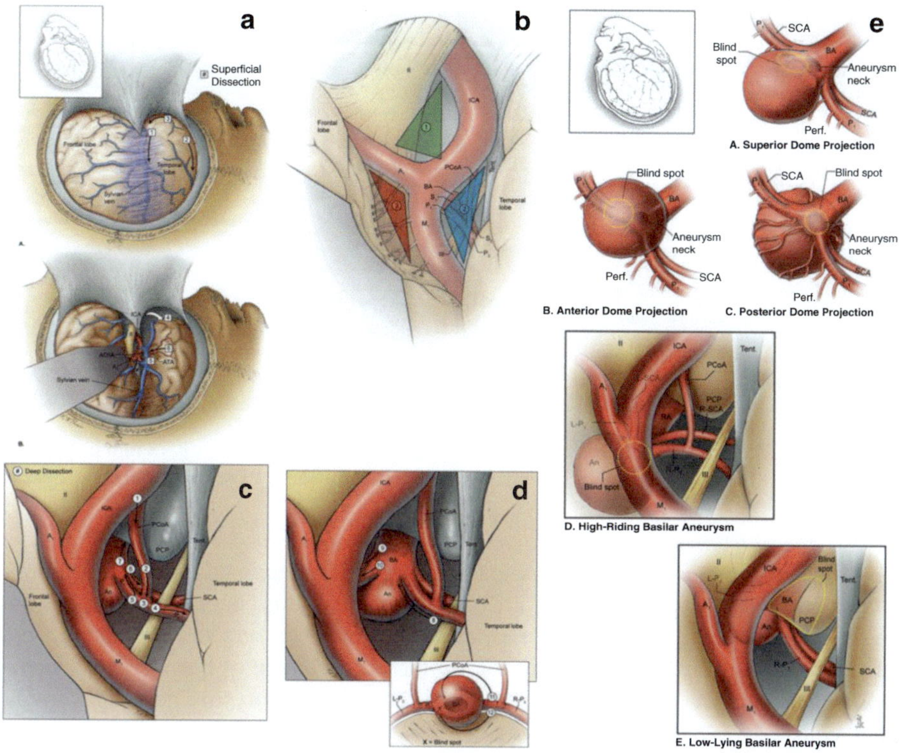

Fig. 7.1 (**a**) Superficial dissection strategy: *1* Splitting Sylvian fissure, *2* Freeing inferior temporal lobe by cutting arachnoid granulations and adhesions, *3* Freeing anterior temporal lobe by dividing temporopolar veins, *4* Opening pretemporal corridor by mobilizing temporal lobe posterolaterally, *5* Dissection along the anterior choroidal artery releases medial temporal lobe, *6*. Dissection along anterior temporal artery allows more posterior mobilization of temporal lobe. (**b**) Anatomic triangles providing access to the basilar bifurcation: *1* Optic-carotid triangle, *2* Carotid-oculomotor triangle, *3* Supracarotid triangle. (**c, d**) Deep dissection strategy: *1* Identify PCoA at its ICA origin, *2* and *3* Follow PCoA to P1-2 junction, *4* Dissect P2 segment laterally over the oculomotor nerve to the tentorial edge, *5* Dissect inferior surface of P1 segment medially through Liliequist's membrane, *6* Identify SCA, *7* Secure proximal control on basilar trunk, *8* Dissect superior surface of P1 segment to aneurysm neck, *9* Identify contralateral SCA across basilar apex, *10* Identify contralateral PCA and distal aneurysm neck, *11* Clear a path across anterior aneurysm neck, *12* Dissect perforators from posterior neck. (**e**) Variations in dome projection: *A* Superiorly projecting hides thalamoperforators behind distal neck, *B* Anterior projecting hides contralateral PCA and SCA, *C* Posteriorly projecting hides thalamoperforators from posterior base of the aneurysm; *D* High-riding aneurysms migrate out of carotid-oculomotor window, *E* Low riding descend out of carotid-oculomotor window and are hidden by posterior clinoid

elected to undergo microsurgical clipping. A right orbitozygomatic-pterional craniotomy was performed (Fig. 7.3). Perforators were identified posterior to the aneurysm and cleared from the neck before clips were applied. Postoperative angiogram confirmed complete obliteration of the aneurysm. The patient was discharged home in good condition with a modified Rankin score of 1.

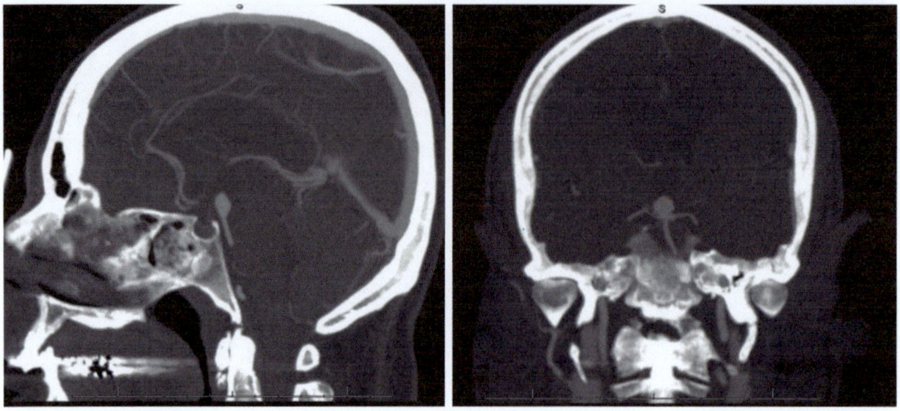

Fig. 7.2 Sagittal and coronal views from CT angiogram demonstrating a 6×8×8 mm irregularly shaped basilar tip aneurysm which partially incorporates the bilateral P1 segments of the posterior cerebral arteries

There are few series directly comparing surgical and endovascular management of posterior circulation aneurysms [18]. The purpose of this chapter is to summarize the best evidence for surgery for basilar aneurysms. The selected reports suggest microsurgery still has an important role in the management of basilar artery aneurysms, particularly for young patients with complex aneurysms needing durable treatment.

Contemporary Surgical Series of Basilar Artery Aneurysms

Samson's 18-year experience is the largest surgical series of basilar aneurysms since Drake (Table 7.1) [35]. Three hundred two aneurysms of the basilar apex were treated microsurgically between 1978 and 1996. The majority of patients presented with subarachnoid hemorrhage ($n=195$), of which the highest proportions were grade III ($n=76$, 39 %). At discharge, 76 % of patients had a good outcome defined

Fig. 7.3 (**a**) Overview of the transsylvian exposure after wide splitting of the Sylvian fissure preserving the temporopolar veins. (**b**) View through the carotid-oculomotor triangle visualizing the basilar apex. Note that only the distal basilar artery, ipsilateral P1 PCA and S1 SCA, and proximal aneurysm neck are visualized through this window. (**c**) The aneurysm is softened with a clip on the distal basilar artery and neck is reconstructed with a tandem clip configuration, with the initial straight fenestrated clip applied first to close the distal neck. (**d**) Before continuing with tandem clipping, perforators on the contralateral P1 PCA are inspected for patency. (**e**) The fenestration on the first clip is closed with a stacked straight clip, and (**f**) mini clips are used to close a remnant within the fenestration. (**g**) Note that redirecting the microscope allows visualization of contralateral anatomy, including the left P1 PCA and oculomotor nerve through the carotid-oculomotor triangle. (**h**) Indocyanine green dye confirms patency of thalamoperforators behind the aneurysm in the interpeduncular fossa

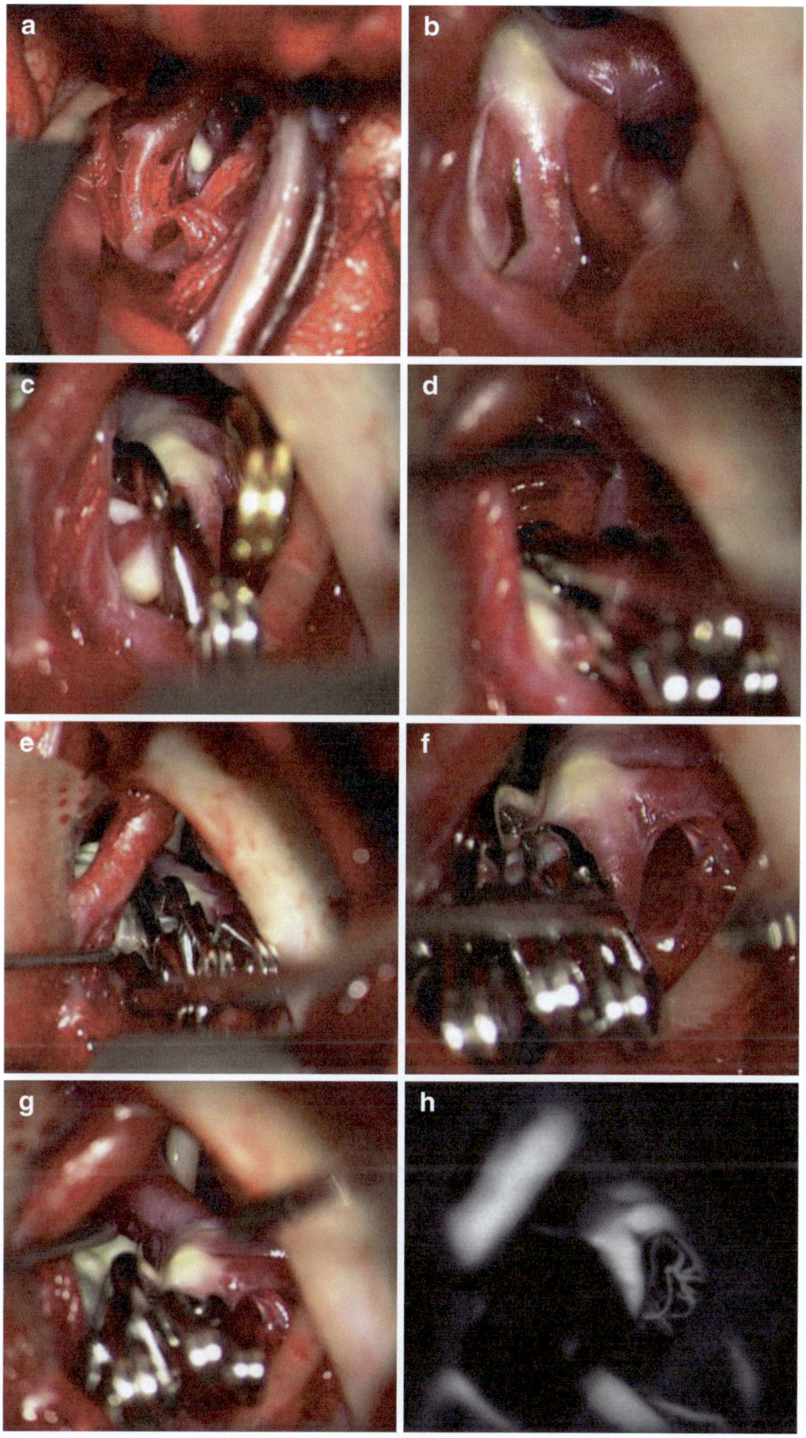
a
b
c
d
e
f
g
h

Table 7.1 Microsurgical clipping of basilar aneurysms

Series	Year	Number	Complete occlusion (%)	Good outcome (%)[b]	Mortality (%)
Sekhar [37]	2005–2012	37	92	76	8
Nanda [26]	1992–2009	62	92	77	8
Lawton [36]	1997–2006	162	98[a]	63	9
Samson [35]	1978–1996	302	94	81	9
Krisht [19]	1998–2006	51	98	90	4
Lawton [21]	1997–2001	56	–	84	9

[a]Includes all posterior circulation aneurysms
[b]Good outcome defined as Glasgow Outcome Scale (GOS) score of 4 or 5 modified Rankin scale (mRS) score of 0–2 depending on study

as Glasgow Outcome Scale (GOS) score of 5 or 4 with a mortality of 7 %. (A GOS score of 5 is defined as low disability and a score of 4 is defined as moderate disability, but independence in daily life [16]). At 6-month follow-up, 81 % had a good outcome and the mortality was 9 %. Complete aneurysm occlusion was demonstrated on follow-up angiography in 94 % of cases. Age, high-grade SAH, and aneurysm size >20 mm were predictors of poor outcome.

At our institution, in an initial experience between 1997 and 2001, 57 basilar apex aneurysms in 56 patients were treated microsurgically by the senior author (MTL) (Table 7.1) [21]. The basilar apex was defined as the basilar bifurcation, P1 PCA, and SCA. Most aneurysms were treated by microsurgical clipping through an orbitozygomatic-pterional craniotomy and transsylvian approach. After surgery, 84 % of patients had good outcomes defined as GOS score of 5 or 4, with a mortality rate of 9 %. Good outcomes increased from 79 % in the first half of the series to 90 % in the second half with a corresponding reduction in mortality attributable to more temporary clipping, better perforator dissection, and more sophisticated clipping techniques [21].

In an updated report including all posterior circulation aneurysms treated between 1997 and 2006, 217 patients with 228 aneurysms, including 106 basilar bifurcation, 27 PCA, 23 SCA, 8 AICA, and 5 basilar trunk aneurysms, underwent microsurgical clipping (Table 7.1) [36]. Aneurysms selected for microsurgical clipping had broad necks, aberrant branches, or fusiform morphology, and patients were younger with lower Hunt and Hess grades and fewer medical comorbidities. Of the 171 aneurysms clipped directly, 167 (98 %) were completely occluded. Sixty-three percent of patients had good outcomes with a mortality rate of 9 % [36].

Krisht et al. reported their results with high-complexity basilar apex aneurysms prone to fail endovascular treatment (Table 7.1) [19]. Between 1998 and 2006, 51 patients with 82 complex basilar apex aneurysms were treated microsurgically using a pretemporal transcavernous approach. Aneurysms were defined as highly complex on the basis of size (large or giant), posterior projecting dome, low bifurcation, wide dysmorphic base, and dolichoectasia. Complete aneurysm occlusion with no residual aneurysm was achieved in 49 aneurysms (98 %). At discharge, 86 % (n=44) of patients had a GOS score of 4 or 5, and at 6-month follow-up, 90 % (n=46) of patients had an mRS score of 0–2 with a mortality of 4 %.

In a more recent series by Sekhar et al. including 100 consecutively treated patients with both ruptured ($n=63$) and unruptured ($n=37$) basilar apex aneurysms, 37 patients were selected for microsurgical clipping (Table 7.1) [37]. All treating physicians had endovascular training and the majority of aneurysms were treated endovascularly. Younger patients with complex aneurysm morphology were more likely to be treated with clip occlusion, while patients with high dome-to-neck and aspect ratios were more likely to be coiled. Over 75 % of patients who underwent microsurgical clipping had a good outcome defined as a modified Rankin Scale (mRS) score of 0–2, and 12 of 13 (92 %) patients with unruptured aneurysms had good outcomes. There were no significant differences in outcomes between clipped and coiled patients. Endovascular treatment was less durable. About 33 % of patients treated endovascularly had residual aneurysm and more than 17 % required additional treatment, while there were no residuals for unruptured clipped aneurysms [37].

In another recent series by Nanda et al., 62 patients underwent microsurgical clipping of basilar apex aneurysms with complete occlusion in 98 % (Table 7.1) [26]. At their institution, since creation of an endovascular unit, the majority of basilar apex aneurysms have been treated endovascularly (25 of 36), while clipping is reserved for large and giant aneurysms, aneurysms with wide necks, or calcified and thrombosed aneurysms. In their series, more than half (33 of 62) of aneurysms were complex. Seventy-seven percent of clipped patients had good outcomes defined as GOS score of 5 or 4. When complex aneurysms were excluded, 82 % of patients had a good outcome.

Discussion

Today, management of basilar aneurysms is dominated by endovascular treatments and microsurgery is performed at few centers. While endovascular treatments are becoming increasingly safe and effective for many aneurysms of the posterior circulation, patients with complex aneurysms, wide-necked, thrombosed, large, or giant aneurysms with vessels arising directly from the aneurysm, are prone to treatment failure and morbidity and should be considered for microsurgical clipping [12, 30]. Flow-diverting stents are associated with substantial morbidity and mortality in these patients [38]. In contrast, surgical results from Samson, Lawton, Krisht, Sekhar, and Nanda demonstrate microsurgical clipping is a safe and durable treatment for highly complex basilar artery aneurysms [19, 21, 26, 35–37]. While aneurysms treated with coils or stents have been shown to recanalize even late [23], aneurysm recurrence is exceedingly rare for aneurysms after clip occlusion [4]. Good outcomes are possible even as cases referred for microsurgical clipping are increasingly technically challenging [26, 37].

Conclusions

Surgery for basilar aneurysms must be cultivated as endovascular treatments increase in sophistication and cerebrovascular neurosurgeons are left with increasingly complex and technically challenging aneurysms. While an increasing number of basilar artery aneurysms are amenable to endovascular treatments, younger patients with complex aneurysms can benefit from microsurgical clipping and its durable cure. The decision to treat endovascularly or microsurgically should be made by a multidisciplinary team, including the neurosurgeon, neurointerventional radiologists, and neurovascular neurologists. Aneurysm size, morphology, neck size, aspect ratio, projection, branch anatomy, intraluminal thrombus, wall calcification, parenchymal hematoma, intracranial pressure, presence of vasospasm, patient age, neurological condition, medical comorbidities, patient preferences, and institutional expertise should influence treatment decision [36]. SCA, P1 PCA, distal AICA, PICA, and some basilar bifurcation aneurysms are often amenable to microsurgical clipping in experienced hands. Treating physicians and patients must weigh higher surgical risks and longer recovery after craniotomy with higher likelihood of residual aneurysm, aneurysm recurrence, the need for ongoing surveillance angiography, and possible re-treatment after endovascular treatment.

References

1. Bavinzski G, Killer M, Gruber A, Reinprecht A, Gross CE, Richling B. Treatment of basilar artery bifurcation aneurysms by using Guglielmi detachable coils: a 6-year experience. J Neurosurg. 1999;90:843–52.
2. Chalouhi N, Tjoumakaris S, Gonzalez LF, Dumont AS, Starke RM, Hasan D, et al. Coiling of large and giant aneurysms: complications and long-term results of 334 cases. AJNR Am J Neuroradiol. 2014;35:546–52. United States.
3. Clajus C, Sychra V, Strasilla C, Klisch J. Stent-assisted coil embolization of intracranial aneurysms using the Solitaire AB neurovascular remodeling device: initial and midterm follow-up results. Neuroradiology. 2013;55:629–38.
4. David CA, Vishteh AG, Spetzler RF, Lemole M, Lawton MT, Partovi S. Late angiographic follow-up review of surgically treated aneurysms. J Neurosurg. 1999;91:396–401.
5. Drake CG. Bleeding aneurysms of the basilar artery. Direct surgical management in four cases. J Neurosurg. 1961;18:230–8.
6. Drake CG. Further experience with surgical treatment of aneurysm of the basilar artery. J Neurosurg. 1968;29:372–92.
7. Drake CG. The surgical treatment of vertebral-basilar aneurysms. Clin Neurosurg. 1969;16: 114–69.
8. Drake CG. The treatment of aneurysms of the posterior circulation. Clin Neurosurg. 1979;26:96–144.
9. Drake CG, Peerless SJ, Hernesniemi J. Surgery of vertebrobasilar aneurysms: London, Ontario, experience on 1767 patients. Wien: Springer; 1996.
10. Gory B, Klisch J, Bonafe A, Mounayer C, Beaujeux R, Moret J, et al. Solitaire AB stent-assisted coiling of wide-necked intracranial aneurysms: mid-term results from the SOLARE Study. Neurosurgery. 2014;75:215–9. discussion 219.
11. Gory B, Klisch J, Bonafe A, Mounayer C, Beaujeux R, Moret J, et al. Solitaire AB stent-assisted coiling of wide-necked intracranial aneurysms: short-term results from a prospective, consecutive, European multicentric study. Neuroradiology. 2013;55:1373–8.
12. Henkes H, Fischer S, Mariushi W, Weber W, Liebig T, Miloslavski E, et al. Angiographic and clinical results in 316 coil-treated basilar artery bifurcation aneurysms. J Neurosurg. 2005;103:990–9.

13. Hernesniemi J, Korja M. At the apex of cerebrovascular surgery – basilar tip aneurysms. World Neurosurg. 2014;82:37–9.
14. Hetts SW, Turk A, English JD, Dowd CF, Mocco J, Prestigiacomo C, et al. Stent-assisted coiling versus coiling alone in unruptured intracranial aneurysms in the matrix and platinum science trial: safety, efficacy, and mid-term outcomes. AJNR Am J Neuroradiol. 2014;35:698–705. United States.
15. Hong Y, Wang YJ, Deng Z, Wu Q, Zhang JM. Stent-assisted coiling versus coiling in treatment of intracranial aneurysm: a systematic review and meta-analysis. PLoS One. 2014;9, e82311. United States.
16. Jennett B, Bond M. Assessment of outcome after severe brain damage. Lancet. 1975;1: 480–4.
17. Klisch J, Eger C, Sychra V, Strasilla C, Basche S, Weber J. Stent-assisted coil embolization of posterior circulation aneurysms using Solitaire ab: preliminary experience. Neurosurgery. 2009;65:258–66. United States, discussion 266.
18. Koivisto T, Vanninen R, Hurskainen H, Saari T, Hernesniemi J, Vapalahti M. Outcomes of early endovascular versus surgical treatment of ruptured cerebral aneurysms. A prospective randomized study. Stroke. 2000;31:2369–77.
19. Krisht AF, Krayenbuhl N, Sercl D, Bikmaz K, Kadri PA. Results of microsurgical clipping of 50 high complexity basilar apex aneurysms. Neurosurgery. 2007;60:242–50. United States, discussion 250–242.
20. Lanzino G, Fraser K, Kanaan Y, Wagenbach A. Treatment of ruptured intracranial aneurysms since the International Subarachnoid Aneurysm Trial: practice utilizing clip ligation and coil embolization as individual or complementary therapies. J Neurosurg. 2006;104:344–9.
21. Lawton MT. Basilar apex aneurysms: surgical results and perspectives from an initial experience. Neurosurgery. 2002;50:1–8. discussion 8–10.
22. Li H, Pan R, Wang H, Rong X, Yin Z, Milgrom DP, et al. Clipping versus coiling for ruptured intracranial aneurysms: a systematic review and meta-analysis. Stroke. 2013;44:29–37. United States.
23. Mericle RA, Wakhloo AK, Lopes DK, Lanzino G, Guterman LR, Hopkins LN. Delayed aneurysm regrowth and recanalization after Guglielmi detachable coil treatment. Case report. J Neurosurg. 1998;89:142–5.
24. Molyneux A, Kerr R, Stratton I, Sandercock P, Clarke M, Shrimpton J, et al. International Subarachnoid Aneurysm Trial (ISAT) of neurosurgical clipping versus endovascular coiling in 2143 patients with ruptured intracranial aneurysms: a randomised trial. Lancet. 2002;360:1267–74. England.
25. Mordasini P, Schroth G, Guzman R, Barth A, Seiler RW, Remonda L. Endovascular treatment of posterior circulation cerebral aneurysms by using Guglielmi detachable coils: a 10-year single-center experience with special regard to technical development. AJNR Am J Neuroradiol. 2005;26:1732–8. United States.
26. Nanda A, Sonig A, Banerjee AD, Javalkar VK. Microsurgical management of basilar artery apex aneurysms: a single surgeon's experience from Louisiana State University, Shreveport. World Neurosurg. 2014;82:118–29.
27. Pandey AS, Koebbe C, Rosenwasser RH, Veznedaroglu E. Endovascular coil embolization of ruptured and unruptured posterior circulation aneurysms: review of a 10-year experience. Neurosurgery. 2007;60:626–36. United States, discussion 636–627.
28. Payner TD, Melamed I, Ansari S, Leipzig TJ, Scott JA, Denardo AJ, et al. Trends over time in the management of 2253 patients with cerebral aneurysms: a single practice experience. Surg Neurol Int. 2011;2:110. India.
29. Peerless SJ, Hernesniemi JA, Gutman FB, Drake CG. Early surgery for ruptured vertebrobasilar aneurysms. J Neurosurg. 1994;80:643–9.
30. Peluso JP, van Rooij WJ, Sluzewski M, Beute GN. Coiling of basilar tip aneurysms: results in 154 consecutive patients with emphasis on recurrent haemorrhage and re-treatment during mid- and long-term follow-up. J Neurol Neurosurg Psychiatry. 2008;79:706–11. England.

31. Phillips TJ, Wenderoth JD, Phatouros CC, Rice H, Singh TP, Devilliers L, et al. Safety of the pipeline embolization device in treatment of posterior circulation aneurysms. AJNR Am J Neuroradiol. 2012;33:1225–31. United States.
32. Qureshi AI, Vazquez G, Tariq N, Suri MF, Lakshminarayan K, Lanzino G. Impact of International Subarachnoid Aneurysm Trial results on treatment of ruptured intracranial aneurysms in the United States. Clinical article. J Neurosurg. 2011;114:834–41.
33. Raymond J, Guilbert F, Weill A, Georganos SA, Juravsky L, Lambert A, et al. Long-term angiographic recurrences after selective endovascular treatment of aneurysms with detachable coils. Stroke. 2003;34:1398–403. United States.
34. Raymond J, Roy D, Bojanowski M, Moumdjian R, L'Esperance G. Endovascular treatment of acutely ruptured and unruptured aneurysms of the basilar bifurcation. J Neurosurg. 1997;86:211–9.
35. Samson D, Batjer HH, Kopitnik Jr TA. Current results of the surgical management of aneurysms of the basilar apex. Neurosurgery. 1999;44:697–702. discussion 702-694.
36. Sanai N, Tarapore P, Lee AC, Lawton MT. The current role of microsurgery for posterior circulation aneurysms: a selective approach in the endovascular era. Neurosurgery. 2008;62:1236–49. United States, discussion 1249–1253.
37. Sekhar LN, Tariq F, Morton RP, Ghodke B, Hallam DK, Barber J, et al. Basilar tip aneurysms: a microsurgical and endovascular contemporary series of 100 patients. Neurosurgery. 2013;72:284–98. discussion 298–289.
38. Siddiqui AH, Abla AA, Kan P, Dumont TM, Jahshan S, Britz GW, et al. Panacea or problem: flow diverters in the treatment of symptomatic large or giant fusiform vertebrobasilar aneurysms. J Neurosurg. 2012;116:1258–66.
39. Spetzler RF, McDougall CG, Albuquerque FC, Zabramski JM, Hills NK, Partovi S, et al. The Barrow Ruptured Aneurysm Trial: 3-year results. J Neurosurg. 2013;119:146–57.
40. Van Rooij WJ, Sluzewski M, Menovsky T, Wijnalda D. Coiling of saccular basilar trunk aneurysms. Neuroradiology. 2003;45:19–21.
41. Wiebers DO, Whisnant JP, Huston 3rd J, Meissner I, Brown Jr RD, Piepgras DG, et al. Unruptured intracranial aneurysms: natural history, clinical outcome, and risks of surgical and endovascular treatment. Lancet. 2003;362:103–10. England.

Craniotomy Is Over for Basilar Artery Aneurysms

8

Leonardo Rangel-Castilla, Stephan A. Munich, and Elad I. Levy

Abbreviations

ANRD	Aneurysm neck reconstruction device
AP	Anteroposterior
BA	Basilar artery
LVIS	Low-profile visualized intraluminal support (device)
mRS	Modified Rankin scale
PCA	Posterior cerebral artery
PED	Pipeline embolization device
SCA	Superior cerebellar artery
VBJ	Vertebrobasilar junction
WEB	Woven EndoBridge

L. Rangel-Castilla, MD • S.A. Munich, MD
Department of Neurosurgery, Jacobs School of Medicine and Biomedical Sciences, University at Buffalo, State University of New York, Buffalo, NY, USA

Department of Neurosurgery, Gates Vascular Institute at Kaleida Health, Buffalo, NY, USA

E.I. Levy, MD, MBA, FACS, FAHA (✉)
Department of Neurosurgery, Gates Vascular Institute at Kaleida Health, Buffalo, NY, USA

Toshiba Stroke and Vascular Research Center, University at Buffalo, State University of New York, Buffalo, NY, USA

Departments of Neurosurgery and Radiology, Jacobs School of Medicine and Biomedical Sciences, University at Buffalo, State University of New York, Buffalo, NY, USA

University at Buffalo Neurosurgery, 100 High Street, Suite B4, Buffalo, NY 14203, USA
e-mail: elevy@ubns.com

E. Veznedaroglu (ed.), *Controversies in Vascular Neurosurgery*,
DOI 10.1007/978-3-319-27315-0_8

Introduction

The management of basilar artery (BA) aneurysms remains one of the most challenging areas of vascular neurosurgery due to the deep location of the BA and its supply to many critical structures. Much of the knowledge surrounding the microsurgical management of BA aneurysms comes from the vast experience of Dr. Charles Drake. In a 1990 update of their experience, Peerless and Drake [1] described 545 patients treated with microsurgical techniques and good outcomes achieved in 87 % of them. Building on this foundation, over the last 50 years, several other vascular neurosurgeons have reported their microsurgical experience with varying results [2–6]. Much of the microsurgical morbidity for the treatment of BA aneurysms results from the need for significant brain retraction, injuring critical temporal lobe structures, and often long duration of temporary arterial occlusion to test the collateral flow to highly sensitive brain stem structures. The complexity and not insignificant morbidity associated with the microsurgical treatment of BA aneurysms have stimulated a shift away from these strategies and toward endovascular techniques [7, 8].

The typically straight course and large caliber of the BA make it particularly favorable to endovascular navigation and catheterization. Depending on the aneurysm shape and associated branch vessels, primary coiling, balloon-assisted coiling, stent-assisted coiling, and flow diversion (with or without adjunctive coiling) may be employed for the endovascular treatment of these aneurysms. As with open microsurgical approaches, the location of the aneurysm on the BA also dictates which techniques are best suited for successful endovascular exclusion of the aneurysm. In this light, we separate the BA into three different anatomical locations: the basilar apex, basilar trunk, and vertebrobasilar junction (VBJ).

Basilar Apex Aneurysms

The basilar apex is the most common location for aneurysms occurring in the posterior circulation [9] (Fig. 8.1). These aneurysms tend to point superiorly in the direction of blood flow and the long axis of the BA [10]. Although the position of the basilar bifurcation is critical to the microsurgical approach to basilar apex aneurysms, it does not influence the endovascular strategy. Rather, associated anomalies and variants (e.g., hypoplastic P1 segment of the posterior cerebral artery [PCA], hypoplastic posterior communicating artery, fetal arrangement) may have a greater impact on endovascular techniques and morbidity.

Narrow-necked basilar apex aneurysms can often be treated with primary coiling. However, approximately 60 % of basilar apex aneurysms are wide necked (e.g., >4 mm) and may involve the PCA origins. In these cases, prevention of coil prolapse and preservation of the parent vessels (i.e., the PCAs) may require adjunctive techniques (balloon remodeling, stent-assisted coiling, multiple catheter techniques, and the application of new devices such as the PulseRider aneurysm neck reconstruction device (ANRD; Pulsar Vascular, San Jose CA) [9, 11–14].

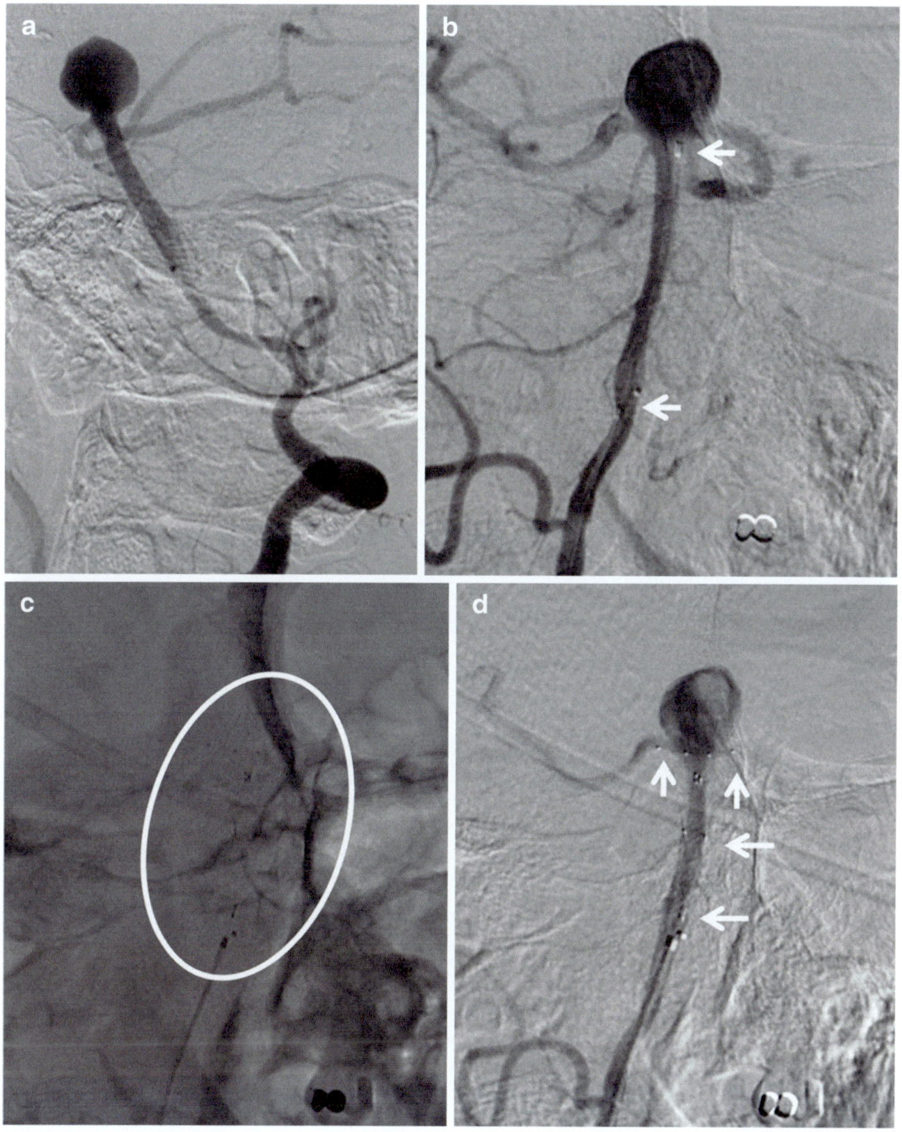

Fig. 8.1 (**a**) An 86-year-old man with a large basilar tip aneurysm treated endovascularly with the PulseRider aneurysm neck reconstruction device (ANRD; Pulsar Vascular, San Jose CA). (**b**) Two microcatheters (*arrows*) in the basilar artery aneurysm, one for device delivery and a second for coil delivery. (**c–e**) Anteroposterior (AP) and lateral views of the ANRD (*circled* in **c** and indicated by *arrows* in **d** and **e**). The T-shape device is situated at the basilar artery and both arms of the "T" are located at the posterior cerebral arteries. (**f–h**) Progressive coiling of the aneurysm. The *arrow* in (**f**) points to the device in the right posterior cerebral artery

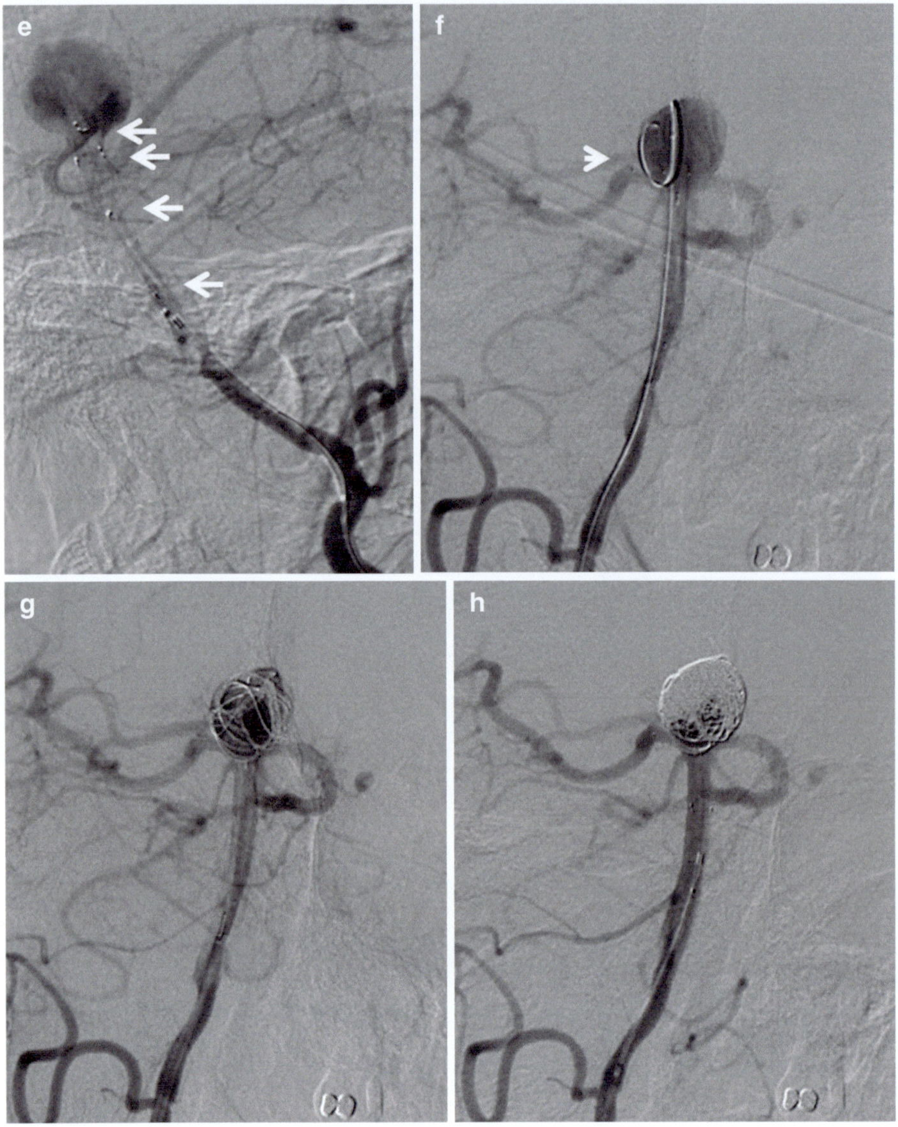

Fig. 8.1 (contiuned)

Balloon remodeling is used to segregate the aneurysm neck from the parent vessel, allowing coil deployment within the aneurysm dome and preventing prolapse into the parent vessel. Typically, the balloon is placed across the aneurysm neck and into the dominant P1. Given the location and morphology of a bifurcation, this technique requires the use of a compliant balloon whose shape can take on that of the parent bifurcation. Balloon-assisted coiling is beneficial in the setting of ruptured aneurysms when stenting (and obligatory dual antiplatelet administration) are not optimal.

Stent-assisted coiling similarly is used to prevent coil prolapse into the BA and PCAs. The stent configuration depends on the aneurysm morphology as well as the local vascular anatomy. For example, incorporation of a P1 PCA segment into the aneurysm neck would require stent placement into that segment for optimal aneurysm exclusion. A single stent, elbowed into the involved PCA segment, is employed when only one of the P1 segments is involved. A very wide-necked aneurysm with involvement of both P1 segments may require a Y-stenting configuration for protection of both PCA segments [15]. The choice of stent is dictated by the local anatomy, as well as surgeon experience. We favor the use of open-cell stents because of their flexibility and good wall apposition. However, it should be noted that the new generation of intracranial stents, such as the low-profile visualized intraluminal support device (LVIS, MicroVention, Tustin, CA) and the LVIS Jr device (MicroVention), has demonstrated advantages over the previous generation with respect to visibility, deployment, and coil mass support [16, 17].

Novel Devices for Bifurcation Aneurysms

New devices such as the aforementioned PulseRider ANRD (Fig. 8.1) or the Woven EndoBridge (WEB; Sequent Medical, Aliso Viejo, CA) are under investigation in clinical trials and are promising adjuncts to endovascular coiling of complex bifurcation aneurysms, including basilar apex aneurysms [13, 18]. The PulseRider ANRD is a novel 0.002-in. laser-cut nitinol self-expanding retrievable device specifically shaped to fit within bifurcated arteries. It is designed to be deployed to abut the aneurysm ostium while remaining outside the aneurysm. The reconstructive scaffold area of the device or "saddle" is oriented by opposing struts that align with the outflow branches to ensure preservation of those branches. Early experience demonstrated that it is a safe and effective adjunct in the treatment of bifurcation aneurysms arising at the basilar apex [13]. Longer follow-up and larger experience are needed to confirm these early results [19]. The WEB is an intrasaccular device designed to disrupt intra-aneurysmal flow at the level of the neck. Initial experience has shown good efficacy, with a high percentage of cases of adequate aneurysm occlusion in the postprocedure period and at short-term follow-up [18]. However, significant neck remnants were observed (56.7 %) [20]. This was due, in part, to the shape of the WEB. The proximal surface of the WEB is not flat but has a recess, which is concave from the direction of the parent artery. Again, long-term results are needed. We await the results from the clinical trials relative to both devices.

Aneurysm Recanalization and Coil Compaction

Due to their anatomic location and morphology, basilar apex aneurysms have an increased risk of coil compaction and recanalization. Traditional treatment strategies seek to obtain 90–100 % angiographic occlusion, which is accepted as protective against hemorrhage. Model studies have shown that complete coil obliteration

Table 8.1 Summary of studies evaluating the endovascular treatment of basilar trunk aneurysms

Study, year	*N*	Technique (no. cases)	Complete or near-complete (90–100 %) angiographic occlusion, no. pts. (%)	Procedure-related morbidity (%)
Peschillo et al. (2014) [39]	3	Flow diversion (3)	3 of 3 (100)	66.6
Chalouhi et al. (2014) [35]	1	Flow diversion (1)	0 of 1 (0 %)	0
Gross et al. (2013) [37]	2	Coiling (2)	2 of 2 (100)	0
Higa et al. (2011) [38]	14	Coiling (14)	14 of 14 (100)	7.1
Chung et al. (2011) [36]	4	Stent-assisted coiling (3) Coiling (1)	4 of 4 (100)	0
Yu et al. (2010) [41]	10	Coiling (7) Balloon-assisted coiling (2) Stent-assisted coiling (1)	10 of 10 (100)	0
Uda et al. (2001) [40]	16	Coiling (16)	14 of 16 (88)	12.5

no. pts. number of patients

of an aneurysm only fills 30 % of the aneurysm with coil mass [21, 22]. Wide-necked aneurysms are at particularly high risk for recanalization, likely related to flow dynamics and stress. Rates of early recanalization have been shown to be significant in wide-necked or partially coil-treated aneurysms [9, 11, 23, 24].

The rate of initial occlusion may be particularly important for long-term obliteration in the setting of basilar apex aneurysms. In their systematic review, Lozier et al. [23] analyzed recanalization rates and found recanalization to occur in 10 % of initially completely coil-occluded, 37 % of nearly completely coil-occluded (90–99 %), and 60 % of incompletely coil-occluded (<90 %) aneurysms. Henkes et al. [9] found coil compaction and residual aneurysm filling in 24 % of patients at their first angiographic follow-up (mean 19.4 months). Their experience provides significant insight into predictors of treatment success – lower occlusion rates during the first treatment session were associated with larger neck widths and fundus diameters, whereas the use of 3D coils correlated with successful occlusion. The degree of occlusion at the time of the initial treatment significantly affected the degree of occlusion at follow-up, with 78.1 % of aneurysms maintaining complete occlusion on follow-up.

The primary benefit of endovascular techniques in the treatment of BA apex aneurysms comes in their reduction in morbidity and mortality. A meta-analysis of 228 endovascularly treated basilar apex aneurysms demonstrated a procedural morbidity of 6.6 % and procedural mortality of 1.3 % [9]. Several other studies have reported even lower morbidity rates, ranging from 0 to 3.7 % [9, 11, 25–30]. These rates stand in stark contrast to those reported in microsurgical series, where even in the best of hands, mortality may approach 10 % and perioperative complications are reported in 40 % [2].

Basilar Trunk Aneurysms

The basilar trunk is typically considered to be the segment of the BA extending from just distal to its origin through the superior cerebellar artery (SCA). Like aneurysms in other locations, basilar trunk aneurysms tend to arise from branch points, most often those formed with the SCA but also with small perforating vessels. Attention to these small brainstem perforators is critical to avoidance of morbidity. Basilar trunk aneurysms are rare, accounting for less than 1 % of intracranial aneurysms and 8 % of vertebrobasilar aneurysms [14].

Microsurgical access to the basilar trunk often requires significant retraction and osseous dissection, including extensive petrosectomies and/or combined supratentorial or infratentorial approaches. Further, it requires navigation through a collection of vital cranial nerves and perforating arteries. Successful occlusion of these aneurysms may require trapping and bypass [31]. In their analysis of management-related morbidity and mortality, Seifert et al. [32] found that aneurysm location at the basilar trunk was associated with poor outcome or death after surgical treatment. Similarly, in their study of surgical or endovascular treatment of large or giant posterior fossa aneurysms, Inamasu et al. [33] found that patients with basilar trunk aneurysms were least amenable to treatment with good outcome.

Flow-diverting stents, such as the Pipeline embolization device (PED; ev3-Covidien, Irvine, CA), provide a new therapeutic option of total intraluminal reconstruction for the treatment of basilar trunk aneurysms. The PED provides 30–35 % metal surface area coverage. The decrease in porosity causes stagnation of blood flow within the aneurysm, thereby promoting its thrombosis while maintaining patency of nearby perforating vessels. The stent scaffold eventually leads to endothelialization of the PED and, therefore, completes intraluminal reconstruction of the diseased vessel. However, due to the increased number of perforating vessels in the posterior circulation and the vital brainstem structures supplied by these perforators, neuroendovascular surgeons have been cautious in their application of the PED in the posterior circulation [34]. A summary of studies in which basilar trunk aneurysms were evaluated is provided in Table 8.1 [35–41].

Saccular Aneurysms

Saccular aneurysms of the basilar trunk are rare lesions, most frequently occurring in patients with multiple intracranial aneurysms or other vascular anomalies [42, 43]. They are most often seen at the level of the SCA; in these cases, there is often a curve at the rostral portion of the BA, such that the hemodynamic thrust is in the direction of the SCA origin, rather than within the long axis of the BA [10]. However, saccular aneurysms may also form at the branch points of small perforating arteries with the BA. Morphologically, these lesions may appear as "side-wall" aneurysms of the BA. The high density of critical perforating arteries and the intimate relationship of basilar trunk aneurysms with them make these particularly formidable lesions.

In contrast to the extensive approaches and variable results of microsurgical strategies, endovascular techniques for the treatment of saccular basilar trunk aneurysms are more technically reliable and associated with better outcomes. Higa et al. [38] report no procedure-related morbidity in their series of 14 patients treated endovascularly. Similarly, Uda et al. [40] report excellent or good clinical results in 89.7 % of patients (35 patients) with basilar trunk aneurysms treated with Guglielmi detachable coils, with complete or near-complete occlusion occurring in 85.4 % (35 aneurysms). The report by van Rooij et al. [14] echoed these excellent clinical results, also noting the mean procedure time of 61 min. This stands in stark contrast to the arduous open surgical techniques needed to effectively treat basilar trunk aneurysms.

Fusiform Aneurysms

Vertebrobasilar fusiform aneurysms (or vertebrobasilar dolichoectasias) comprise a distinct disease entity that may cause a wide range of clinical symptoms, including embolic ischemic strokes, cranial nerve palsies, brain stem compression, obstructive hydrocephalus, and intraparenchymal or subarachnoid hemorrhage. Passero and Rossi [44] found that, without treatment, 43 % of patients experienced anatomical (i.e., radiographic) progression and 60 % experienced new symptoms. Though rare, rupture of a basilar fusiform aneurysm is associated with a particularly poor prognosis and high mortality rate within the first 48 h [45, 46]. The higher frequency of giant fusiform aneurysms in the basilar trunk compared with those in the anterior circulation may reflect segmental vulnerability of the basilar arterial system.

Microsurgical management of these lesions is challenging because of difficult surgical access, circumferential involvement of the vessel, and frequent incorporation of the perforating branches of the BA in the aneurysm. The introduction of flow-diverting stents to the endovascular armamentarium has revolutionized treatment of these formidable lesions. Chalouhi et al. [47] recently reported favorable outcomes in three patients with vertebrobasilar fusiform aneurysms treated with the PED. Similarly, Munich et al. [12] demonstrated effective parent vessel reconstruction (90 %) and good neurologic outcome (modified Rankin Scale [mRS] scores of 0–3) in 75 % of patients with vertebrobasilar dolichoectasia treated with the PED.

Endovascular techniques other than flow diversion may also provide effective, minimally invasive treatment strategies for these lesions (Fig. 8.2). Chen et al. [48] demonstrated good neurologic outcomes in nine of ten patients with large and giant vertebrobasilar fusiform aneurysms treated with a variety of endovascular techniques (e.g., stenting, stent-assisted coiling, and proximal vessel occlusion). These techniques, offered through a femoral arteriotomy, stand in stark contrast to the extensive skull base approaches and parent vessel bypass and/or reconstructions required to treat these lesions surgically.

We have learned that patient selection is extremely important [34]. Patients presenting with acute ischemic symptoms from brainstem infarction and compression may not be good candidates for endovascular treatment because they may then

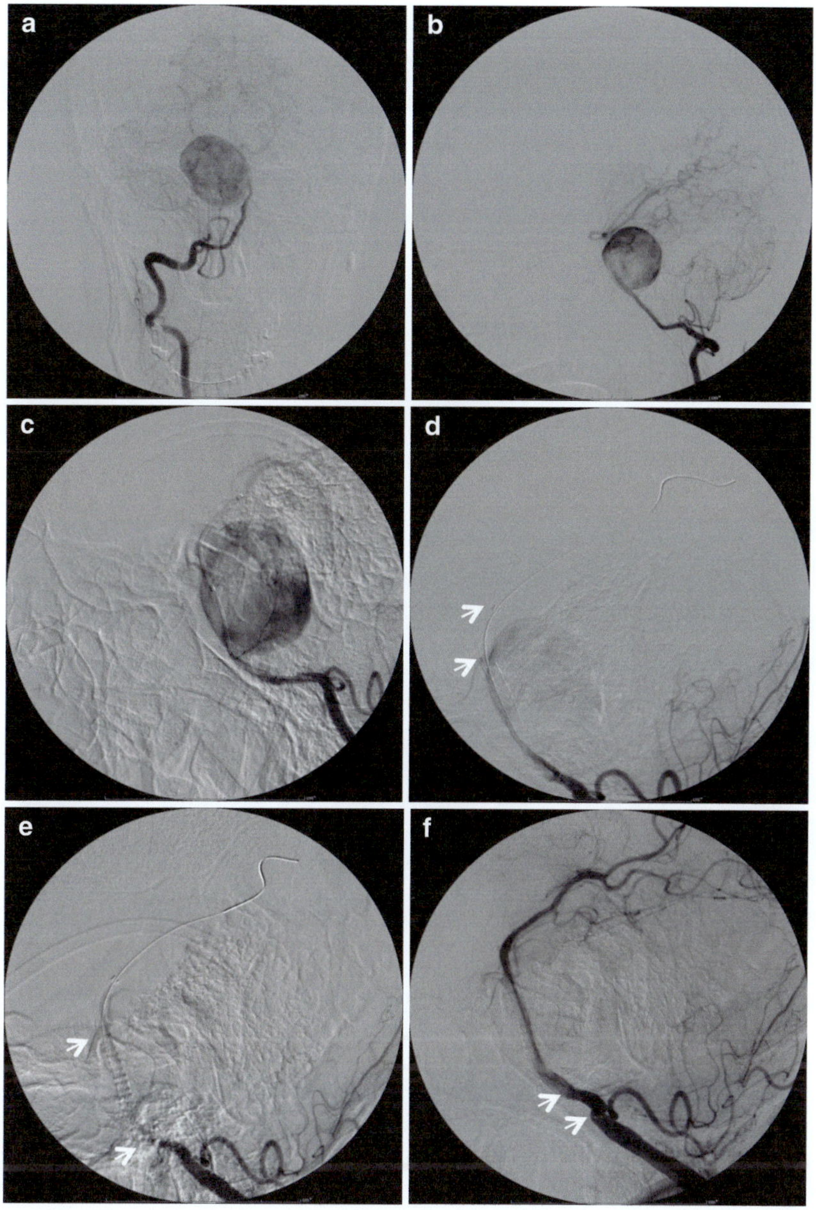

Fig. 8.2 A 36-year-old man presented with severe headaches, dysmetria, and gait ataxia. Noninvasive neuroimaging showed a large posterior fossa aneurysm. AP (**a**) and lateral (**b**) angiograms, right vertebral artery injection, demonstrate a giant basilar trunk aneurysm. After discussing different treatment options, the patient underwent endovascular treatment. (**c**) Lateral angiogram demonstrating access into the left posterior cerebellar artery and basilar artery. Progressive stenting reconstruction of the basilar artery with a Neuroform stent (Stryker Neurovascular, Kalamazoo, Michigan) (**d**), two covered stents (JOSTENTS, Abbott Vascular, Santa Clara, California) (**e**), and a Wingspan stent (Stryker Neurovascular) (**f**). Six-month follow-up AP (**g**) and lateral (**h**) angiograms demonstrating complete aneurysm thrombosis. Sagittal CT angiogram (**i**) demonstrating patency of the stents and no evidence of aneurysm recurrence at 1 year

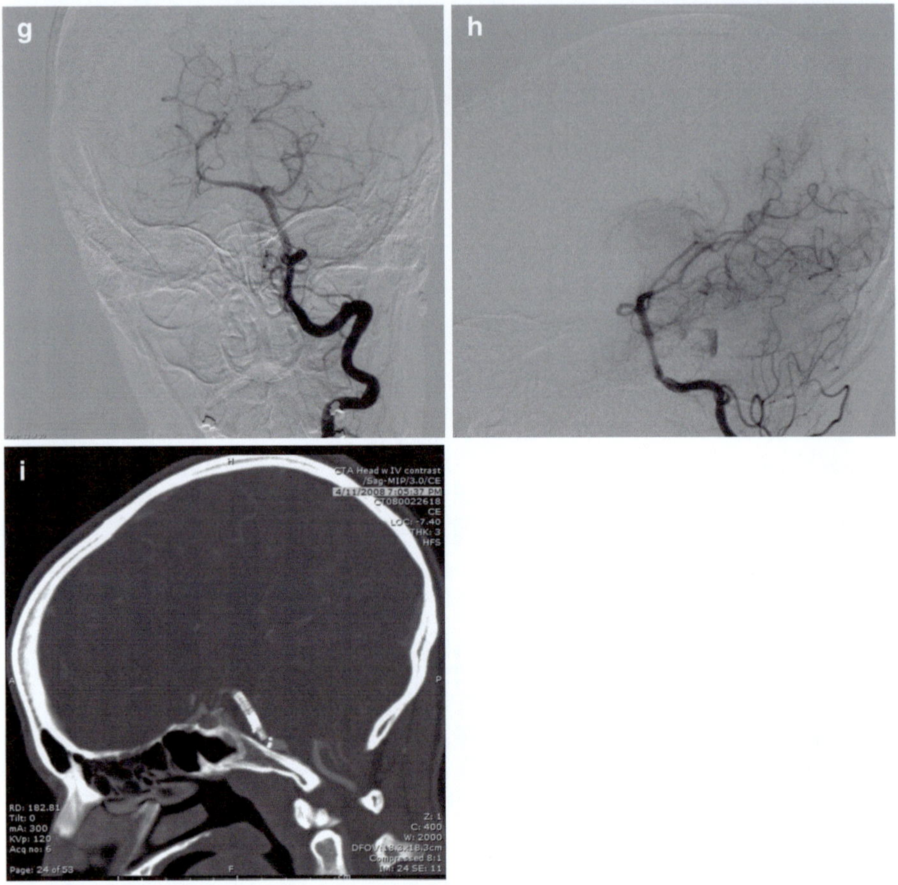

Fig. 8.2 (contiuned)

progress to have brain stem strokes. This may be reflective of already compromised ostia of affected perforators as well as the large number of devices. Aneurysms in perforator-rich regions, especially fusiform mid-BA aneurysms, have a higher chance of perforator infarcts after flow diversion. Patients with partially thrombosed aneurysms with significant clot burden also have a higher risk of perforator strokes. We do not believe flow diversion in its current iteration is an option for giant holobasilar fusiform dolichoectatic aneurysms with major branch points coming off opposite walls of the aneurysm. We also believe that the use of PED should be limited to one device only, when possible. A second device could be used solely to ensure adequate coverage of the aneurysm neck. This is mostly in the case of giant aneurysms where one device is not long enough to provide adequate coverage of the aneurysm and a long enough anchor segment in the normal segments proximal or distal to the aneurysm. We do not use a second device to achieve aneurysm stasis or better flow diversion.

Vertebrobasilar Junction Aneurysms

The natural history of aneurysms located at the VBJ is one of the most ominous of all intracranial aneurysms (Fig. 8.3). Although their incidence is low (0.17–0.76 % [49, 50]), the mortality associated with these lesions approaches 30 %. These aneurysms have a significant male predominance (70 %) [51]. In more than half of the cases, the aneurysm is associated with a fenestration [52, 53]. Similar to dolichoectatic BA aneurysms, VBJ aneurysms may cause mass symptoms of mass effect (on the brainstem, cranial nerves, and/or cerebellum), hydrocephalus, ischemia from thrombus formation and emboli (Fig. 8.4), and subarachnoid hemorrhage. Their

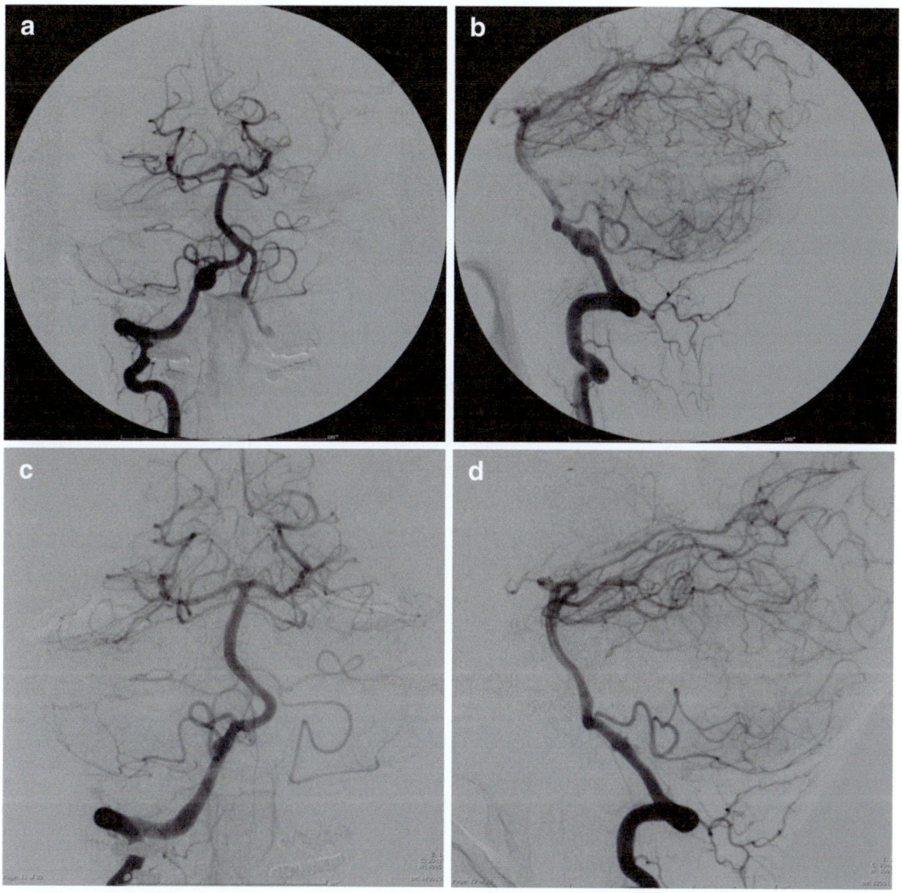

Fig. 8.3 A 40-year-old man with a history of migraines underwent magnetic resonance imaging and magnetic resonance angiography that revealed a right vertebral artery aneurysm. AP (**a**) and lateral (**b**) angiograms demonstrate a fusiform right vertebral artery aneurysm. The aneurysm was treated with two Enterprise stents (Codman, Raynham, MA). The patient was treated in 2007 before the flow-diverter era. The 1-year follow-up angiographic images (**c**, AP; **d**, lateral) show complete obliteration of the aneurysm with preservation of the related posteroinferior cerebellar artery

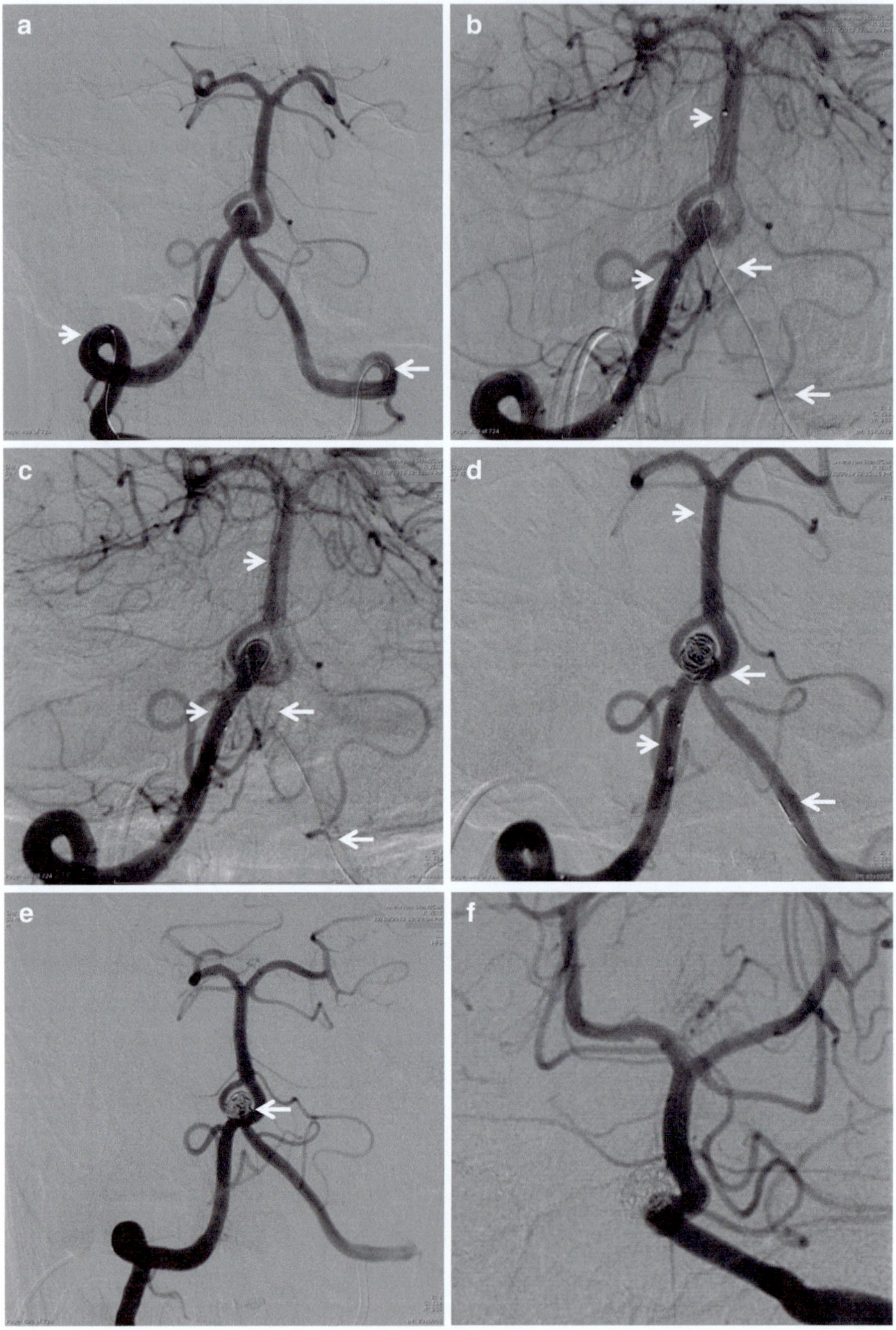

Fig. 8.4 A 50-year-old man who experienced a transient ischemic attack was found to have a fenestrated basilar artery aneurysm on diagnostic angiography (**a**). (**b–e**) The patient underwent stent-assisted coiling through both vertebral arteries. Right vertebral artery with microcatheter for stent delivery (*arrow*) and left vertebral artery microcatheter for coil delivery (*long arrow*). (**f**) 6-month follow-up angiogram showing complete aneurysm obliteration

clinical course is slowly progressive but often is punctuated by stuttering episodes of abrupt exacerbation, corresponding to intramural hemorrhage or microdissection [54]. Ischemia is the most common presentation, occurring in 45 % of patients and ranging from transient ischemic attack to large pontine infarctions. When infarctions occur, they preferentially affect the pons (33–50 %), thalamus (4.5–11 %), and lateral medulla (9 %) [51].

Similar to the microsurgical techniques needed for the treatment of basilar trunk aneurysms, microsurgical techniques for VBJ aneurysms often require extensive skull base approaches with or without parent vessel occlusion and bypass, thereby necessitating their treatment at specialized neurosurgical centers. With the advent of endovascular techniques, and particularly the development of flow-diverting stents, endovascular strategies have become the preferred method for the treatment of these lesions (Fig. 8.3). Graziano et al. [52] published their series of the endovascular treatment of ten patients with VBJ aneurysms, finding all to have good neurologic outcome (mRS) at last follow-up. We refer readers to that article, which includes a meta-analysis of the endovascular treatment of VBJ aneurysms since 2004. The success of endovascular techniques extends to ruptured VBJ aneurysms – Peluso et al. [53] demonstrated successful endovascular treatment of ten patients with VBJ, with complete or near-complete (90 %) occlusion in all patients.

The use of flow-diverting stents in the posterior circulation remains controversial. As previously mentioned, apprehension toward the application of this technique in this location rests on the concern surrounding critical basilar perforating arteries. Marinkovic and Gibo [55] have demonstrated a particularly high density of perforating vessels in the rostral BA. Therefore, the use of flow-diverting stents may be better tolerated at the VBJ than rostral to the VBJ. Indeed, in a clinical series of patients with vertebrobasilar fusiform aneurysms in which the use of flow-diverting stents was restricted to caudal to the anterior inferior cerebellar artery, the mean mRS score at follow-up was 1.9 [12]. Meckel et al. [56] demonstrate good angiographic outcome in nine of ten patients, with one patient requiring the addition of another flow-diverting stent.

The aforementioned techniques were performed with preservation of the parent vessel. However, some complex VBJ aneurysms require parent vessel occlusion and/or flow reversal. As Steinberg et al. [57] documented in their series, Hunterian ligation resulted in excellent outcome in 74 % of patients with VBJ aneurysms. However, even these strategies may be employed endovascularly (Fig. 8.4) (e.g., with coiling with or without liquid embolic material) without the need for extensive surgical approaches or techniques.

References

1. Peerless SJ, Drake CG. Management of aneurysms of the posterior circulation. In: Youmans J, editor. Neurological surgery. A comprehensive reference guide to the diagnosis and management of neurosurgical problems. 3rd ed. Philadelphia: WB Saunders; 1990. p. 1764–806.
2. Nanda A, Sonig A, Banerjee AD, et al. Microsurgical management of basilar artery apex aneurysms: a single surgeon's experience from Louisiana State University, Shreveport. World Neurosurg. 2014;82:118–29.

3. Shi X, Qian H, Singh KC, et al. Surgical management of vertebral and basilar artery aneurysms: a single center experience in 41 patients. Acta Neurochir (Wien). 2013;155:1087–93.
4. Kalani MY, Zabramski JM, Nakaji P, et al. Bypass and flow reduction for complex basilar and vertebrobasilar junction aneurysms. Neurosurgery. 2013;72:763–75; discussion 75–6.
5. Lozier AP, Kim GH, Sciacca RR, et al. Microsurgical treatment of basilar apex aneurysms: perioperative and long-term clinical outcome. Neurosurgery. 2004;54:286–96; discussion 96–9.
6. Bendok BR, Getch CC, Parkinson R, et al. Extended lateral transsylvian approach for basilar bifurcation aneurysms. Neurosurgery. 2004;55:174–8; discussion 78.
7. Abla AA, Lawton MT, Spetzler RF. The art of basilar apex aneurysm surgery: is it sustainable in the future? World Neurosurg. 2014;82:e51–3.
8. Hernesniemi J, Korja M. At the apex of cerebrovascular surgery – basilar tip aneurysms. World Neurosurg. 2014;82:37–9.
9. Henkes H, Fischer S, Mariushi W, et al. Angiographic and clinical results in 316 coil-treated basilar artery bifurcation aneurysms. J Neurosurg. 2005;103:990–9.
10. Rhoton Jr AL. Aneurysms. Neurosurgery. 2002;51:S121–58.
11. Bavinzski G, Killer M, Gruber A, et al. Treatment of basilar artery bifurcation aneurysms by using Guglielmi detachable coils: a 6-year experience. J Neurosurg. 1999;90:843–52.
12. Munich SA, Tan LA, Keigher KM, et al. The pipeline embolization device for the treatment of posterior circulation fusiform aneurysms: lessons learned at a single institution. J Neurosurg. 2014;121:1077–84.
13. Spiotta AM, Chaudry MI, Turk AS, et al. Initial experience with the PulseRider for the treatment of bifurcation aneurysms: report of first three cases in the USA. J Neurointerv Surg. 2016;8:186–9.
14. Van Rooij WJ, Sluzewski M, Menovsky T, et al. Coiling of saccular basilar trunk aneurysms. Neuroradiology. 2003;45:19–21.
15. Fargen KM, Mocco J, Neal D, et al. A multicenter study of stent-assisted coiling of cerebral aneurysms with a Y configuration. Neurosurgery. 2013;73:466–72.
16. Cho YD, Sohn CH, Kang HS, et al. Coil embolization of intracranial saccular aneurysms using the Low-profile Visualized Intraluminal Support (LVIS) device. Neuroradiology. 2014;56:543–51.
17. Poncyljusz W, Bilinski P, Safranow K, et al. The LVIS/LVIS Jr. stents in the treatment of wide-neck intracranial aneurysms: multicentre registry. J Neurointerv Surg. 2015;7:524–9.
18. Gherasim DN, Gory B, Sivan-Hoffmann R, et al. Endovascular treatment of wide-neck anterior communicating artery aneurysms using WEB-DL and WEB-SL: short-term results in a multicenter study. AJNR Am J Neuroradiol. 2015;36:1150–4.
19. Turk A, Turner RD, Tateshima S, et al. Novel aneurysm neck reconstruction device: initial experience in an experimental preclinical bifurcation aneurysm model. J Neurointerv Surg. 2013;5:346–50.
20. Pierot L, Klisch J, Cognard C, et al. Endovascular WEB flow disruption in middle cerebral artery aneurysms: preliminary feasibility, clinical, and anatomical results in a multicenter study. Neurosurgery. 2013;73:27–34; discussion 34–5.
21. Kawanabe Y, Sadato A, Taki W, et al. Endovascular occlusion of intracranial aneurysms with Guglielmi detachable coils: correlation between coil packing density and coil compaction. Acta Neurochir (Wien). 2001;143:451–5.
22. Piotin M, Mandai S, Murphy KJ, et al. Dense packing of cerebral aneurysms: an in vitro study with detachable platinum coils. AJNR Am J Neuroradiol. 2000;21:757–60.
23. Lozier AP, Connolly Jr ES, Lavine SD, et al. Guglielmi detachable coil embolization of posterior circulation aneurysms: a systematic review of the literature. Stroke. 2002;33:2509–18.
24. McDougall CG, Halbach VV, Dowd CF, et al. Endovascular treatment of basilar tip aneurysms using electrolytically detachable coils. J Neurosurg. 1996;84:393–9.
25. Eskridge JM, Song JK. Endovascular embolization of 150 basilar tip aneurysms with Guglielmi detachable coils: results of the Food and Drug Administration multicenter clinical trial. J Neurosurg. 1998;89:81–6.

26. Mordasini P, Schroth G, Guzman R, et al. Endovascular treatment of posterior circulation cerebral aneurysms by using Guglielmi detachable coils: a 10-year single-center experience with special regard to technical development. AJNR Am J Neuroradiol. 2005;26:1732–8.
27. Pandey AS, Koebbe C, Rosenwasser RH, et al. Endovascular coil embolization of ruptured and unruptured posterior circulation aneurysms: review of a 10-year experience. Neurosurgery. 2007;60:626–36; discussion 36–7.
28. Peluso JP, van Rooij WJ, Sluzewski M, et al. Coiling of basilar tip aneurysms: results in 154 consecutive patients with emphasis on recurrent haemorrhage and re-treatment during mid- and long-term follow-up. J Neurol Neurosurg Psychiatry. 2008;79:706–11.
29. Tateshima S, Murayama Y, Gobin YP, et al. Endovascular treatment of basilar tip aneurysms using Guglielmi detachable coils: anatomic and clinical outcomes in 73 patients from a single institution. Neurosurgery. 2000;47:1332–9; discussion 39–42.
30. Vallee JN, Aymard A, Vicaut E, et al. Endovascular treatment of basilar tip aneurysms with Guglielmi detachable coils: predictors of immediate and long-term results with multivariate analysis 6-year experience. Radiology. 2003;226:867–79.
31. Terasaka S, Itamoto K, Houkin K. Basilar trunk aneurysm surgically treated with anterior petrosectomy and external carotid artery-to-posterior cerebral artery bypass: technical note. Neurosurgery. 2002;51:1083–7; discussion 87–8.
32. Seifert V, Raabe A, Stolke D. Management-related morbidity and mortality in unselected aneurysms of the basilar trunk and vertebrobasilar junction. Acta Neurochir (Wien). 2001;143:343–8; discussion 48–9.
33. Inamasu J, Suga S, Sato S, et al. Long-term outcome of 17 cases of large-giant posterior fossa aneurysm. Clin Neurol Neurosurg. 2000;102:65–71.
34. Natarajan SK, Lin N, Sonig A, et al. The safety of Pipeline flow diversion in fusiform vertebrobasilar aneurysms: a consecutive case series with longer-term follow-up from a single US center. J Neurosurg epub [ahead of print] December 11, 2015. DOI: 10.3171/2015.6.JNS1565.
35. Chalouhi N, Jabbour P, Starke RM, et al. Treatment of a basilar trunk perforator aneurysm with the Pipeline embolization device: case report. Neurosurgery. 2014;74:E697–701; discussion 01.
36. Chung J, Park H, Lim YC, et al. Endovascular treatment of basilar artery trunk aneurysms. Acta Neurochir (Wien). 2011;153:2137–45.
37. Gross BA, Puri AS, Du R. Basilar trunk perforator artery aneurysms. Case report and literature review. Neurosurg Rev. 2013;36:163–8; discussion 68.
38. Higa T, Ujiie H, Kato K, et al. Endovascular treatment of basilar trunk saccular aneurysms. Neuroradiol J. 2011;24:687–92.
39. Peschillo S, Caporlingua A, Cannizzaro D, et al. Flow diverter stent treatment for ruptured basilar trunk perforator aneurysms. J Neurointerv Surg. 2014. doi:10.1136/neurintsurg-2014-011511 (epub December 16 2014).
40. Uda K, Murayama Y, Gobin YP, et al. Endovascular treatment of basilar artery trunk aneurysms with Guglielmi detachable coils: clinical experience with 41 aneurysms in 39 patients. J Neurosurg. 2001;95:624–32.
41. Yu JL, Wang HL, Xu N, et al. Endovascular treatment of aneurysms arising from the basilar artery trunk and branches. Interv Neuroradiol. 2010;16:369–83.
42. Higa T, Ujiie H, Kato K, et al. Basilar artery trunk saccular aneurysms: morphological characteristics and management. Neurosurg Rev. 2009;32:181–91; discussion 91.
43. Saliou G, Sacho RH, Power S, et al. Natural history and management of basilar trunk artery aneurysms. Stroke. 2015;46:948–53.
44. Passero SG, Rossi S. Natural history of vertebrobasilar dolichoectasia. Neurology. 2008;70:66–72.
45. Rinkel GJ, Djibuti M, Algra A, et al. Prevalence and risk of rupture of intracranial aneurysms: a systematic review. Stroke. 1998;29:251–6.
46. van Oel LI, van Rooij WJ, Sluzewski M, et al. Reconstructive endovascular treatment of fusiform and dissecting basilar trunk aneurysms with flow diverters, stents, and coils. AJNR Am J Neuroradiol. 2013;34:589–95.

47. Chalouhi N, Tjoumakaris S, Dumont AS, et al. Treatment of posterior circulation aneurysms with the pipeline embolization device. Neurosurgery. 2013;72:883–9.
48. Chen Z, Yang Y, Miao H, et al. Endovascular treatment for large and giant fusiform aneurysms of the vertebrobasilar arteries. Clin Imaging. 2013;37:227–31.
49. Pia HW. Classification of vertebro-basilar aneurysms. Acta Neurochir (Wien). 1979;47:3–30.
50. Yu YL, Moseley IF, Pullicino P, et al. The clinical picture of ectasia of the intracerebral arteries. J Neurol Neurosurg Psychiatry. 1982;45:29–36.
51. Flemming KD, Wiebers DO, Brown Jr RD, et al. The natural history of radiographically defined vertebrobasilar nonsaccular intracranial aneurysms. Cerebrovasc Dis. 2005;20:270–9.
52. Graziano F, Ganau M, Iacopino DG, et al. Vertebro-basilar junction aneurysms: a single centre experience and meta-analysis of endovascular treatments. Neuroradiol J. 2014;27:732–41.
53. Peluso JP, van Rooij WJ, Sluzewski M, et al. Aneurysms of the vertebrobasilar junction: incidence, clinical presentation, and outcome of endovascular treatment. AJNR Am J Neuroradiol. 2007;28:1747–51.
54. Serrone JC, Gozal YM, Grossman AW, et al. Vertebrobasilar fusiform aneurysms. Neurosurg Clin N Am. 2014;25:471–84.
55. Marinkovic SV, Gibo H. The surgical anatomy of the perforating branches of the basilar artery. Neurosurgery. 1993;33:80–7.
56. Meckel S, McAuliffe W, Fiorella D, et al. Endovascular treatment of complex aneurysms at the vertebrobasilar junction with flow-diverting stents: initial experience. Neurosurgery. 2013;73:386–94.
57. Steinberg GK, Drake CG, Peerless SJ. Deliberate basilar or vertebral artery occlusion in the treatment of intracranial aneurysms. Immediate results and long-term outcome in 201 patients. J Neurosurg. 1993;79:161–73.

Treatment of Basilar Artery Aneurysms: Natural Selection and Propagation of Endovascular Techniques

9

Aditya S. Pandey, Joseph J. Gemmete, Neeraj Chaudhary, and B. Gregory Thompson

Introduction

While 3–5 % of the general population harbors cerebral aneurysms, only 10–15 % of these are located within the basilar artery circulation, and most of these are at the basilar apex [1, 3]. Rupture of aneurysms located within this region leads to significant morbidity as the aneurysms are located in close proximity to the brainstem. In addition, ruptured basilar artery aneurysms may lead to obstructive hydrocephalus secondary to blood reaching the intraventricular space via direct rupture into the third ventricle as well as via foramen of Luschka into the fourth ventricle. Both endovascular and microsurgical techniques have been utilized in managing these complex lesions, and treatment paradigms vary based on anatomical considerations as well as operator experience.

Both authors have done an elegant job of presenting the respective risks and nuances of each treatment modality. Risks associated with microsurgery for basilar aneurysms are related to the location of such aneurysms. Rutledge et al. cite the presence and manipulation of cranial nerves, basilar artery perforators, as well as a small corridor for visualization of affected vessels as the reasons for poor outcome associated with microsurgery. The basilar trunk region represents the toughest location for clip ligation as it requires skull base approaches including petrosectomies, extensive cerebral retraction, as well as manipulation of numerous perforating vessels. In addition, the lack of proximal control if intraprocedural rupture were to occur may add significant morbidity as well as cause of higher mortality rates for patients undergoing microsurgery. The rich vascularity of the brainstem, the

A.S. Pandey, MD (✉) • B.G. Thompson, MD
Department of Neurosurgery, University of Michigan, Ann Arbor, MI 48109, USA
e-mail: adityap@med.umich.edu

J.J. Gemmete, MD • N. Chaudhary, MD
Department of Radiology, University of Michigan, Ann Arbor, MI, USA

E. Veznedaroglu (ed.), *Controversies in Vascular Neurosurgery*,
DOI 10.1007/978-3-319-27315-0_9

presence of 10–15 perforators along the basilar artery, places perforating vessels at risk with endovascular as well as microsurgical treatment [4].

Rutledge et al. summarize their treatment paradigm as follows: "At our center, microsurgery is considered a competitive alternative to endovascular therapy for P1 PCA, SCA, distal AICA, PICA, and some basilar bifurcation aneurysms. Conversely, endovascular treatment is preferred for P2 PCA, proximal AICA, basilar trunk, vertebrobasilar junction, and vertebral artery aneurysms, as these often require extensive cranial base approaches and carry a high risk of perforator infraction and cranial neuropathy." We would agree that anteriorly pointing BA apex aneurysms which are above the level of the posterior clinoid as well as SCA aneurysms may be amenable to microsurgical techniques secondary to the fact that these aneurysms can be clipped utilizing common approaches. It becomes important to perform a frontotemporal craniotomy with a wide sylvian fissure dissection as well as drilling the lesser wing of the sphenoid. This allows the operator to retract the temporal lobe without moving the frontal lobe and thus access the interpeduncular fossa. The PCOM artery can be followed to the PCA and then onto the basilar artery. As pointed out by Rutledge et al., the optico-carotid, carotid-oculomotor, and supracarotid spaces serve as corridors to BA apex and SCA aneurysms. Nonetheless, we agree with the authors that most other BA apex aneurysms (posteriorly pointing or those located below the posterior clinoid) and BT and VB junction aneurysms are better treated with endovascular techniques given the complexities and morbidity associated with access.

On the other hand, Rangel-Castilla et al. describe endovascular methods for treating basilar aneurysms. The authors eloquently describe that BA aneurysms are well suited for coil embolization as the dome of the aneurysm is directed in the same direction as the parent vessel. This allows easy catheterization as well as a more stable micro-catheter position within the aneurysm. Endovascular techniques have made significant advances since the arrival of the GDC coil [5]. Adjunct technologies such as balloons and stents allow for coil embolization of wide-necked aneurysms as well as allowing for increased packing density (Fig. 9.1a–c). In addition, flow diverters act as intravascular clips as they divert flow away from the aneurysm without the need of placing thrombotic material within the aneurysm. The authors caution that flow diversion of holo-ectatic aneurysms of the basilar artery is related to significant morbidity and mortality associated with post-procedure infarction as well as delayed rupture. In addition, intra-saccular devices such as the WEB allow for endovascular management of wide-necked aneurysm without placing metallic material within the parent vessel [6]. Such devices could be ideal candidates to compete with microsurgery in the treatment of ruptured wide-necked cerebral aneurysms.

Discussion

The debate of microsurgery vs. endovascular methods has raged in the past; however, now operators realize that both are effective treatment modalities leading to great clinical outcome. However, over the past 10 years, endovascular techniques

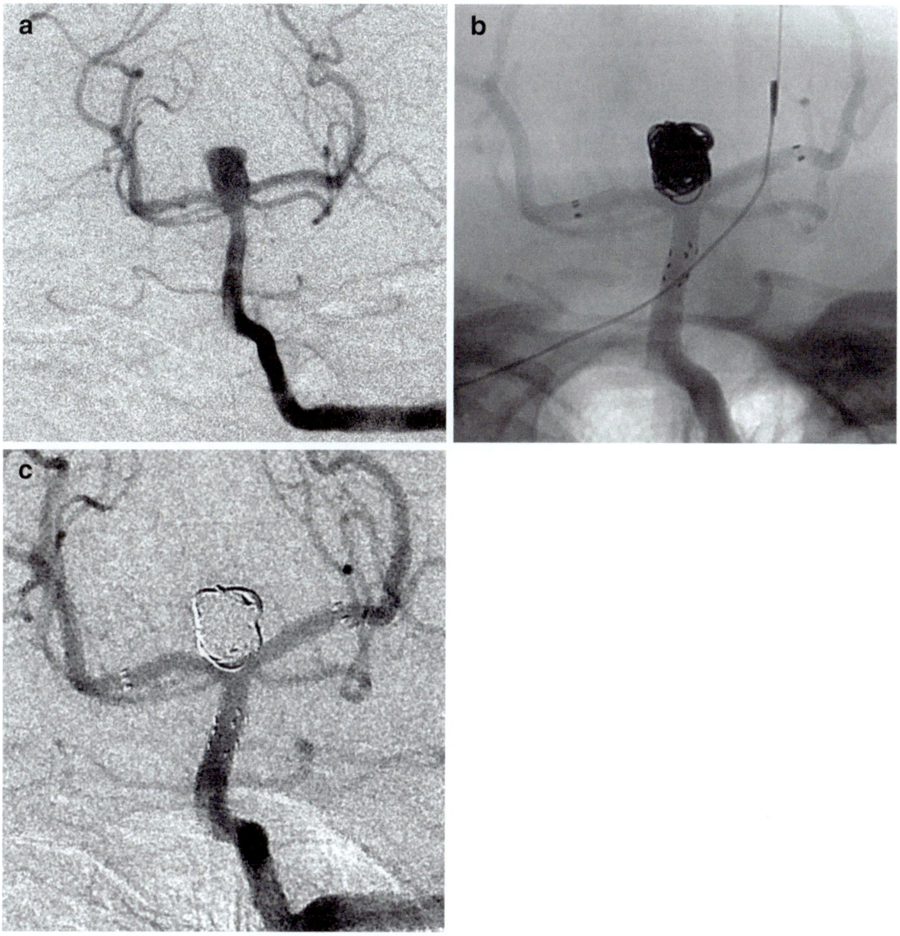

Fig. 9.1 (**a**) A 43-year-old female presenting with worsening headaches and found to have a 6 mm BA apex aneurysm. Left vertebral artery injection in the AP plane delineating a wide-necked BA apex aneurysm. (**b**) Y-stenting technique with jailed micro-catheter and coil embolization of BA apex aneurysm. Left vertebral artery injection in the AP plane – unsubtracted image. (**c**) Post-embolization – left vertebral artery injection in the AP projection revealing 100 % obliteration of BA apex aneurysm

are supplanting microsurgical techniques in the treatment of cerebral aneurysms based on the results of the ISAT [7]. This is truly exemplified in the management of basilar artery aneurysms where the benefits of endovascular techniques have always been realized and recently been documented with the publication of the BRAT. Rutledge et al. and Rangel-Castilla et al. do a superb job of documenting the pros and cons of each technique as well as eloquently stating the support of microsurgical techniques or endovascular techniques, respectively. Nonetheless, the treatment modality chosen is based on a combination of patient clinical factors, aneurismal angioarchitectural factors, as well as operator experience.

Morbidity and Mortality of Treatment

When comparing two techniques jockeying for pole position, one must evaluate the morbidity and mortality associated with each therapy. Both authors have performed thorough study of the literature documenting published morbidity and mortality rates in large series of patients undergoing treatment for basilar artery aneurysms. The inherent risks associated with the microsurgical treatment of BA aneurysms were well established by Drake et al. as well as Sampson et al. – reporting a 7–9 % morality in their respective series [8–10]. This is further exemplified as Rutledge et al. report a 9 % mortality when utilizing microsurgical approaches of treating BA aneurysms (including SCA aneurysms) [11, 12]. The six largest series of patients undergoing microsurgical treatment of basilar aneurysms report serious morbidity rates ranging from 10 to 37 % while mortality rates ranging from 4 to 9 % [13–17]. The increased risk of microsurgical treatment of posterior circulation aneurysms has been further exemplified in the powerful randomized control trial performed at the Barrow Neurological Institute (BNI) – BRAT (Barrow Ruptured Aneurysm Trial). Randomizing SAH patients to either microsurgical treatment or endovascular treatment, the BRAT has a much better representation of the posterior circulation aneurysms (17 %) as opposed to the ISAT (2.7 %) [2, 7]. The proportion of SAH patients harboring posterior circulation aneurysms and with poor outcome (mRS >2) was significantly higher in the microsurgery group as compared to coiling group (58.3 % vs. 26.9 %, $p=0.01$). The same difference continued to exist in favor of coiling (mRS >2–62.1 % vs. 29.6 %, $p=0.01$). Based on past retrospective studies as well as the BRAT, endovascular management of posterior circulation aneurysms is the first line of treatment.

Angioarchitectural Features Favoring Microsurgery

Nonetheless, there continues to be debate on the treatment modality of choice for smaller as well as giant and holo-basilar dolichoectatic aneurysms. Smaller aneurysms tend to have risk with endovascular management as there is smaller area for micro-catheterization as well as less micro-catheter stability within the aneurysm. Brinjikji et al. (2010) performed a meta-analysis of patients undergoing endovascular management of small aneurysms (<3 mm) and reported a much higher periprocedural rupture rate (8.3 %) than for larger cerebral aneurysms [18]. In addition, coiling of such small aneurysms led to significant morbidity and mortality (7.3 %) [18]. In addition, ruptured basilar aneurysms which are wide necked prevent the use of stents, and thus balloon-assisted coiling is the only option of definitive treatment. While flow diverters may be utilized by some operators, it does not lead to immediate therapeutic occlusion and does require treating patients with antiplatelets thus increasing morbidity [19]. Thus such cases represent ideal cases for the potential of microsurgical treatment. Clipping of small BA apex aneurysms potentially requires less cerebral retraction as well as easier visualization of surrounding perforating vessel and thus should be entertained.

Giant posterior circulation aneurysms pose significant risk of rupture with a 5 year cumulative rate of rupture of 50 % as based on the International Study of Unruptured Intracranial Aneurysms (ISUIA) [20]. Such aneurysms tend to not only pose risk of rupture but also lead to brainstem compression, while microsurgery in these instances is extremely challenging as circumferential portions of the vessel are involved within the aneurysm. In addition, perforators may be emanating from the neck of the aneurysm thus leading to increased risk associated with either endovascular or microsurgery. Nonetheless, one other option is for flow reversal and subsequent thrombosis. Patients can undergo balloon test occlusion (BTO) of each vertebral artery and subsequent endovascular or microsurgical vessel deconstruction leading to reversal of flow across the basilar artery. Killu et al. describe such a case example harboring a giant BA apex aneurysm with the P1s incorporated into the neck of the aneurysm [21]. Patient subsequently underwent occlusion of the basilar artery below the superior cerebellar arteries (SCA) for reversal of flow through the posterior communicating (PCOM) artery and subsequent thrombosis of the aneurysm. Of note precise occlusion of the basilar artery is more feasible with microsurgery as exemplified in the previous case as opposed to endovascular means.

Endovascular techniques of filling such aneurysms with coils tend to lead to a high rate of recurrence and retreatments as well as potential for further brainstem compression. Rooij et al. (2007) reported that endovascular treatment of large BA apex aneurysms (>15 mm in diameter) led to 20 % of patients needing to be coiled more than six times, while flow diversion represents an ideal treatment modality as it leads to a minimally invasive method of diverting flow away from the aneurysm leading to endothelialization across the neck of the aneurysm while maintaining flow within perforator vessels [22]. In addition, flow diverters may actually lead to less mass effect from the giant aneurysm as Moon et al. reported that 75 % of patients with cranial neuropathies reported improvement in symptoms post-pipeline deployment [23]. We present a case of a patient presenting with transient ischemic attack who was found to have a giant basilar trunk aneurysm. Given the fact that this aneurysm did not involve the entirety of the basilar artery, we proceeded with coil embolization and flow diversion (Fig. 9.2a–d). This patient had no complications and has continued to show no radiographic signs of recurrence. However, there has been an increased incidence of brainstem infarction and posttreatment hemorrhage when treating giant posterior circulation aneurysms which involve majority of the basilar artery. Siddiqui et al. had reported that two of seven patients undergoing flow diversion of large posterior circulation aneurysms had delayed aneurismal rupture and death [24]. Treatment of giant BA aneurysms poses significant risk to the patient whether choosing natural history, microsurgical, or endovascular treatment paradigms. Future developments in flow-diverting technology represent the best option for treatment in this patient population.

Endovascular methods certainly lead to better outcomes in the short term; however, durability of such treatment continues to be an area of concern. We have previously reported that 15–25 % of all posterior circulation aneurysms treated with endovascular means recur [3]. The risks of invasive radiographic follow-up

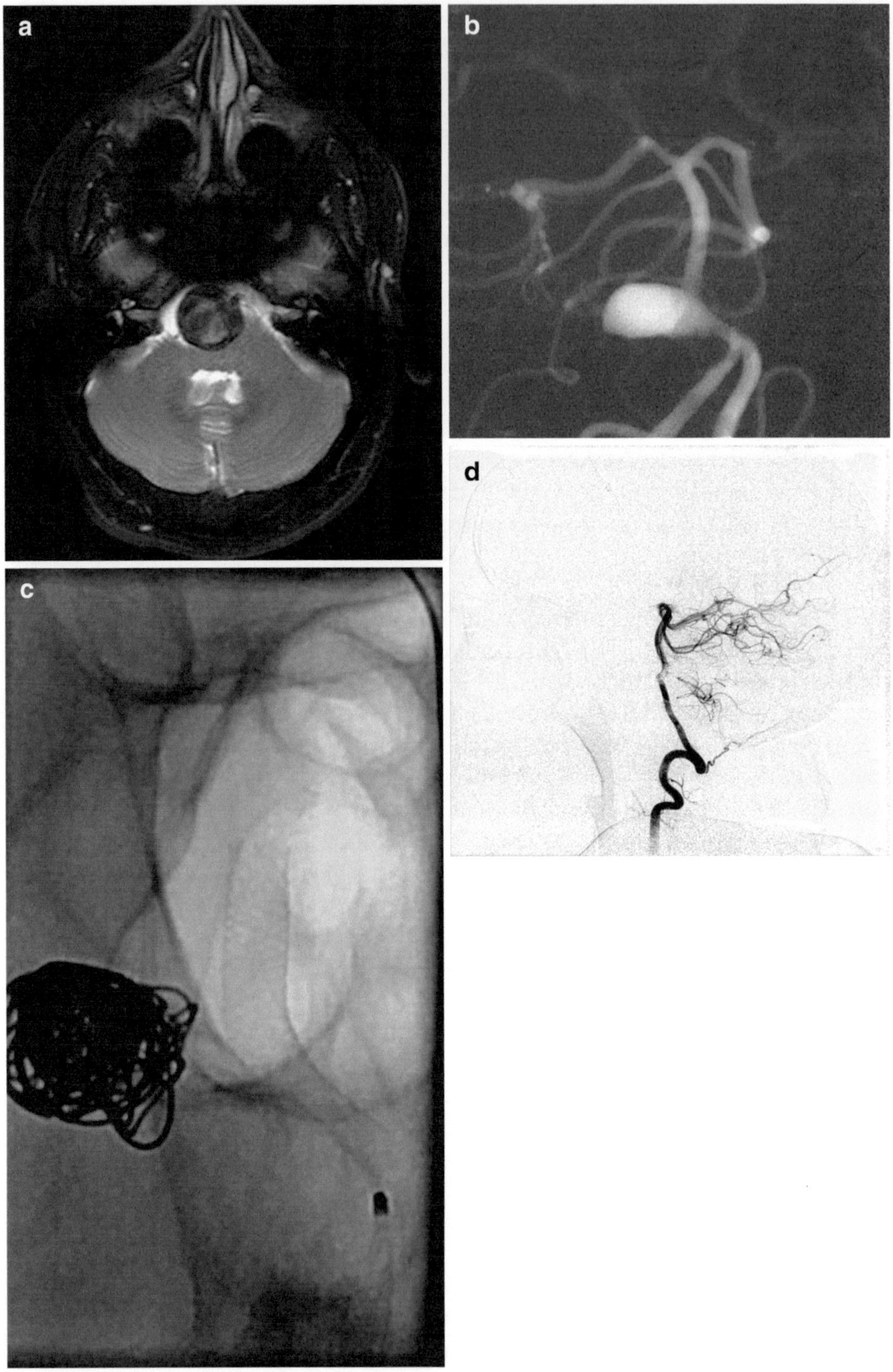
a
b
c
d

as well as retreatment must be considered when choosing endovascular techniques. Ringer et al. reported that routine cerebral angiographic follow-up of coiled aneurysms carries minimal risk (0.43 %) [25]. In addition, they also reported that endovascular treatment of recurrent aneurysm carries a 1.13 % risk of death or disability [26]. In our experience, patients with previous history of SAH and large recurrences tend to undergo retreatment, while others are followed with routine radiography. Our own data show that retreatment of recurrent aneurysms does not lead to significant risk; however it does lead to increased costs (in publication). Nonetheless, current developments of stents and specifically flow diverters are leading to more durable results.

Intraprocedural Complications and Management

When choosing a modality of treatment, one always evaluates the safety and ability to counteract the most devastating complications. During aneurysm treatment, the most complicating feature is intraprocedural rupture (IPR) as well as vessel thrombosis. The morbidity and mortality associated with intraprocedural rupture are significantly higher during endovascular treatment as compared to microsurgery. During microsurgery the cranial opening prevents rise in intracranial pressure (ICP) as compared to endovascular methods where IPR leads to severe rise in ICP leading to devastating neurological disability [27]. As for thrombotic complications, they occur infrequently during microsurgery as compared to endovascular techniques; however, management of such complications during endovascular techniques is simpler as patients can be anticoagulated without the risk of hemorrhage within the cranial surgical cavity. We have a protocol for managing with IPR: continue coiling, balloon occlusion of the neck if a balloon has been prepared, reversal of anticoagulant agents (protamine for heparin and platelet transfusion for antiplatelet use), burst suppression, mannitol and Lasix, immediate CTH, and then subsequent ventriculostomy. While balloon use could serve as temporary clips, its presence requires further intravascular manipulation leading to theoretical risk of thromboembolic complications. Endovascular techniques will need to continue evolving and improving methods of managing devastating complications such as IPR.

Fig. 9.2 (**a**) A 40-year-old male presenting with left extremity numbness and found to have an ovoid mass at the pontomedullary junction. Axial T2-weighted image revealing a large flow void at the pontomedullary junction. (**b**) Subtracted oblique projection image acquired via a left vertebral artery injection – revealing a partially thrombosed giant aneurysm of the proximal basilar trunk.(**c**) Unsubtracted AP projection image revealing coil embolization of aneurysm and deployment of a Pipeline embolization device (PED). (**d**) Subtracted AP projection image revealing complete obliteration of aneurysm and patency of BA

Treatment Decisions Based Upon Neurocognitive Outcome

The goal of any surgical modality is to return the patient to their baseline functioning and quality of life. This requires that we not only perform global clinical assessments but also focus on neurocognitive outcomes. Good clinical outcome on global assessment scales does not always translate to good neurocognitive functioning. This has been well documented as some series have reported that greater than 50 % of patients with good clinical outcome may harbor neurocognitive deficits [28, 29]. Based on the ISAT, 32.1 % of all patients who had good clinical outcome, mRS <2 at 12 months posttreatment, were diagnosed with significant cognitive impairment at 1 year post-procedure. Patients undergoing endovascular occlusion were significantly less likely to have cognitive decline as compared to those undergoing clip ligation (26.7 % vs. 38.7 %, $p=0.0055$) [30]. While the proportion of patients in the ISAT was dominated by anterior circulation aneurysms, the approaches to most BA apex aneurysms do utilize supratentorial approaches with microdissection and retraction. Our own study evaluating neurocognitive outcome in patients undergoing microsurgery vs. coiling for unruptured aneurysms demonstrated that there was significant decline in memory and executive functioning within the first 3 months of the procedure. However, the clipping and coiling groups achieved similar neurocognitive results at the 6 month mark (unpublished results). Both of these studies show benefit in neurocognitive outcome in favor of patients undergoing endovascular treatments as compared to microsurgery.

Future Treatment Paradigms and Surgical Training

While microsurgery is a reasonable option for treatment of aneurysms on the basilar artery at UCSF, large-volume surgical experiences do not exist at most centers, and thus such paradigm cannot be extrapolated to other centers unless neurosurgeons have extensive experience in clipping basilar artery aneurysms. Most certainly volume outcome relationships exist for complex diseases requiring surgical intervention, and certainly this relates to microsurgery of basilar artery aneurysms. In fact, Rutledge et al. report that the proportion of patients having a good outcome increased from 79 % in the first half of the series to 90 % in the second half of the series. They attribute this change to improved techniques gained through increased surgical volume experience. We have shown that as volumes of SAH patients increase from 20 per year to 100 per year, mortality rates decline from 28.4 to 18.7 % as based on evaluation of the National Inpatient Sample (NIS) [31]. While the mediators of better outcome at high-volume centers are not well defined, it is plausible that high-volume centers have high-volume surgical experiences and thus better surgical outcome.

Given that 35,000 patients present with SAH and that 10–15 % of these are within the posterior circulation, this leaves 3,500 patients with cerebral aneurysms within this location. Even if 50 % of these patients are clipping candidates secondary to angioarchitecture of cerebral aneurysms, this would lead to 1,750 patients as potential candidates for microsurgery. There are over 100 neurosurgical training programs within the United States thus allowing for 17 basilar aneurysm candidates for microsurgery in 1 year. While such aneurysm numbers may be barely enough for an attending neurosurgeon to maintain surgical skill set, such numbers are insufficient in teaching resident surgeons or fellows to clip ligate such aneurysms. The involvement of non-neurosurgical interventionalists in the management of cerebral aneurysms leads to fewer aneurysms referred to neurosurgeons that have the capability of offering both microsurgical and endovascular treatment options. Thus in all actuality, that number of 17 posterior circulation aneurysms needing clip ligation is actually much smaller.

Coiling of anterior and posterior circulation aneurysms requires similar techniques, and thus coiling of any such aneurysms can be translated and taught to treat aneurysms anywhere within the cerebral vasculature. This is not the case with microsurgery as most anterior circulation aneurysms can be clipped via a frontal temporal approach, while basilar artery aneurysms require skull base approaches and instances when proximal control is not achievable. In addition, there are more non-neurosurgeon practitioners treating cerebral aneurysms, thus decreasing the possible number of aneurysms requiring microsurgery. Combination of these factors is leading to natural selection forces guiding the survival and dominance of endovascular techniques.

Conclusion

The selection of appropriate treatment of these complex aneurysms should be made in a multidisciplinary team where microsurgical and endovascular options are discussed. Each team must determine what technique at each particular center will minimize risk and maximize benefit. There continues to be necessity of treating ruptured small wide-necked BA apex aneurysms utilizing microsurgical technique. These aneurysms are more challenging to treat with endovascular techniques given that the risk of intraprocedural rupture and associated morbidity increases. The challenge for neurosurgical operators is to continue to maintain microsurgical skill sets while mastering the ever changing and evolving endovascular techniques. Extrapolating from the success and advances since the arrival of the GDC coil, we expect that established treatment of the smaller wide necked and the giant aneurysms via endovascular techniques is a matter of time. Rutledge et al. state that "Microsurgical clipping of appropriately selected basilar artery aneurysms by well trained and experienced cerebrovascular neurosurgeons is safe and effective and offers a durable cure." Unfortunately, the dynamics of today's cerebrovascular arena poses a significant threat in developing well-trained and experienced cerebrovascular neurosurgeons. Future strategies of simulation-based training as well as evaluation of volume outcome relationship by policy makers are necessary in making sure that our patients continue to have the best options of treatment for their posterior circulation aneurysm.

References

1. Vlak MH, et al. Prevalence of unruptured intracranial aneurysms, with emphasis on sex, age, comorbidity, country, and time period: a systematic review and meta-analysis. Lancet Neurol. 2011;10(7):626–36.
2. Spetzler RF, et al. The Barrow Ruptured Aneurysm Trial: 6-year results. J Neurosurg. 2015;123(3):609–17.
3. Pandey AS, et al. Endovascular coil embolization of ruptured and unruptured posterior circulation aneurysms: review of a 10-year experience. Neurosurgery. 2007;60(4):626–36; discussion 636–7.
4. Marinkovic SV, Gibo H. The surgical anatomy of the perforating branches of the basilar artery. Neurosurgery. 1993;33(1):80–7.
5. Murayama Y, et al. Endovascular treatment of incidental cerebral aneurysms. Report on 115 cases treated with guglielmi detachable coils. Interv Neuroradiol. 1999;5 Suppl 1:79–81.
6. Behme D, Berlis A, Weber W. Woven EndoBridge intrasaccular flow disrupter for the treatment of ruptured and unruptured wide-neck cerebral aneurysms: report of 55 cases. AJNR Am J Neuroradiol. 2015;36(8):1501–6.
7. Molyneux AJ, et al. International subarachnoid aneurysm trial (ISAT) of neurosurgical clipping versus endovascular coiling in 2143 patients with ruptured intracranial aneurysms: a randomised comparison of effects on survival, dependency, seizures, rebleeding, subgroups, and aneurysm occlusion. Lancet. 2005;366(9488):809–17.
8. Nanda A, et al. Microsurgical management of basilar artery apex aneurysms: a single surgeon's experience from Louisiana State University, Shreveport. World Neurosurg. 2014;82(1–2):118–29.
9. Steinberg GK, Drake CG, Peerless SJ. Deliberate basilar or vertebral artery occlusion in the treatment of intracranial aneurysms. Immediate results and long-term outcome in 201 patients. J Neurosurg. 1993;79(2):161–73.
10. Hernesniemi J, Korja M. At the apex of cerebrovascular surgery – basilar tip aneurysms. World Neurosurg. 2014;82(1–2):37–9.
11. Sanai N, et al. The current role of microsurgery for posterior circulation aneurysms: a selective approach in the endovascular era. Neurosurgery. 2008;62(6):1236–49; discussion 1249–53.
12. Lawton MT. Basilar apex aneurysms: surgical results and perspectives from an initial experience. Neurosurgery. 2002;50(1):1–8; discussion 8–10.
13. Krisht AF, Kadri PA. Surgical clipping of complex basilar apex aneurysms: a strategy for successful outcome using the pretemporal transzygomatic transcavernous approach. Neurosurgery. 2005;56(2 Suppl):261–73; discussion 261–73.
14. Krisht AF, et al. Results of microsurgical clipping of 50 high complexity basilar apex aneurysms. Neurosurgery. 2007;60(2):242–50; discussion 250–2.
15. Drake CG, Peerless SJ, Ferguson GG. Hunterian proximal arterial occlusion for giant aneurysms of the carotid circulation. J Neurosurg. 1994;81(5):656–65.
16. Peerless SJ, et al. Early surgery for ruptured vertebrobasilar aneurysms. J Neurosurg. 1994;80(4):643–9.
17. Samson D, Batjer HH, Kopitnik Jr TA. Current results of the surgical management of aneurysms of the basilar apex. Neurosurgery. 1999;44(4):697–702; discussion 702–4.
18. Brinjikji W, et al. Endovascular treatment of very small (3 mm or smaller) intracranial aneurysms: report of a consecutive series and a meta-analysis. Stroke. 2010;41(1):116–21.
19. Cruz JP, et al. Pipeline embolization device in aneurysmal subarachnoid hemorrhage. AJNR Am J Neuroradiol. 2013;34(2):271–6.
20. Wiebers DO, et al. Unruptured intracranial aneurysms: natural history, clinical outcome, and risks of surgical and endovascular treatment. Lancet. 2003;362(9378):103–10.
21. Killu AM, Lanzino G. Images in clinical medicine: giant basilar-artery aneurysm. N Engl J Med. 2012;367(19):e28.

22. Alderazi YJ, et al. Flow diverters for intracranial aneurysms. Stroke Res Treat. 2014;2014:415653.
23. Moon K, et al. Resolution of cranial neuropathies following treatment of intracranial aneurysms with the Pipeline Embolization Device. J Neurosurg. 2014;121(5):1085–92.
24. Siddiqui AH, et al. Panacea or problem: flow diverters in the treatment of symptomatic large or giant fusiform vertebrobasilar aneurysms. J Neurosurg. 2012;116(6):1258–66.
25. Ringer AJ, et al. Does angiographic surveillance pose a risk in the management of coiled intracranial aneurysms? A multicenter study of 2243 patients. Neurosurgery. 2008;63(5):845–9; discussion 849.
26. Ringer AJ, et al. Defining the risk of retreatment for aneurysm recurrence or residual after initial treatment by endovascular coiling: a multicenter study. Neurosurgery. 2009;65(2):311–5; discussion 315.
27. Zhang X, et al. Factors responsible for poor outcome after intraprocedural rerupture of ruptured intracranial aneurysms: identification of risk factors, prevention and management on 18 cases. Eur J Radiol. 2012;81(1):e77–85.
28. Hutter BO, Gilsbach JM. Which neuropsychological deficits are hidden behind a good outcome (Glasgow = I) after aneurysmal subarachnoid hemorrhage? Neurosurgery. 1993;33(6):999–1005; discussion 1005–6.
29. Hutter BO, Gilsbach JM, Kreitschmann I. Quality of life and cognitive deficits after subarachnoid haemorrhage. Br J Neurosurg. 1995;9(4):465–75.
30. Scott RB, et al. Improved cognitive outcomes with endovascular coiling of ruptured intracranial aneurysms: neuropsychological outcomes from the International Subarachnoid Aneurysm Trial (ISAT). Stroke. 2010;41(8):1743–7.
31. Pandey AS, et al. High subarachnoid hemorrhage patient volume associated with lower mortality and better outcomes. Neurosurgery. 2015;77(3):462–70.

Surgical and Radiologic Intervention for Prevention of Ischemic Stroke

10

Andrew J. Ringer

Stroke is now the fourth leading cause of death in the United States, down from its previously third ranking place [1]. Approximately 88 % of all strokes are ischemic, 9 % are intracerebral hemorrhages, and 3 % are subarachnoid hemorrhages [2]. The etiology of ischemic strokes can be broadly categorized into several subtypes as cardioembolic, extracranial atherosclerotic, intracranial atherosclerotic, lacunar, traumatic (e.g., dissections), inflammatory (e.g., moyamoya, vasculitis), and cryptogenic. A population-based study of incidence (per 100,000 population) for ischemic stroke subtype identified 40 cardioembolic, 27 intracranial and extracranial atherosclerosis, 25 lacunar, 4 other or uncommon cause (i.e., traumatic, inflammatory), and 52 cryptogenic [3]. This chapter focuses on thromboembolic strokes that develop from extracranial carotid atherosclerosis, identifies the preferred tools useful in the process of diagnosis and surgical or endovascular planning, and discusses particular indications for each treatment.

Extracranial Athero-occlusive Disease

Clinical Presentation and Natural Evolution of the Disease

Carotid disease encompasses several disorders, including, but not limited to, atherosclerosis, fibromuscular dysplasia, dissections, cystic medial necrosis, radiation vasculopathy, and arteritis [4]. By far, the most common etiology is atherosclerosis

A.J. Ringer, MD
Department of Neurosurgery, University of Cincinnati (UC) College of Medicine, ML 0515, Cincinnati, OH 45267-0515, USA

Comprehensive Stroke Center, UC Neuroscience Institute, Cincinnati, OH, USA

Mayfield Clinic, Cincinnati, OH, USA
e-mail: aringer@mayfieldclinic.com; mary.kemper@uc.edu

E. Veznedaroglu (ed.), *Controversies in Vascular Neurosurgery*,
DOI 10.1007/978-3-319-27315-0_10

defined as a chronic, slowly developing condition that causes narrowing of the arteries [4–6]. The symptoms of atherosclerotic disease depend on the extent of vessel narrowing and can result from thrombosis, embolism, or occlusion of the involved artery [6]. Of note, many patients may remain asymptomatic during their life. Other important risk factors for the disease include smoking, dyslipidemia, diabetes mellitus, and hypertension [6–8].

Carotid atherosclerotic disease is a common pathology, especially among elderly patients with peripheral and coronary arterial disease. Carotid artery stenosis is believed to account for 20–30 % of strokes [9, 10] with the risk related to the symptomatology and severity of stenosis [6]. Patients presenting with stroke or transient ischemic attack (TIA) are at higher risk than asymptomatic patients. Additionally, increased severity of stenosis incurs a higher risk of stroke, even among asymptomatic patients [11–13]. In their 2009 publication, Ois et al. reported that 27.6 % of patients with symptomatic carotid stenosis of 70 % or more developed recurrence of neurological symptoms, 20.9 % presented within the first 72 h, 6.7 % between 72 h and 7 days, and 3.7 % at 14 days [14].

Atheroma of the carotid artery causing some degree of intimal thickening is not uncommon, found in 65 % of men and 75 % of women over age 70 years [9, 10, 15]. These mild lesions are universally asymptomatic. More severely stenotic lesions, although less common, incur a higher stroke risk. In the Rotterdam Study of cardiovascular determinants of carotid artery disease in people over 55 years of age, Bots et al. noted that reduction in lumen diameter of the internal carotid artery ranged from 16 % to 49 % in 3 % of patients and in severe stenosis (≥50 %) in 1.4 % of patients [5]. In a population-based study of volunteers aged 50–79 years, the prevalence of asymptomatic carotid stenosis of ≥50 % was 6.4 %, whereas severe stenosis was detected in only 0.4 % of the subjects examined [16].

Most studies agree that the prevalence of stenosis of the carotid artery is affected largely by age and sex. In their cardiovascular health study of men and women ages 65 years or more, O'Leary et al. found that a stenosis range of 50–74 % occurred in 7 % of men and 5 % of women [17]. Mathiesen et al. reported that the prevalence of carotid stenosis increased with age and was significantly higher in men 4.2 % than women 2.7 % [7]. Thus, male sex and advanced age are associated with a higher incidence of moderate or severe carotid atherosclerotic disease.

Occlusion of the internal carotid artery (ICA) is the cause of 10 % of transient ischemic attacks (TIAs) and 15–25 % of ischemic strokes of the carotid territory [18]. Recurrent stroke risk increases with time and may be as high as 70 % in patients with poor cerebral hemodynamics [18, 19]. However, in asymptomatic patients, carotid occlusion carries a very low risk of subsequent ischemic stroke and a low incidence of cerebral hemodynamic compromise [20]. The risk of recurrent stroke in patients with ICA occlusion on medical therapy determined by the Carotid Occlusion Surgery Study (COSS) was 5–7 % per year for all strokes and 2–6 % per year for ipsilateral ischemic stroke for the first 2 years [18]. The authors noted that this stroke risk was dramatically reduced from earlier estimates, possibly related to the increased use of clopidogrel and statins. However, Johansson et al. noted the risk of ipsilateral ischemic stroke recurrence was higher if the presenting event was a stroke or TIA compared with amaurosis fugax [13]. Unlike carotid stenosis, occlusion of the carotid artery should only be treated if symptoms and/or other clinical proof of hemodynamic instability are present. Based on COSS results of 30-day rates for ipsilateral ischemic stroke of 14.4 % in the surgical group and 2.0 % in the nonsurgical group – a 12.4 % difference, aggressive medical management, and habit changes must be the initial therapy for asymptomatic patients with carotid occlusion [18].

Patient Evaluation

Given that patients with extracranial carotid disease may or may not have symptoms, clinical evaluation is of utmost importance, serving to unveil not only the presence of symptoms but the cardiovascular risk factors. The extent of stenosis is another risk factor that influences the natural history and management approach of this disease [9, 10]. Because of the proven superiority of carotid endarterectomy compared with medical therapy for symptomatic high-grade carotid stenosis, it is important to clarify if the carotid is completely occluded and not just highly stenotic in symptomatic patients [18].

Except for its use in differentiating severe stenosis from carotid occlusion, the conventional contrast angiogram, once considered as the gold standard for diagnosis, is used rarely today. Rather, the advent of noninvasive axial imaging for diagnosing carotid stenosis has evolved as a more reliable and inexpensive method. For the initial serial imaging of the carotid bifurcation, carotid duplex ultrasonography remains an essential component in the management of carotid bifurcation disease [9, 21]. Duplex ultrasonography of the carotid artery when aided with other noninvasive modalities (i.e., CT angiography, contrast-enhanced magnetic resonance angiography) can better determine the stroke risk and guide treatment decisions [21]. Magnetic resonance (MR) angiography is noninvasive and does not require an iodinated contrast medium. However, it overestimates the degree of stenosis, is susceptible to artifacts, and is problematic for people who feel claustrophobic. According to some authors, contrast-enhanced MR angiography is the best MR imaging modality for carotid stenosis. Its sensitivity and specificity rates in detecting ICA stenosis exceeding 70 % are as high as 97 % and 96 %, respectively. Additionally, it has proven to be an effective tool in demonstrating ulcerated plaques. Yet, MR angiography with contrast is not innocuous and may lead to significant dermatologic and renal damage [9, 10, 22].

Computerized tomographic (CT) angiography is a promising diagnostic and planning tool that is more often used to delineate the extent of the disease and aid the surgical planning [9]. It is fast, widely available, and less susceptible to artifact. Its sensitivity ranges from 70 % to 90 % in the detection of severe ICA artery stenosis, and its specificity achieves 90–97 % [10]. We find that this technique is very helpful for surgical planning because of its ability to use bony landmarks (e.g., angle of the mandible, cervical spinal level) in determining the accessibility to the lesion. However, CT angiography is expensive, is software dependent, has risks related to contrast media, is limited by technical personnel expertise, and may show artifacts from calcified plaques [9, 10].

Digital subtraction angiography (DSA) continues to be the gold standard for treatment planning [10]. It precisely defines the degree of arterial narrowing, does not have the artifact dilemma of other diagnostic tools, and may serve as the first step to endovascular therapy. Given these attributes, this technique could be considered the preferred method for diagnosis of near-carotid occlusion [23]. However, compared with noninvasive diagnostic methods, DSA requires contrast, has relatively higher costs, is invasive, and may be restricted at times by availability of the angiography suite and personnel.

Measurement of the hemodynamic status of the distal circulation to the occluded vessel can identify a subgroup of patients with poor circulation who are at particularly high risk for recurrent stroke [6]. The validity of methods for measurement has been criticized because of variability in reporting methods and baseline measurements between centers. Measurement of oxygen extraction fraction with positron emission tomography (PET) and quantitative measurement of cerebral blood flow with xenon-133 single photon emission computed tomography (SPECT) before and after administration of acetazolamide have the best evidence base to support stroke predictive accuracy in symptomatic patients [24]. We recommend evaluation of hemodynamic status in patients with completely occlusive lesions whom might be considered for bypass surgery.

In our practice, we use techniques such as carotid ultrasound, MR angiography, or CT angiography as the first tools in the process of diagnosis and surgical or endovascular planning. When considering surgical or endovascular interventions, duplex ultrasound should complement whatever technique is used. DSA should be an option when findings of the noninvasive methods still are inconclusive in differentiating between high-grade stenosis and complete occlusion or when artifact is a limitation preventing an adequate calculation of the extent of carotid narrowing [18].

Management and Treatment

During the last three decades, the management of carotid artery disease has become increasingly standardized, especially since the studies of the 1980s and 1990s [25]. These later studies separated the management of carotid disease based on the presence or absence of symptoms and the extent of carotid lumen narrowing [10–12, 25–27]. However, this treatment approach has been criticized recently on the grounds of the methodologies used by these 1990s studies. In comparison, today's approaches offer better diagnostic tools, more effective management of risk factors associated with carotid stenosis, and improved medical management [27].

The initial management of patients with carotid stenosis should include lifestyle modifications, such as smoking cessation, daily exercise, and a healthy diet [4, 6]. Blood pressure should be targeted to 140/90 mmHg or less for patients with neither renal disease nor diabetes or below 130/80 mmHg for those with either or both conditions [10]. Medical management should also include restricting

Table 10.1 Maximum medical therapy for stroke or TIA caused by intracranial atherosclerosis is identical to that used in the medical arm of SAMMPRIS [33]

Strategy	Target
Aspirin	325 mg daily
Plavix	75 mg daily for 90 days after symptoms
Smoking cessation	By patient preference
Blood pressure control	(<140 mmHg in nondiabetics, <130 in diabetics)
Statins	Aim for fasting LDL of <70 mg/dL
Fenofibrate	Achieve triglyceride <200 mg/dL
Weight loss	Body mass index <25 kg/m^2
Blood glucose in diabetics	Goal HbA1c <7 %

cholesterol and saturated fats and administering statin medications to target LDL levels below 100 mg/dL in patients without history of diabetes mellitus and below 70 mg/dL in those with diabetes [4, 9, 28, 29]. Antiplatelet therapy plays an important part of the management of atherosclerotic disease [4, 6]. Aspirin doses between 75 and 325 mg daily are recommended for patients with occlusive or nonocclusive atherosclerosis [6].

Controversy on the need for tight glycemic control persists for patients at risk of stroke or with history of TIA [30–32]. A reasonable option is to maintain the glycated hemoglobin (Hb_{A1c}) <7 % [6]. Because of the concomitant presence of coronary artery disease in patients with carotid stenosis, a cardiovascular work-up is prudent, especially in those with known risks for coronary artery disease [9]. Many practitioners might argue that the ideal medical management for all atherosclerotic disease should mirror the SAMMPRIS protocol used for patients with symptomatic intracranial atherosclerosis. Management of intracranial athero-occlusive disease depends on whether the patient is symptomatic, the extent of stenosis, and whether maximum medical therapy succeeded or failed. Maximum medical therapy for stroke or TIA caused by intracranial atherosclerosis is identical to that used in the medical arm of SAMMPRIS [33] and is summarized (Table 10.1). In our practice, this protocol is our choice for the medical management of all symptomatic patients with carotid, intracranial, or vertebrobasilar atherosclerosis whether or not intervention is planned.

Carotid stenosis can be treated by carotid endarterectomy (CEA) or carotid artery stenting (CAS). Moderate asymptomatic carotid stenosis of 50–70 % is associated with a low risk of ischemic stroke and does not warrant treatment. A population with severe stenosis (>70 %) sees a marginal benefit with CEA [34]. In the Asymptomatic Carotid Atherosclerosis Study, authors concluded that for patients with >60 % stenosis, a 5.9 % absolute risk reduction was obtained over 5 years with CEA compared with maximum medical management (11 % vs. 5.1 %, respectively).

Symptomatic patients should be evaluated in a timely manner because of the high risk of recurrent strokes [10, 14, 35, 36]. With confirmation that the carotid disease is the cause of the patient's symptoms, invasive treatment should be considered unless compelling contraindications exist. The absolute risk reduction of stroke or death for CEA in moderate (50–70 %) and severe (>70 %) stenosis is 10.1 % at 5 years and 16.5 % at 2 years, respectively. The method of intervention is best defined in a multispecialty practice that considers medical comorbidities, life expectancy, surgical risks, surgeon experience, neurological status of the patients, and other individual factors [4].

Age and sex are important considerations when working up patients to undergo endarterectomy. According to Rothwell et al., the benefits of surgery were greatest in men, patients aged 75 years or older, and those randomized within 2 weeks after their last ischemic event [36]. They specified for patients with ≥50 % stenosis that the number of patients needed to undergo surgery to prevent one ipsilateral stroke in 5 years was 9 for men and 36 for women, 5 for patients age 75 years or older and 18 for patients younger than 65 years, and 5 for those randomized within 2 weeks after their last ischemic event versus 125 for patients randomized after 12 weeks.

Carotid artery stenting has been proposed as an equivalent to endarterectomy. However, results from a recent randomized controlled trial called CREST failed to establish this equivalency [4]. Specifically, patients randomized to CEA had fewer periprocedural strokes, fewer strokes out to 4 years of follow-up, and fewer deaths. Perioperative myocardial infarction was elevated in the CEA group perhaps because 90 % of patients were under general anesthesia; however, long-term impact clinically was minimal because events were included even for asymptomatic cardiac enzyme elevation. CREST also showed greater benefits in younger patients from stenting and older patients from CEA, with the crossover point at 70 years old. This finding was also confirmed in a 2011 systematic review that found that octogenarian patients had a major adverse event rate of 6.9 % after carotid stenting (CAS) versus 4.2 % after CEA [37].

In summary, patients with symptomatic carotid artery stenosis must be worked up and managed expeditiously to prevent symptom recurrence. Currently, I believe that CEA is superior to CAS, which is superior to best medical management. Accordingly at our institution, we recommend CEA to all patients with asymptomatic carotid stenosis >70 % or symptomatic stenosis of >50 % in the absence of relative high-risk features. Several factors may increase the perioperative risk of CEA, specifically local or anatomic factors and medical comorbidities. These factors include contralateral carotid artery occlusion, high carotid bifurcation or lesion extent above the angle of the mandible, prior carotid endarterectomy with recurrent stenosis, previous head and neck dissection or radiation, and New York Heart classification three cardiac disease (angina at rest or ejection fraction <30 %). Each risk factor is associated with an increased risk of complications from CEA including perioperative stroke, cranial nerve injury, or myocardial infarction.

Management of atherosclerotic carotid occlusion begins by performing an adequate clinical and imaging evaluation of the patient. Ideally, the case can be managed by a dedicated multidisciplinary neurovascular center [18, 38]. Asymptomatic carotid occlusion carries a very low rate of stroke and should only be managed by optimization of medical therapy [20]. Pertaining to symptomatic carotid occlusion, various Class I studies have unsuccessfully tried to prove superiority of bypass surgery over medical therapy for the prevention of further stroke events in symptomatic carotid occlusion [38, 39]. Although the results proved nonsuperiority or futility of bypass surgery, other factors could include (1) ineffective patient selection, (2) strict aggressiveness of medical management that does not meet the reality of the current medical system, or (3) inexperience of the surgeons performing the procedures. Indications for bypass surgery for patients are chronic low cerebral blood flow associated to ischemic clinical events, compliance issues related to medical therapy, or medical therapy failed to prevent symptoms. In summary, aggressive medical therapy is the initial approach to symptomatic carotid occlusion, and surgical bypass should be reserved for symptomatic patients when best medical management has failed.

Conclusions

Our approach to carotid athero-occlusive disease is based on, but not limited to, whether the patient is clinically affected by the stenosis, adequacy of medical therapy, life expectancy, and existence of additional risk factors for stroke (i.e., normal hemodynamics, comorbid disease, collateralization of the affected territory). In symptomatic patients, a prompt assessment will be performed to rule out amaurosis fugax, TIA, or stroke. If this is evidenced by the history and clinical exam, the next step will be to rule out other causes of stroke. Once the carotid stenosis (at least 50 %) has been confirmed as the culprit for the patient's symptoms, an assessment of the surgical benefits and the timing for intervention will be discussed by the stroke neurologist and neurosurgeon. Patients with no history of neck surgery or radiation therapy, satisfactory anatomy, and imaging convincing of nonocclusive disease will be considered for endarterectomy. Endovascular management will be performed in those with high surgical risk as described above and suitable vascular anatomy (e.g., mild or no tortuosity). The approach for the asymptomatic carotid stenosis is to initially screen for other cardiovascular risk factors, initiate changes in lifestyle habits, and start the patient in validated medical management. Surgery is reserved for severe disease (>70 %) in asymptomatic carotid stenosis. For carotid occlusive disease, aggressive medical management must be prompt. We reserved bypass surgery for patients with proven low cerebral blood flow accompanied by episodes of ischemic symptoms.

References

1. Towfighi A, Saver JL. Stroke declines from third to fourth leading cause of death in the United States: historical perspective and challenges ahead. Stroke. 2011;42(8):2351–5.
2. Thom T, Haase N, Rosamond W, Howard VJ, Rumsfeld J, Manolio T, et al. Heart disease and stroke statistics – 2006 update: a report from the American Heart Association Statistics Committee and Stroke Statistics Subcommittee. Circulation. 2006;113(6):e85–151.
3. Petty GW, Brown Jr RD, Whisnant JP, Sicks JD, O'Fallon WM, Wiebers DO. Ischemic stroke subtypes: a population-based study of incidence and risk factors. Stroke. 1999;12:2513–6.
4. Brott TG, Hobson 2nd RW, Howard G, Roubin GS, Clark WM, Brooks W, et al. Stenting versus endarterectomy for treatment of carotid-artery stenosis. N Engl J Med. 2010;363(1):11–23.

5. Bots ML, Breslau PJ, Briët E, de Bruyn AM, van Vliet HH, van den Ouweland FA, et al. Cardiovascular determinants of carotid artery disease. The Rotterdam Elderly Study. Hypertension. 1992;6(2):717–20.
6. European Stroke Organisation, Tendera M, Aboyans V, Bartelink ML, Baumgartner I, Clément D, Collet JP, et al. ESC Guidelines on the diagnosis and treatment of peripheral artery diseases: document covering atherosclerotic disease of extracranial carotid and vertebral, mesenteric, renal, upper and lower extremity arteries: the Task Force on the Diagnosis and Treatment of Peripheral Artery Diseases of the European Society of Cardiology (ESC). Eur Heart J. 2011;32(22):2851–906.
7. Mathiesen EB, Joakimsen O, Bønaa KH. Prevalence of and risk factors associated with carotid artery stenosis: the Tromsø Study. Cerebrovasc Dis. 2001;12(1):44–51.
8. Bos D, van der Rijk MJ, Geeraedts TE, Hofman A, Krestin GP, Witteman JC, et al. Intracranial carotid artery atherosclerosis: prevalence and risk factors in the general population. Stroke. 2012;43(7):1878–84.
9. Saha SP, Whayne Jr TF, Mukherjee D. Evidence-based management of carotid artery disease. Int J Angiol. 2010;19(1):e21–4.
10. Lanzino G, Rabinstein AA, Brown Jr RD. Treatment of carotid artery stenosis: medical therapy, surgery, or stenting? Mayo Clin Proc. 2009;84(4):362–87.
11. North American Symptomatic Carotid Endarterectomy Trial Collaborators. Beneficial effect of carotid endarterectomy in symptomatic patients with high-grade carotid stenosis. N Engl J Med. 1991;325(7):445–53.
12. European Carotid Surgery Trialists' Collaborative Group. Randomised trial of endarterectomy for recently symptomatic carotid stenosis: final results of the MRC European Carotid Surgery Trial (ECST). Lancet 1998;351(9113):1379–87.
13. Johansson EP, Arnerlöv C, Wester P. Risk of recurrent stroke before carotid endarterectomy: the ANSYSCAP study. Int J Stroke. 2013;8(4):220–7.
14. Ois A, Cuadrado-Godia E, Rodríguez-Campello A, Jimenez-Conde J, Roquer J. High risk of early neurological recurrence in symptomatic carotid stenosis. Stroke. 2009;40(8):2727–31.
15. Ebrahim S, Papacosta O, Whincup P, Wannamethee G, Walker M, Nicolaides AN, et al. Carotid plaque, intima media thickness, cardiovascular risk factors, and prevalent cardiovascular disease in men and women: the British Regional Heart Study. Stroke. 1999;30(4):841–50.
16. Mineva PP, Manchev IC, Hadjiev DI. Prevalence and outcome of asymptomatic carotid stenosis: a population-based ultrasonographic study. Eur J Neurol. 2002;9(4):383–8.
17. O'Leary DH, Polak JF, Kronmal RA, et al. Distribution and correlates of sonographically detected carotid artery disease in the Cardiovascular Health Study. The CHS Collaborative Research Group. Stroke. 1992;3(12):1752–60.
18. Powers WJ. Management of patients with atherosclerotic carotid occlusion. Curr Treat Options Neurol. 2011;13(6):608–15.
19. Grubb Jr RL, Derdeyn CP, Fritsch SM, Carpenter DA, Yundt KD, Videen TO, et al. Importance of hemodynamic factors in the prognosis of symptomatic carotid occlusion. JAMA. 1998;280(12):1055–60.
20. Powers WJ, Derdeyn CP, Fritsch SM, et al. Benign prognosis in never-symptomatic carotid occlusion. Neurology. 2000;54(4):878–82.
21. Byrnes KR, Ross CB. The current role of carotid duplex ultrasonography in the management of carotid atherosclerosis: foundations and advances. Int J Vasc Med. 2012;2012:187872. doi:10.1155/2012/187872.
22. Chappell FM, Wardlaw JM, Young GR, et al. Carotid artery stenosis: accuracy of noninvasive tests – individual patient data meta-analysis. Radiology. 2009;1(2):493–502.
23. Thanvi B, Robinson T. Complete occlusion of extracranial internal carotid artery: clinical features, pathophysiology, diagnosis and management. Postgrad Med J. 2007;83(976):95–9.
24. Ogasawara K, Ogawa A, Terasaki K, Shimizu H, Tominaga T, Yoshimoto T. Use of cerebrovascular reactivity in patients with symptomatic major cerebral artery occlusion to predict 5-year outcome: comparison of xenon-133 and iodine-123-IMP single-photon emission computed tomography. J Cereb Blood Flow Metab. 2002;22(9):1142–8.

25. Meschia JF, Brott TG, Hobson 2nd RW. Diagnosis and invasive management of carotid atherosclerotic stenosis. Mayo Clin Proc. 2007;82(7):851–8.
26. Hobson 2nd RW, Weiss DG, Fields WS, Goldstone J, Moore WS, Towne JB, et al. Efficacy of carotid endarterectomy for asymptomatic carotid stenosis. The Veterans Affairs Cooperative Study Group. N Engl J Med. 1993;328(4):221–7.
27. Chatzikonstantinou A, Wolf ME, Schaefer A, Hennerici MG. Asymptomatic and symptomatic carotid stenosis: an obsolete classification? Stroke Res Treat. 2012;12:340798. doi:10.1155/2012/340798. Epub 2012 Jan 23.
28. Amarenco P, Bogousslavsky J, Callahan 3rd A, Goldstein LB, Hennerici M, Rudolph AE, et al. High-dose atorvastatin after stroke or transient ischemic attack. N Engl J Med. 2006;355(6):549–59.
29. Ballantyne CM. Cholesterol, lipids, and statins. Tex Heart Inst J. 2005;32(3):378–9.
30. Patel A, MacMahon S, Chalmers J, Neal B, Billot L, Woodward M, ADVANCE Collaborative Group. Intensive blood glucose control and vascular outcomes in patients with type 2 diabetes. N Engl J Med. 2008;358(24):2560–72.
31. Gerstein HC, Miller ME, Byington RP, Goff Jr DC, Bigger JT, Buse JB, Action to Control Cardiovascular Risk in Diabetes Study Group, et al. Effects of intensive glucose lowering in type 2 diabetes. N Engl J Med. 2008;358(24):2545–59.
32. Boussageon R, Bejan-Angoulvant T, Saadatian-Elahi M, Lafont S, Bergeonneau C, Kassaï B, et al. Effect of intensive glucose lowering treatment on all cause mortality, cardiovascular death, and microvascular events in type 2 diabetes: meta-analysis of randomised controlled trials. BMJ. 2011;343:d4169. doi:10.1136/bmj.d4169.
33. Chimowitz MI, Lynn MJ, Derdeyn CP, Turan TN, Fiorella D, Lane BF, et al. Stenting versus aggressive medical therapy for intracranial stenosis. N Engl J Med. 2011;365(11):993–1003.
34. Endarterectomy for asymptomatic carotid artery stenosis. Executive Committee for the Asymptomatic Carotid Atherosclerosis Study. JAMA. 1995;273(18):1421–8.
35. Johnston SC, Rothwell PM, Nguyen-Huynh MN, Giles MF, Elkins JS, Bernstein AL, et al. Validation and refinement of scores to predict very early stroke risk after transient ischaemic attack. Lancet. 2007;369(9558):283–92.
36. Rothwell PM, Eliasziw M, Gutnikov SA, Warlow CP, Barnett HJ, Carotid Endarterectomy Trialists Collaboration. Endarterectomy for symptomatic carotid stenosis in relation to clinical subgroups and timing of surgery. Lancet. 2004;363(9413):915–24.
37. Reichmann BL, van Lammeren GW, Moll FL, de Borst GJ. Is age of 80 years a threshold for carotid revascularization? Curr Cardiol Rev. 2011;7(1):15–21.
38. Powers WJ, Clarke WR, Grubb Jr RL, Videen TO, Adams Jr HP, Derdeyn CP, COSS Investigators. Extracranial-intracranial bypass surgery for stroke prevention in hemodynamic cerebral ischemia: the Carotid Occlusion Surgery Study randomized trial. JAMA. 2011;306(18):1983–92.
39. Awad IA, Spetzler R. Extracranial-intracranial bypass surgery: a critical analysis in light of the International Cooperative Study. Neurosurgery. 1986;19(4):655–64.

Whom I Stent

11

Keith DeSousa, Erez Nossek, Matthew Potts, and Howard Riina

Introduction

Carotid angioplasty and stenting (CAS) is a common and increasingly selected option for treating cervical carotid atherosclerotic disease. It is essential that the neurointerventionalist is familiar with the indications for selecting patients for this therapy. This section aims to serve as a review of the current literature to help guide clinicians to determine which patients are likely to have a favorable outcome with CAS. As with any interventional procedure, reducing morbidity is possible only with careful consideration of each patient's risk factor profile.

Background

According to the World Health Organization, nearly six million people die from stroke annually [1]. Specifically, around 7–10% of ischemic strokes are due to carotid atherosclerosis [2]. The Northern Manhattan Stroke Study (NOMASS) found that extracranial artery atherosclerosis was the cause of ischemic stroke in 17% of black patients, 9% of Hispanic patients, and 5% of white patients [3]. Extracranial atherosclerosis resulting in stroke is most commonly found at the level

K. DeSousa, MD
Division NeuroInterventional Radiology, NYU School of Medicine, NYU Langone Medical Center, New York, NY, USA

E. Nossek, MD
Department of Neurosurgery, Maimonides Medical Center, Brooklyn, NY, USA

M. Potts, MD
Assistant Professor, Department of Neurosurgery, Northwestern University, Illinois, USA

H. Riina, MD, FACS, FAANS (✉)
Director Neurosurgery Residency Program, Department of Neurosurgery, New York University School of Medicine, New York University Langone Medical Center, 530 First Ave, Suite 8R, New York, NY 10016, USA

E. Veznedaroglu (ed.), *Controversies in Vascular Neurosurgery*,
DOI 10.1007/978-3-319-27315-0_11

of the common carotid bifurcation, by the origin of the internal carotid artery. Ischemia results due to impairment of blood flow distal to the narrowing. Atherosclerotic plaque rupture with resultant distal emboli is thought to play a significant role in the disease process as well [4]. According to the Framingham Heart Study, carotid stenosis was attributable to common vascular risk factors such as advanced age, smoking, high cholesterol, and hypertension [5].

The symptoms generally caused by carotid disease include hemispheric cerebral infarctions or transient ischemic attacks (TIAs), retinal infarctions, and transient monocular vision loss otherwise known as amaurosis fugax. Generally speaking, patients with these symptoms during the last 6 months are defined as having symptomatic carotid disease.

Current Evidence for Carotid Revascularization

Although the data supporting surgical revascularization is beyond the scope of this paper, a basic understanding of the landmark trials is necessary to make an evidence-based recommendation to patients. Surgical treatment for carotid stenosis is well established and has been studied primarily during the 1980s and 1990s. Many trials have looked at preventing stroke in patients with symptomatic carotid stenosis. The most commonly quoted study is the North American Symptomatic Endarterectomy Trial (NASCET), which aimed to identify stroke risk after carotid endarterectomy (CEA) in patients with symptomatic carotid disease. This trial found that patients with carotid stenosis of 70 % or greater had a 17 % lower incidence of stroke when treated with CEA versus medical treatment alone. There was no benefit in treating patients with less than 50 % stenosis [6].

The European Carotid Surgery Trial (ECST), while slightly different in design from NASCET, also randomized patients to CEA versus medical management. Patients with greater than 80 % stenosis experienced major ipsilateral stroke or death at a rate of 26.5 % after 3 years. CEA reduced that rate to 14.9 % for an absolute benefit of 11.6 % favoring surgery [7].

Treatment of patients with asymptomatic carotid disease has been studied as well. The Asymptomatic Carotid Stenosis Study (ACAS) enrolled 721 patients with at least 60 % carotid stenosis. This trial estimated that the 5-year risk for stroke in medically treated patients was 11 % versus 5.1 % in patients treated with CEA [8].

After several trials showed the benefit of CEA for both symptomatic and asymptomatic patients, the next question was how to minimize perioperative risk for stroke in these patients. Later subgroup analysis from these and other major trials identified risk factors for surgical complications such as contralateral carotid stenosis, use of local anesthesia, and higher degree of stenosis (including string sign) [9]. In NASCET, 115 patients (8.1 %) experienced some sort of medical complication. These included myocardial infarctions (1 %), other cardiovascular disorders (7.1 %), respiratory complications (0.8 %), transient confusions (0.4 %), and other complications (0.7 %) [10]. With this in mind, the less invasive endovascular option seemed to be a possible alternative to CEA.

Carotid Angioplasty and Stenting

Treatment of carotid stenosis via the endovascular route involves accessing the femoral artery at the level of the groin and threading a catheter up to the level of stenosis. During the formative years of endovascular treatment, balloon angioplasty was used to dilate the vessel and improve the degree of stenosis. Recently, the placement of a stent in the carotid artery has replaced angioplasty as the treatment of choice. Such treatment provides a minimally invasive alternative to surgery as well as an option for patients with surgical contraindications, such as surgically inaccessible carotid arteries (i.e., high bifurcations) or those on anticoagulant or antiplatelet medications which carry high risk when stopping these medications.

The drawbacks to CAS are that, unlike surgery, the atherosclerotic plaque is not removed during stenting. Crossing the lesion with a guidewire, catheter, or placement of the stent itself may dislodge plaque material sending distal emboli into the brain. It has been shown multiple times that CAS results in a higher rate of periprocedural strokes, whereas CEA has a higher risk of cranial nerve palsies and myocardial infarction [11]. Therefore, further studies were necessitated to determine which patients may benefit from stenting.

The Carotid Angioplasty and Stenting Trials

There have been many trials examining endovascular treatment of carotid disease with the goal of identifying the particular subset of patients who would most likely benefit. In 2001, the Carotid and Vertebral Artery Transluminal Angioplasty Study (CAVATAS) was published. It enrolled 504 patients from 1992 to 1997. It compared balloon angioplasty alone with CEA. Additional stenting was performed in 26 % of the angioplasty patients. High-risk surgical patients were excluded from this trial including those with recent MI, uncontrolled hypertension, diabetes, renal disease, respiratory failure, difficult to access carotid stenosis, and severe cervical spondylosis. No statistically significant difference was seen in the rate of disabling stroke or death within 30 days between treatment arms (6.4 % for CAS vs. 5.9 % for CEA). There was also no statistically significant difference in the 3-year risk of stroke or death between the groups [12].

The Carotid Revascularization using Endarterectomy or Stenting Systems (CaRESS) trial was a multicenter, randomized prospective study comparing CAS with distal embolic protection to CEA in both symptomatic and asymptomatic patients with or without high surgical risk. This was one of the first trials to use distal protection. Again, no significant difference in 30-day (2.1 % CAS vs. 3.6 % CEA) and 1-year stroke rates was found (10.0 % CAS vs. 13.6 % CEA).

The Stenting and Angioplasty with Protection in Patients at High Risk for Endarterectomy (SAPPHIRE) trial was a multicenter randomized trial in which the primary intent was to prove noninferiority of CAS to CEA in high-risk patients. The risk of 30-day MI, stroke, or death was 4.8 % for CAS versus 9.8 % for CEA [13]. A second trial, Stent-Supported Percutaneous Angioplasty of the Carotid Artery versus Endarterectomy (SPACE), was started to demonstrate noninferiority of CAS in low-risk patients. It was halted early when an interim analysis showed that the initial planned enrollment was not sufficient for the trial to reach significance. It should be noted that in SPACE, distal protection was not required in the CAS group. It was only used in a very small proportion of cases [14].

In 2006, the Endarterectomy Versus Angioplasty in Patients with Symptomatic Severe Carotid Stenosis (EVA-3S) results was published. The trial enrolled 527 patients. It was stopped early because the 30-day stroke or death rate was significantly higher in the endovascular group than the endarterectomy group (9.6 % vs. 3.9 % $P=0.01$). Once again, distal embolic protection was not required [15].

With all of the conflicting data and multiple trials with various standards of quality, another more rigorous trial was carried out by the National Institutes of Health (NIH). Published in 2010, the Carotid Revascularization Endarterectomy vs. Stenting trial (CREST) provided the most comprehensive data on this subject. Quality of the proceduralists was ensured by strict standards. The primary endpoint was ipsilateral stroke, death, or MI for up to 4 years. Symptomatic patients with more than 50 % stenosis and asymptomatic patients with more than 60 % stenosis were included. Among the 2,502 patients followed, no statistically significant difference between the two groups for the primary endpoint was seen (7.2 % with CAS vs. 6.8 % with CEA, hazard ratio 1.11, 95 % confidence interval 0.81–1.51). In the symptomatic group, the rates were 8.0 % and 6.4 %, respectively (hazard ratio 1.37, $P=0.14$). In the asymptomatic group, the rates were 4.5 % and 2.7 %, respectively (hazard ratio 1.86, $P=0.07$). Subgroup analysis found the rate of periprocedural stroke was higher in CAS, but the rate of MI was higher in the CEA arm. Patients older than 70 did better in the CEA arm and younger than 70 did better with CAS [11].

Embolic Protection Options During Stenting Procedure

Given the findings of the aforementioned clinical trials, one thought is that embolic protection devices may reduce the incidence of embolic complications during CAS. There are two generally accepted methods in use: proximal protection devices or distal protection devices. Proximal protection generally involves deploying a balloon in the common carotid artery to arrest antegrade flow. A second balloon is often deployed in the external carotid artery to prevent retrograde flow through the external carotid artery into the carotid bifurcation that could send embolic material up the internal carotid artery. The stenting and/or angioplasty procedure is completed, and the blood is aspirated from the common carotid artery to remove any possible debris which could have been formed as a result of the intervention.

Distal protection involves crossing the lesion with a guidewire and deploying a retrievable filter basket distal to the location of the stenosis. In theory, the filter should trap any debris lost during the CAS procedure. The filter is carefully removed as to not lose any retained material within the device.

There is scarce literature comparing the efficacy of CAS using either proximal or distal protection. One retrospective study looked at 287 cases performed with either proximal or distal protection. Two hundred eight patients were treated with distal protection and 79 with proximal flow arrest. Patients with higher degrees of stenosis were treated with proximal protection (82.5 % vs. 74.5 %, $p<0.001$). Death rates were 1.9 % for proximal and 1.3 % for distal protection, while stroke rates were 4.3 % and 3.8 %, respectively, and MI rates were 1.4 % and 1.3 %, respectively. All differences did not reach statistical significance [16].

Consensus Recommendations for Treatment of Carotid Disease

The following recommendations are based on findings from consensus panels regarding symptomatic and asymptomatic patients with carotid stenosis. CEA is recommended for patients with TIA or stroke within the past 6 months with ipsilateral 70–99 % carotid stenosis (Class I, level of evidence: A). CEA and CAS are not recommended in patients with stenosis less than 50 % (Class III, level of evidence: A). Surgery should be performed within 2 weeks if treatment is warranted (Class IIa, level of evidence: B). CAS is an alternative to CEA if the anticipated perioperative stroke/death rate is <6 % (Class IIa, level of evidence: B). In asymptomatic patients, CAS can be considered if the risk of perioperative stroke/death is <3 % (Class IIb, level of evidence: B) [2, 17–19].

Future of Therapy

The endovascular technique for treating carotid disease is continually improving. Operators are gaining more experience as well. Interestingly, medical therapy alone has made advances as more insight is gained into the optimal regimen for treating atherosclerosis. As a result, there is renewed interest in clinical trials for carotid disease in order to reevaluate medical treatment option. The Carotid Revascularization Endarterectomy Stenting Trial 2 (CREST 2) is enrolling patients with carotid stenosis greater than 70 % (measured by Doppler) and randomizing them to optimal medical therapy (OMT) as was used in the SAMMPRIS [20] (Stenting and Aggressive Medical Management for the Prevention of Recurrent Ischemic Stroke) trial or to OMT and CAS or CEA. The European Carotid Surgery Trial 2 (ECST-2) trial is investigating both symptomatic and asymptomatic patients with severe carotid stenosis and randomizing them to OMT or OMT plus either stenting or endarterectomy.

Summary

Navigating the somewhat tortuous and confusing data of CAS vs. CEA has proven challenging. Despite so much conflicting evidence, a consistently higher risk of periprocedural stroke has been shown in patients treated with CAS versus CEA. These are usually minor strokes. Most of the CAS stroke complications occur in elderly patients who most likely have more unstable plaque. In younger patients, CAS appears to be as safe as CEA. MI is shown to be less frequent in CAS patients

[11]. For this reason, in patients with cardiac disease, stenting may be a more favorable option. Timing of treatment should also be taken into account. Carotid revascularization should be delayed at least 2 weeks in patients with a large stroke to minimize the risk of reperfusion injury or in patients with hemorrhage given the need for dual antiplatelet therapy and short period of anticoagulation during the procedure. In patients with difficult aortic arches, tortuous carotid anatomy, or inability to tolerate short periods of anticoagulation may be better candidates for CEA. In patients who have restenosis of a previously treated carotid artery, contralateral carotid occlusion or severe stenosis, surgically inaccessible carotid bifurcations, prior neck radiation, or need to remain on antiplatelet or anticoagulation therapy may be better candidates for stenting. While these may be high-risk patients, the decision to treat should be undertaken only if the patient stands to benefit from revascularization. In the end, the decision to offer carotid stenting to a patient should only be made after thorough, careful, and thoughtful analysis of each individual's risk factor profile.

References

1. Organization WS. 2015. [cited 7 Jul 2015]; Available from: http://www.world-stroke.org.
2. Chaturvedi S, Sacco RL. How recent data have impacted the treatment of internal carotid artery stenosis. J Am Coll Cardiol. 2015;65(11):1134–43.
3. White H, et al. Ischemic stroke subtype incidence among whites, blacks, and Hispanics: the Northern Manhattan Study. Circulation. 2005;111(10):1327–31.
4. Szabo K, et al. Acute stroke patterns in patients with internal carotid artery disease: a diffusion-weighted magnetic resonance imaging study. Stroke. 2001;32(6):1323–9.
5. Fine-Edelstein JS, et al. Precursors of extracranial carotid atherosclerosis in the Framingham Study. Neurology. 1994;44(6):1046–50.
6. Beneficial effect of carotid endarterectomy in symptomatic patients with high-grade carotid stenosis. N Engl J Med. 1991;325(7): 445–53.
7. Randomised trial of endarterectomy for recently symptomatic carotid stenosis: final results of the MRC European Carotid Surgery Trial (ECST). Lancet. 1998;351(9113):1379–87.
8. Rothwell PM, Goldstein LB. Carotid endarterectomy for asymptomatic carotid stenosis: asymptomatic carotid surgery trial. Stroke. 2004;35(10):2425–7.
9. Ferguson GG, et al. The North American Symptomatic Carotid Endarterectomy Trial: surgical results in 1415 patients. Stroke. 1999;30(9):1751–8.
10. Paciaroni M, et al. Medical complications associated with carotid endarterectomy. North American Symptomatic Carotid Endarterectomy Trial (NASCET). Stroke. 1999;30(9): 1759–63.
11. Brott TG, et al. Stenting versus endarterectomy for treatment of carotid-artery stenosis. N Engl J Med. 2010;363(1):11–23.
12. Endovascular versus surgical treatment in patients with carotid stenosis in the Carotid and Vertebral Artery Transluminal Angioplasty Study (CAVATAS): a randomised trial. Lancet. 2001;357(9270):1729–37.
13. Yadav JS, et al. Protected carotid-artery stenting versus endarterectomy in high-risk patients. N Engl J Med. 2004;351(15):1493–501.
14. Eckstein H-H, et al. Results of the Stent-Protected Angioplasty versus Carotid Endarterectomy (SPACE) study to treat symptomatic stenoses at 2 years: a multinational, prospective, randomised trial. Lancet Neurol. 2008;7(10):893–902.

15. Mas J-L, et al. Endarterectomy versus stenting in patients with symptomatic severe carotid stenosis. N Engl J Med. 2006;355(16):1660–71.
16. Hernandez-Fernandez F, et al. Comparison between proximal versus distal protection devices in 287 cases of carotid revascularization using angioplasty and stenting: periprocedure complications, morbidity, and mortality. Cardiovasc Intervent Radiol. 2014;37(3):639–45.
17. Kernan WN, et al. Guidelines for the prevention of stroke in patients with stroke and transient ischemic attack: a guideline for healthcare professionals from the American Heart Association/American Stroke Association. Stroke. 2014;45(7):2160–236.
18. Meschia JF, et al. Guidelines for the primary prevention of stroke: a statement for healthcare professionals from the American Heart Association/American Stroke Association. Stroke. 2014;45(12):3754–832.
19. Brott TG, et al. 2011 ASA/ACCF/AHA/AANN/AANS/ACR/ASNR/CNS/SAIP/SCAI/SIR/SNIS/SVM/SVS guideline on the management of patients with extracranial carotid and vertebral artery disease: executive summary: a report of the American College of Cardiology Foundation/American Heart Association Task Force on Practice Guidelines, and the American Stroke Association, American Association of Neuroscience Nurses, American Association of Neurological Surgeons, American College of Radiology, American Society of Neuroradiology, Congress of Neurological Surgeons, Society of Atherosclerosis Imaging and Prevention, Society for Cardiovascular Angiography and Interventions, Society of Interventional Radiology, Society of NeuroInterventional Surgery, Society for Vascular Medicine, and Society for Vascular Surgery. J Am Coll Cardiol. 2011;57(8):1002–44.
20. Chimowitz MI, et al. Stenting versus aggressive medical therapy for intracranial arterial stenosis. N Engl J Med. 2011;365(11):993–1003.

Distal Protection for Carotid Artery Stenting: Where Is the Evidence?

12

Mandy J. Binning

Introduction

Carotid artery stenting (CAS) has achieved clinical equipoise to carotid endarterectomy (CEA) for most patient populations [1] and has gained acceptance as a treatment for cervical internal carotid artery (ICA) stenosis. CEA was long thought to be superior to CAS, in part, due to the ability to achieve flow arrest to prevent distal embolization of plaque particles from plaque disruption. In order to prevent or minimize embolic showering from balloon angioplasty and stenting and to improve the safety profile of CAS, embolic protection devices were developed. As a result, embolic protection devices (EPDs), specifically distal protection devices (filters), have become the standard of care in CAS. Despite multiple retrospective and prospective reviews of techniques, to date, there is not a randomized trial comparing and showing superiority of protected to unprotected CAS. Despite a lack of class 1 evidence supporting lower incidence of cerebral ischemia with EPDs and even evidence to the contrary, EPDs have become the standard of care in CAS.

Distal Embolic Protection

To date, there has not been a randomized control trial comparing CAS with and without EPD. Most of the evidence has come from studies using historical controls for the unprotected arm.

Kastrup et al. performed one of the earliest literature reviews in 2003 comparing studies of protected to unprotected CAS [2]. They evaluated the results of 40 unprotected and 14 protected studies. These were primarily retrospective, single-center groups with no consistency in protection type (balloon versus filter), and stent type

M.J. Binning, MD
Drexel Neurosciences Institute, Philadelphia, PA, USA
e-mail: mbinning@gnineuro.org

E. Veznedaroglu (ed.), *Controversies in Vascular Neurosurgery*,
DOI 10.1007/978-3-319-27315-0_12

or operator experience. However, the authors concluded that in early analysis, the use of cerebral protection devices appeared to reduce thromboembolic complications during CAS.

In 2005, Ouriel et al. looked at a series of 261 patients who underwent CAS [3]. EPDs were used toward the latter stages of this study in 90 patients. Debris was reported to be found in roughly half of patients and there were fewer major ipsilateral strokes in the EPD group.

Similarly, Cossotini et al. reported on their series of 52 patients who underwent CAS, 30 with EPD and 22 without EPD [4]. Magnetic resonance (MR) diffusion-weighted imaging (DWI) was performed in both groups of patients following stenting. The authors found a 30 % incidence of ischemic lesions in all comers, with 26 % and 36 % in the protected and unprotected groups, respectively. In addition the protected group was found to have fewer DWI lesions on MRI. The number of contralateral lesions was not different between the groups. This finding led to a recommendation that distal protection for carotid stenting may decrease the ipsilateral risk of stroke from CAS.

As a result of some of the early evidence, carotid stenting trials began using EPDs in an effort to show equipoise to CEA. The Stenting and Angioplasty with Protection in Patients at High Risk for Endarterectomy (SAPPHIRE) trial mandated the use of EPDs in the stenting group in patients who were high risk for CEA [5]. Enrollment in the CEA arm was very low, so instead of an active control, outcomes were compared to surgical and medical data in similar patient populations. Interestingly, the lead author of SAPPHIRE invented the EPD used for the trial, and the majority of the remaining authors either worked for Cordis at the time or had financial relationships with the company [6].

Similarly, the ACCULINK for Revascularization of Carotids in High-Risk Patients (ARCHeR) trial was a positive trial for showing non-inferiority to CEA [7]. The Food and Drug Administration (FDA) based their approval of the ACCULINK stent and ACCUNET EPD on the ARCHeR data [8]. It should be stressed, however, that the FDA does not require use of EPDs with carotid stents. SAPPHIRE and ARCHeR were able to show non-inferiority to CEA and hence the trend for the use of EPDs in all future trials began. In addition, the Centers for Medicare and Medicaid Services (CMS) based their reimbursement criteria for CAS on these trials and began requiring the use of EPDs during CAS procedures. The rest is history, and to date there has not been a randomized trial comparing protected and unprotected CAS that shows an advantage to EPD use.

The Evidence Against Distal Embolic Protection

Intuitively, EPDs sound like a simple solution to an obvious problem. Why are some interventionalists concerned about the routine use of EPDs? The arguments against the routine use of filter-protected CAS include the fact that the lesion has to be crossed with the wire and filter device, a step in the procedure that is unprotected. The filter device can be difficult to navigate through tortuous anatomy and tight stenosis causing dissections and possible embolic complications. The filter is bulky as it is passed across the plaque in an unprotected fashion. Filter design has not significantly evolved since most of these studies were published. In addition, filter devices do not have ideal wall apposition, allowing material to embolize around the filter. Furthermore, thrombus can form on the filter itself and embolize around the filter. Recapturing the filter can fail and embolic material can become dislodged during this step. Finally, EPDs add expense to the CAS procedure, a fact that no one would mind, if there was proof of their efficacy.

Pro-CAS is a prospective registry of CAS procedures in Germany [9]. During the same time period in the registry, 4,709 patients were treated with (3,543) and without (1,166) the use of EPDs. Analysis of the registry revealed no difference in stroke and death rate between the two groups of patients.

These results were concordant with the Stent-Supported Percutaneous Angioplasty of the Carotid Artery versus Endarterectomy (SPACE) trial in which secondary analysis of their data compared patients who underwent protected versus unprotected CAS and even factored in whether the stent design was open or closed cell [10]. Five hundred and sixty-three patients were treated with a stent, 145 with and 418 without EPDs, respectively. There was found to be no difference in stroke or major stroke between the two groups. There were significantly fewer events in patients who underwent stenting with a closed-cell stent and no significant difference in events with the use of EPDs in different stent design groups.

The Endarterectomy Versus Angioplasty in Patients with Symptomatic Carotid Stenosis (EVA-3S) trial stopped allowing unprotected CAS after 80 patients were enrolled [11]. This decision was made after it was found that the 30-day risk of stroke was three times higher in patients undergoing unprotected CAS. However, the lower limits of the confidence interval were compatible with an absence of difference between protected and unprotected CAS. In addition, most of the patients who underwent unprotected CAS and had an event did so in the 30 days following the procedure and not during the procedure, casting doubt if cerebral protection was truly a factor in the event.

The International Carotid Stenting Study looked at a subgroup of patients who underwent MRI before and after CAS and CEA. The CAS group was further subdivided into patients who underwent stenting with and without EPDs. Interestingly, more patients had new ischemic lesions on MRI diffusion-weighted imaging (DWI) after stenting with cerebral protection devices than without [12]. In addition, the rate of stroke was higher in the EPD group (5.1 %) than the unprotected group (2.4 %).

Furthermore, Tietke and Jansen pooled data from multiple studies including SPACE, EVA-3S, and ICSS [13]. Again, they evaluated CAS with and without EPD and again found that most recent data at that time from prospective multicenter trials support the thought that EPDs do not reduce, but may increase the perioperative complication rate.

Macdonald et al. showed in a small randomized trial that patients undergoing filter-protected CAS had significantly higher rates of microembolism on transcranial Doppler studies and more new lesions on diffusion-weighted MRI [14].

These findings were similar to those found in another small randomized study by Barbato et al. 2 years prior, in which, new MRI lesions were noted in 72 % of the cerebral protection group compared with 44 % in the no cerebral protection group ($P=0.09$) [15].

In 2011, Tallarita et al. reviewed their series of unprotected versus protected CAS [16]. They reviewed 357 CAS patients, 105 who underwent unprotected CAS and 252 who underwent filter-protected CAS, and found no significant difference in the primary end points of perioperative stroke, death, or MI between the two groups.

Pandey et al. retrospectively reviewed a series of 108 CAS without the use of EPD and reported a perioperative stroke and death rate of 2.85 % [17]. The authors mention in their technique that most patients did not undergo post-stenting angioplasty but did not discuss the possible importance of this nuance. Each step of CAS carries a potential risk of causing embolic complications, from crossing the lesions with either the wire and balloon or the wire and filter, followed by pre-stenting angioplasty, stenting, and post-stenting angioplasty. Especially with open-cell stent designs, there is a concern that post-stenting angioplasty can cause a "cheese grater" effect of plaque between the cells of the stent. Pandey showed that eliminating this step allowed for low complication rates with unprotected CAS.

Similarly, in our institution, CAS is performed without the use of EPDs and without post-stenting angioplasty. A review of our data, although retrospective, shows a 0 % perioperative stroke and death rate and 2 % rate of perioperative non-ST elevation myocardial infarction (MI). The stroke, death, and MI rate in CREST was 5.2 %, 4.1 % for minor stroke and 0.9 % for major stroke [1]. In SAPPHIRE< the perioperative stroke and death rate was 3.6 % [5]. Our myocardial infarction rate is similar to the carotid endarterectomy (CEA) group in CREST [1]. This is likely due to the fact that many of our cases are performed under general anesthesia.

Almost 80 % of our patients had symptomatic lesions and 75 % of those had greater than 80 % stenosis, making it more comparable to the CREST population. Most patients were treated with a closed-cell design stent. Despite the fact that we did not perform post-stenting angioplasty, the rate of restenosis requiring retreatment was 2.8 %. This is less than the restenosis rate in CREST in which post-stenting angioplasty was performed in most cases [1].

The avoidance of post-stenting angioplasty may be one explanation why one of the earlier carotid trials, Carotid and Vertebral Artery Transluminal Angioplasty Study (CAVATAS), was non-inferior for endovascular treatment, despite the lack of distal protection [18]. Most of the carotid procedures in this trial consisted of angioplasty only, avoiding any further embolic risk of stenting or post-stenting angioplasty. While angioplasty alone is no longer advocated, the low complication rate in an unprotected trial is of interest.

Multiple single and multicenter studies have found no difference in ischemic events with the use of embolic protection. To the contrary, many of these papers reveal the safety of unprotected CAS with results that exceed large trials utilizing a filter-protected technique.

Looking Beyond Distal Protection

Few physicians who perform carotid intervention would argue the fact that CAS carries a risk of causing embolic complications. CEA has long been the standard to treat carotid atherosclerotic disease due to its ability to achieve flow arrest and prevent the embolization of debris. While CREST was able to show clinical equipoise of CAS to CEA, concerns about the true efficacy of EPDs have led to the development of proximal protection devices to create flow arrest and even flow reversal during CAS procedures by simultaneous balloon occlusion of the external and common carotid arteries.

Mokin et al. reported a series of 70 patients treated with proximal protection devices compared to matched patients treated with distal protection [19]. The authors found no difference in 30-day adverse events between the two groups, although they treated more morphologically high-risk lesions using proximal protection.

Three additional studies showed a reduction of MRI-DWI lesions with the use of proximal protection when compared to distal EPDs, but the number of adverse clinical or symptomatic events was not different [20–22].

Conclusions

Multiple single and multicenter studies have found no difference between protected and unprotected CAS, distally or proximally protected CAS, and some larger registries, and trials actually show worse outcomes with the use of distal EPDs. It is clear that current distal filters are unlikely to be the final answer when it comes to making CAS as safe as possible. As technology advances, distal EPDs may improve, or more evidence may show that proximal protection is superior. The most current trials will also require comparison to today's best medical therapy as well as CEA to truly decide the overall best management for carotid disease.

The use of distal filter embolic protection devices for CAS has been handed down as a directive despite the lack of adequate evidence as to their benefit and efficacy. However, there is doubt regarding the efficacy of EPDs in preventing thromboembolic complications during carotid stenting procedures. Many institutions and multiple studies have shown that unprotected CAS can be performed safely and effectively. The current "standard" to perform CAS with EPD should be reexplored with a randomized trial, and until then, distal filter-protected CAS should be considered optional and at the operator's discretion.

References

1. Mantese VA, Timaran CH, Chiu D, Begg RJ, Brott TG, CREST investigators. The Carotid Revascularization Endarterectomy Versus Stenting Trial (CREST) stenting versus carotid endarterectomy for carotid disease. Stroke. 2010;41:S31–4.
2. Kastrup A, Gröschel K, Krapf H, Brehm BR, Dichgans J, Schulz JB. Early outcome of carotid angioplasty and stenting with and without cerebral protection devices: a systematic review of the literature. Stroke. 2003;34:813–9.

3. Ouriel K, Wholey MH, Fayad P, Katzen BT, Whitlow P, Frentzko M, et al. Feasibility trial of carotid stenting with and without an embolus protection device. J Endovasc Ther. 2005; 12:525–37.
4. Cosottini M, Michelassi MC, Puglioli M, Lazzarotti G, Orlandi G, Marconi F, et al. Silent cerebral ischemia detected with diffusion-weighted imaging in patients treated with protected and unprotected carotid artery stenting. Stroke. 2005;36:2389–93.
5. Yadav JS, Wholey MH, Kuntz RE, Fayad P, Katzen BT, Mishkel GJ, Stenting and Angioplasty with Protection in Patients at High Risk for Endarterectomy Investigators, et al. Protected carotid-artery stenting versus endarterectomy in high risk patients. N Engl J Med. 2004;351:1493–501.
6. Thomas DJ. Protected carotid artery stenting versus endarterectomy in high-risk patients: reflections from SAPPHIRE. Stroke. 2005;36:912–3.
7. Gray WA, Hopkins LN, Yadav S, Davis T, Wholey M, Atkinson R, ARCHeR Trial Collaborators, et al. Protected carotid stenting in high-surgical-risk patients: the ARCHeR results. J Vasc Surg. 2006;44:258–68.
8. Toor SA, Cavanaugh KJ, Lim LM. Regulation of carotid artery stents and embolic protection devices in the United States. A history of, and perspectives on, FDA regulation of carotid stents and associated embolic protection devices over the years. Endovasc Today. 2013; 44–58.
9. Theiss W, Hermanek P, Mathias K, Bruckmann H, Dembski J, Hoffmann FJ, et al. Predictors of death and stroke after carotid angioplasty and stenting: a subgroup analysis of the PRO-CAS data. Stroke. 2008;39:2325–30.
10. Jansen O, Fiehler J, Hartmann M, Bruckmann H. Protection or nonprotection in carotid stent angioplasty the influence of interventional techniques on outcome data from the SPACE trial. Stroke. 2009;40:841–6.
11. EVA-3S Investigators. Carotid angioplasty and stenting with and without cerebral protection clinical alert from the endarterectomy versus angioplasty in patients with symptomatic severe carotid stenosis (EVA-3S) trial. Stroke. 2004;35:e18–21.
12. Bonati LH, Jongen LM, Haller S, Flach HZ, Dobson J, Nederkoorn PJ, ICSS-MRI Study Group. New ischaemic brain lesions on MRI after stenting or endarterectomy for symptomatic carotid stenosis: a substudy of the International Carotid Stenting Study (ICSS). Lancet Neurol. 2010;9(4):353–62.
13. Tietke M, Jansen O. Cerebral protection vs no cerebral protection: timing of stroke with CAS. J Cardiovasc Surg (Torino). 2009;50(6):751–60.
14. Macdonald S, Evans DH, Griffiths PD, et al. Filter-protected versus unprotected carotid artery stenting: a randomised trial. Cerebrovasc Dis. 2010;29:282–9.
15. Barbato JE, Dillavou E, Horowitz MB, et al. A randomized trial of carotid artery stenting with and without cerebral protection. J Vasc Surg. 2008;47:760–5.
16. Tallarita T, Rabinstein AA, Cloft H, et al. Are distal protection devices 'protective' during carotid angioplasty and stenting? Stroke. 2011;42:1962–6.
17. Pandey AS, Koebbe CJ, Liebman K, Rosenwasser RH, Veznedaroglu E. Low incidence of symptomatic strokes after carotid stenting without embolization protection devices for extracranial carotid stenosis: a single-institution retrospective review. Neurosurgery. 2008;63: 867–73.
18. Endovascular versus surgical treatment in patients with carotid stenosis in the Carotid and Vertebral Transluminal Angioplasty Study (CAVATAS): a randomised trial. Lancet. 2001; 357:1729–37.
19. Mokin M, Dumont TM, Chi JM, Manhan CJ, Kass-Hout T, Sorkin G, et al. Proximal versus distal protection during carotid artery stenting: analysis of the two treatment approaches and associated clinical outcomes. World Neurosurg. 2014;81(3/4):543–8.
20. Leal I, Orgaz A, Flores A, Gil J, Rodriguez R, Peinado J, et al. A diffusion-weighted magnetic resonance imaging-based study of transcervical carotid stenting with flow reversal vs transfemoral filter protection. J Vasc Surg. 2012;56:1585–90.

21. Bijuklic K, Wandler A, Hazizi F, Schofer J. The PROFI study (prevention of cerebral embolization by proximal balloon occlusion compared to filter protection during carotid artery stenting): a prospective randomized trial. J Am Coll Cardiol. 2012;59:1383–9.
22. Cano MN, Kambara AM, de Cano SJF, Portela LAP, Paes AT, Costa JR. Randomized comparison of distal and proximal cerebral protection during carotid artery stenting. J Am Coll Cardiol Intv. 2013;6:1204–9.

Carotid Artery Stenosis: Discussion

13

Badih Daou and Pascal Jabbour

Introduction

Despite recent advances in the diagnosis and management, stroke remains one of the most common causes of death and the leading cause of disability in adulthood in developed countries. More than 700,000 new and recurrent strokes occur in the United States each year [1]. Carotid atherosclerotic disease is an important cause of stroke and is responsible for up to 30 % of acute cerebrovascular accidents. Effective prevention remains the best option for reducing the burden of stroke. Therapeutic options include medical treatment, carotid endarterectomy (CEA), and carotid artery stenting (CAS). To choose the appropriate treatment strategy, the risks, benefits, and costs of each option should be assessed. CEA has been established as an effective management strategy in patients with high-grade carotid stenosis and is considered the standard of care for the primary and secondary prevention of stroke related to carotid artery stenosis [2]. With technological advancements in balloon catheter and stent technology, CAS has become widely used, both in the management of symptomatic and asymptomatic patients with carotid disease. However, the debate regarding the best treatment of carotid stenosis has led to the development of a multitude of randomized controlled trials that compared the safety and efficacy of CEA and CAS and their roles in the management of carotid atherosclerotic disease. In patients undergoing CAS, the most important acute complication is related to the

B. Daou, MD
Department of Neurosurgery, Thomas Jefferson University Hospital, Philadelphia, Pennsylvania, USA

P. Jabbour, MD (✉)
Division of Neurovascular Surgery and Endovascular Neurosurgery, Department of Neurosurgery, Thomas Jefferson University Hospital, Philadelphia, Pennsylvania, USA
e-mail: pascal.jabbour@jefferson.edu

E. Veznedaroglu (ed.), *Controversies in Vascular Neurosurgery*,
DOI 10.1007/978-3-319-27315-0_13

distal embolization of particles generated during the endovascular procedure. Another debate has emerged questioning the use of embolic protection devices (EPD) in patients treated with CAS and the role of these devices in preventing the occurrence of thromboembolic events. In this chapter, we aim to shed the light on the major clinical trials dealing with CAS and CEA and compare the safety and efficacy of these two interventions in the management of carotid stenosis.

Carotid Endarterectomy

Several trials have clearly established the benefit of CEA over medical therapy alone in the management of symptomatic carotid stenosis (≥70 %). The NASCET (North American Symptomatic Carotid Endarterectomy Trial) randomized 328 patients with symptomatic carotid stenosis to CEA and 331 symptomatic patients to medical treatment alone [3]. The trial was stopped after 18 months of follow-up for patients with 70–99 % stenosis after a significant benefit was clearly established in patients who underwent CEA. The trial reported a 2-year cumulative risk of ipsilateral stroke of 9 % with CEA versus 26 % with medical therapy alone with an absolute risk reduction of ipsilateral stroke of 17 % in patients treated with CEA. Further results of the NASCET trial demonstrated a moderate advantage of CEA in patients with 50–69 % stenosis (risk of ipsilateral stroke was 15.7 % at 5 years with CEA versus 22.2 % with medical treatment). Patients with stenosis of less than 50 %, however, were not found to benefit from CEA [4]. The ECST (European Carotid Surgery Trial) compared 1,811 patients who underwent CEA for symptomatic carotid stenosis and 1,213 patients who did not have surgical management (a total of 2,518 patients) with a mean follow-up period of 6.1 years [5]. The investigators found that a major stroke or death occurred in 26.5 % of the control group and 14.9 % of the surgery group at 3 years, an absolute benefit from surgery of 11.6 %. They concluded that the benefits of CEA outweigh the risks with extreme degrees of stenosis (≥80 %), while the benefit decreases with mild stenosis. In the ECST the benefit of CEA was reported in patients with symptomatic carotid stenosis of ≥80 %, whereas in the NASCET the benefit of surgery was observed with stenosis ≥70 %. This discrepancy was due to differences in measuring the degree of stenosis on angiography. Rothwell et al. conducted a pooled analysis of 6,092 patients with symptomatic carotid disease who underwent CEA and found that surgery was highly beneficial in patients with 70 % stenosis or greater ($p<0.001$), whereas CEA was not beneficial in patients with <50 % stenosis and only of marginal benefit in those with 50–69 % stenosis [6].

The ACAS trial (Asymptomatic Carotid Atherosclerosis Study) recruited a total of 1,662 patients with asymptomatic carotid stenosis and randomized patients to either medical treatment alone or medical treatment in addition to CEA [7]. The median follow-up period was 2.7 years. The trial reported that in asymptomatic patients with ≥60 % stenosis, the 5-year risk of ipsilateral stroke, perioperative stroke, and death was 5.1 % in patients who had CEA versus 11 % in patients placed on medical treatment alone (risk reduction of 53 %). The benefit of CEA in asymptomatic patients was found to be more significant in men than in women in this study. In 2004, the ACST (Asymptomatic Carotid Surgery Trial) enrolled 3,120 patients with asymptomatic carotid stenosis (>60 %) with an average follow-up of 3.4 years and reported similar results [8]. They reported a 6.4 % rate of stroke or death over 5 years in the surgery group versus 11.7 % in the group initiated on medical treatment. In 2010, the ACST-1 further showed that CEA for asymptomatic patients younger than 75 years of age reduces the 10-year risk of stroke (13.4 % versus 17.9 %) [9]. The results of the ACAS and ACST led to major increases in rates of endarterectomy for asymptomatic stenosis. Overall, CEA provides a marked benefit over medical management in terms of stroke prevention for patients with ≥70 % stenosis with a persistent but less striking benefit in those with less severe stenosis (50–70 %). In 2010, an estimated 100,000 CEAs were performed in the United States. Carotid endarterectomy is the most frequently performed surgical procedure to prevent stroke [1].

Carotid Artery Stenting

Despite its proven efficacy in the management of carotid stenosis, CEA is an invasive procedure, usually requires general anesthesia, and carries a nonnegligible risk of cardiovascular events, wound complications, and cranial nerve damage. CAS has been proposed as a valid, minimally invasive alternative to CEA with several advantages that include fewer cardiovascular complications, need for only mild sedation, decreased risk of cranial nerve palsy, ability to perform the procedure in patients with severe cardiac and pulmonary disease, and suitability for patients with anatomically challenging lesions or history of neck radiation. The major limitation of CAS appears to be related to the higher risk of perioperative embolic strokes as compared to CEA. The use of carotid stenting has increased dramatically from <3 % of all carotid artery revascularization procedures in 1998 to 13 % in 2008 [1]. According to the recommendations of the ASA/AHA, CAS is indicated as an alternative to CEA for symptomatic patients at average or low risk of complications associated with endovascular intervention in the presence of carotid stenosis ≥70 % as documented by noninvasive imaging or ≥50 % as documented by angiography if the anticipated rate of periprocedural stroke or mortality is less than 6 %. CAS may also be considered for asymptomatic patients with carotid stenosis ≥70 %. CAS is also important in patients with unfavorable neck anatomy, previous ipsilateral CEA, contralateral vocal cord paralysis, open tracheostomy, contralateral carotid occlusion, radical surgery, and irradiation [10].

Carotid Endarterectomy Versus Carotid Artery Stenting

Stroke and Death

The ICSS trial (International Carotid Stenting Study) enrolled 1,713 patients with symptomatic carotid stenosis of whom stenting was performed in 855 patients and CEA in 858 patients [11]. Patients who were managed with CAS had worse outcomes than patients who underwent CEA with a higher rate of disabling stroke or death at 120 days in the stenting group (4 %) compared with the CEA group (3.2 %), higher incidence of stroke, death, or procedural myocardial infarction (MI) in the stenting group (8.5 %) compared with the endarterectomy group (5.2 %) ($p=0.006$) and higher risk of any stroke and all-cause death in the stenting group. However, in 2015, the ICSS trial published their long-term results and reported that stenting is as effective as endarterectomy in preventing fatal or disabling stroke in patients with symptomatic carotid stenosis up to 10 years after treatment [12]. The cumulative 5-year risk was similar between CAS and CEA (6.4 % versus 6.5 %). The occurrence of any stroke was more frequent in the stenting group than in the CEA group (5-year cumulative risk 15.2 % versus 9.4 %) but was mainly nondisabling strokes. The EVA-3S (Endarterectomy Versus Stenting in Patients with Symptomatic Severe Carotid Stenosis trial) enrolled 527 patients with symptomatic carotid disease ≥60 % but was stopped early in 2005 because of a higher rate of stroke and adverse events in patients who underwent CAS [13]. The 30-day incidence of any stroke or death was 3.9 % after endarterectomy and 9.6 % after stenting. The 30-day incidence of disabling stroke or death was 1.5 % after endarterectomy and 3.4 % after stenting. This study was mainly criticized for not using EPDs in all patients and for excluding MI from the primary endpoint. A secondary analysis of the long-term outcomes of the EVA-3S trial showed that the 4-year differences in outcomes between CAS and CEA were mainly due to a higher periprocedural risk of stenting compared with endarterectomy [14]. After the periprocedural period, the risk of ipsilateral stroke was low and similar in both treatment groups. They concluded that carotid stenting is as effective as carotid endarterectomy after long-term follow-up. The SPACE trial (Stent-Protected Angioplasty versus Carotid Endarterectomy in Symptomatic Patients trial) randomly assigned 1,214 patients with symptomatic stenosis ≥50 % to CEA or CAS and reported that there was no significant difference in the rate of ipsilateral ischemic stroke or death between the two groups at 30 days and after 2 years of follow-up (9.5 % with CAS versus 8.8 % with CEA, $p=0.62$) [15, 16]. The SAPPHIRE trial (Stenting and Angioplasty with Protection in Patients at High Risk for Endarterectomy trial) compared CAS with EPD against CEA [17]. The trial included 334 high-risk patients with symptomatic stenosis ≥50 % or asymptomatic stenosis ≥80 %. High-risk patients were defined as those having at least one of the following criteria: clinically significant cardiac disease, contralateral carotid occlusion, severe pulmonary disease, contralateral laryngeal nerve palsy, previous radical neck surgery or radiation therapy to the neck, recurrent stenosis after endarterectomy, and age >80 years. The investigators found similar outcomes with possibly a modest benefit for CAS at 1 year (primary endpoint of stroke or death at 1 year was 12.2 % with CAS versus 20.1 % with CEA, $p=0.004$). Longer follow-up showed that death or ipsilateral stroke after 3 years occurred in 24.6 % of patients in the stenting group and 26.9 % of patients in the endarterectomy group [18]. No significant difference could be shown in long-term outcomes between patients who underwent CAS with an embolic protection device and those who underwent CEA. CREST (Carotid Revascularization Endarterectomy versus Stenting Trial) which reported its results in 2010 was one of the largest trials that directly compared CEA and CAS [19]. The mean follow-up period was

2.5 years. The study enrolled 2,502 symptomatic and asymptomatic patients of whom 1,262 patients underwent CAS and 1,240 patients underwent CEA. The trial found no significant difference between CAS and CEA in the composite outcome of stroke, myocardial infarction, or death at 30 days (5.2 % with CAS versus 4.5 % with CEA, $p=0.38$) or at 4 years (7.2 % with CAS versus 6.8 % with CEA, $p=0.51$) [19]. However, the risk of periprocedural stroke was found to be significantly higher with CAS compared with CEA (4.1 % versus 2.3 %, $p=0.01$). Success of treatment was significantly affected by age. Carotid artery stenting was best in patients who were ≤70 years old, and CEA had the greatest benefit in patients who were ≥70 years of age. Bonati et al. conducted a Cochrane systematic review of 16 major trials that included 7,572 patients [20]. They reported that in patients with symptomatic carotid stenosis at standard surgical risk, endovascular treatment was associated with a higher short-term risk of death or any stroke (OR 1.72; $p=0.0003$). The rate of death or major disabling stroke did not differ significantly between treatments (OR 1.28; $p=0.13$) [20]. Similarly, Economopoulos et al. reported in a meta-analysis that included 3,723 patients who were managed with CEA and 3,754 patients with CAS that short-term finding showed that CAS was associated with elevated risk of death or stroke [21]. Concerning long-term outcomes, CAS was associated with higher rates of death or stroke only in patients >68 years old. In younger patients, outcomes after both treatments were similar. Bangalore et al. assessed the long-term differences in outcome after CAS and CEA and found no difference after 3 years of follow-up in the rates of death or stroke (CAS, 26.9 %, versus CEA, 24.6 %; $p=0.71$) [22]. To sum up, CAS is associated with an increased risk of perioperative stroke compared with endarterectomy. However, this excess risk appears to be limited to older patients (≥70 years old). The long-term risk of stroke and death is similar with the use of either CAS or CEA.

Myocardial Infarction

The rate of MI was 0.4 % for CAS and 0.8 % for CEA in the EVA-3S trial, 0.4 % for CAS and 0.6 % for CEA in the ICSS trial, and 0 % for both CAS and CEA in the SPACE study [11, 13, 16]. The SAPPHIRE trial incorporated systematic collection of CK and CK-MB and reported higher overall rates of MI with a 5.9 % rate in patients managed with CEA and 2.4 % in patients treated with CAS [17]. In CREST, 1.1 % of patients who had stenting had an MI as compared to 2.3 % of patients who underwent CEA ($p=0.032$) [19]. Similarly, Bonati et al. reported in their systematic review that endovascular treatment was associated with lower risks of myocardial infarction (OR 0.44; $p=0.02$) [20].

Restenosis

A secondary analysis of the CREST showed similar rates of restenosis of ≥70 % after CAS (6 %) and CEA (6.3 %) during a 2-year follow-up period [23]. The SPACE trial reported that the rate of restenosis of ≥70 % at 2 years was 10.7 %

versus 4.6 % for CEA ($p = 0.0009$) [15]. The EVA-3S investigators reported that the rate of ≥50 % restenosis at 2 years was significantly higher with CAS than with CEA (12.5 % after CAS and 5 % after CEA) [24]. They concluded that the short-term rate of carotid restenosis of ≥50 % or occlusion is around 2.5 times more common after CAS than after CEA. Compared to the other studies, the CAVATAS trial reported higher rates of restenosis. The rate of restenosis of ≥50 % was 36.6 % with CAS versus 31.5 % with CEA, and rate of restenosis of ≥70 % was 16.6 % with CAS versus 10.5 % with CEA [25]. In general, restenosis during follow-up is more common in patients receiving endovascular treatment than in patients assigned to CEA.

Other Complications

The risk of perioperative adverse events ranges from 2.5 % to 6 % with either CEA or CAS. Possible complications of CEA include stroke, MI, hemorrhage, hypertension, hypotension, acute arterial occlusion, venous thromboembolism, infection, cranial nerve palsy, hematomas, restenosis, and death. Complications of CAS include stroke, access-site complications, target vessel perforation and dissection, external carotid artery occlusion, device malfunction, restenosis, and death. In CREST, the risk of cranial nerve palsy was reported to be significantly lower with CAS than with CEA (0.3 % versus 4.8 %; $p < 0.05$) [19]. The ICSS trial reported that cranial nerve palsies were almost completely avoided by stenting and that there were fewer hematomas of any severity in the stenting group than in the endarterectomy group [11]. The EVA-3S investigators reported that there were more major local complications after stenting and more systemic complications (mainly pulmonary) after endarterectomy [13]. Cranial nerve injury was more common after endarterectomy than after stenting. They added that median duration of the hospital stay was shorter after stenting. Bonati et al. reported that cranial nerve palsy and access-site hematomas were significantly more common with CEA [12].

Cost-Effectiveness

Studies have shown that CAS is associated with better quality of life (e.g., less physical limitations and pain) during the early recovery period as compared with CEA, but the differences are not evident with longer-term follow-up [26]. A sub-analysis of the SAPPHIRE trial showed that the procedural costs of CAS are considerably higher than CEA, but the difference in total hospital costs is less significant as a result of reduction in the hospital stay length and procedural complications [27]. Similarly, the CREST showed that although initial procedural costs were higher with CAS, post-procedure costs and physician costs were lower such that total costs were similar with CAS and CEA [28].

Embolic Protection Devices

The greatest concern with endovascular management of atherosclerotic carotid disease is the risk of thromboembolic complications. Diffuse cerebral embolization has been confirmed to occur during CAS by transcranial Doppler (TCD) studies and diffusion-weighted magnetic resonance imaging (DWI). Crawley et al. examined patients with TCD during CEA and unprotected CAS and reported that CAS was associated with four times the number of embolic signals on TCD [29]. Such studies have confirmed that embolization during CAS occurs more frequently than during CEA [30]. With the accumulating experience and technical advancements, several studies have reported that it is possible to decrease CAS-related embolic complications with the use of embolic protection devices. However, whether the use of EPDs will enhance the safety of CAS is a continuing debate. In 2004, the EVA-3S investigators decided to change their protocol to use embolic protection devices during all CAS procedures because they found evidence of lower 30-day risk of stroke or death in patients treated with an EPD device (7.9 % versus 25 %; $p<0.03$) [13]. On the other hand, the SPACE trial did not find any significant difference in the periprocedural complication rate between patients with and without EPD (7 % in both groups of patients) [16]. Currently there is no level I evidence from randomized controlled trials proving the necessity of EPDs in all cases; however, there is level III and IV data from case series that suggest that the use of EPDs has improved the results of CAS with lower rates of neurologic complications. Cremonesi et al. reported a low overall complication rate (3.4 %) and ipsilateral stroke rate (1.1 %) after protected CAS [31]. Cosottini et al. reported that embolic cerebral lesions detected on DWI are more frequent with unprotected than with protected CAS, although they can still occur with the use of cerebral protection devices [32]. These results are further supported by several review studies. A systematic review that included 11 trials compared CAS with EPD in 839 patients and CAS without EPD in 2,537 patients and found the risk of perioperative stroke and death to be 5.5 % in patients treated without embolic protection versus only 1.8 % in those treated with cerebral protection with a decrease in both minor strokes (3.7 % without cerebral protection versus 0.5 % with cerebral protection, $P<0.001$) and major strokes (1.1 % without cerebral protection versus 0.3 % with cerebral protection, $P<0.05$) [33]. The authors concluded that the use of embolic protection devices seemed to reduce thromboembolic complications. In another systematic review of 32 studies comprising 1,363 patients who underwent CAS, Schnaudigel et al. reported that the incidence of new DWI lesions was significantly lower with the use of EPDs (33 %) than without EPDs (45 %; $p<0.01$). Other studies failed to show the benefit of using EPDs in patients undergoing CAS. A subanalysis of the ICSS trial showed that there were more lesions on DWI after CAS with the use of EPD than after unprotected stenting [34]. These findings were also demonstrated in two small trials. Macdonald et al. reported that new lesions on DWI and TCD occurred more often with the use of EPDs [35]. Barbato et al. reported that new MRI lesions occurred in 72 % of patients with EPD compared with 44 % in patients without EPD ($P=0.09$) [36].

Although some studies have argued against the use of EPD and despite the lack of randomized controlled trials that support its use, EPDs have become widely used in patients being managed with CAS. The types of embolic protection devices include temporary distal balloon occlusion devices, intravascular filter devices, or flow reversal devices. Several studies have attempted to compare different EPDs, proximal versus distal and individual types of EPDs, but most studies found a comparable safety and efficacy with the different devices [37, 38].

Conclusion

In conclusion, the management of carotid disease has greatly evolved in recent years. CEA remains the standard procedure for carotid revascularization, but CAS has emerged as a valid and reasonable alternative for many patients. CEA promises a lower risk of perioperative stroke and restenosis but higher risk of myocardial infarction and other perioperative complications. Both CEA and CAS have great safety and efficacy profiles that are constantly improving with technical advancements and higher level of operator experience, and both interventions promise comparable long-term outcomes.

References

1. Mozaffarian D, Benjamin EJ, Go AS, et al. Heart disease and stroke statistics – 2015 update: a report from the American Heart Association. Circulation. 2015;131(4):e29–322.
2. Biller J, Feinberg WM, Castaldo JE, et al. Guidelines for carotid endarterectomy: a statement for healthcare professionals from a special writing group of the Stroke Council, American Heart Association. Stroke; J Cereb Circ. 1998;29(2):554–62.
3. Beneficial effect of carotid endarterectomy in symptomatic patients with high-grade carotid stenosis. N Engl J Med. 1991;325(7):445–53.
4. Barnett HJ, Taylor DW, Eliasziw M, et al. Benefit of carotid endarterectomy in patients with symptomatic moderate or severe stenosis. North American Symptomatic Carotid Endarterectomy Trial Collaborators. N Engl J Med. 1998;339(20):1415–25.
5. Randomised trial of endarterectomy for recently symptomatic carotid stenosis: final results of the MRC European Carotid Surgery Trial (ECST). Lancet. 1998;351(9113):1379–87.
6. Rothwell PM, Eliasziw M, Gutnikov SA, et al. Analysis of pooled data from the randomised controlled trials of endarterectomy for symptomatic carotid stenosis. Lancet. 2003;361(9352):107–16.
7. Endarterectomy for asymptomatic carotid artery stenosis. Executive committee for the asymptomatic carotid atherosclerosis study. JAMA: J Am Med Assoc. 1995;273(18):1421–8.
8. Halliday A, Mansfield A, Marro J, et al. Prevention of disabling and fatal strokes by successful carotid endarterectomy in patients without recent neurological symptoms: randomised controlled trial. Lancet. 2004;363(9420):1491–502.
9. Halliday A, Harrison M, Hayter E, et al. 10-year stroke prevention after successful carotid endarterectomy for asymptomatic stenosis (ACST-1): a multicentre randomised trial. Lancet. 2010;376(9746):1074–84.
10. Brott TG, Halperin JL, Abbara S, et al. ASA/ACCF/AHA/AANN/AANS/ACR/ASNR/CNS/SAIP/SCAI/SIR/SNIS/SVM/SVS guideline on the management of patients with extracranial carotid and vertebral artery disease. A report of the American College of Cardiology Foundation/American Heart Association Task Force on Practice Guidelines, and the American Stroke Association, American Association of Neuroscience Nurses, American Association of

Neurological Surgeons, American College of Radiology, American Society of Neuroradiology, Congress of Neurological Surgeons, Society of Atherosclerosis Imaging and Prevention, Society for Cardiovascular Angiography and Interventions, Society of Interventional Radiology, Society of NeuroInterventional Surgery, Society for Vascular Medicine, and Society for Vascular Surgery. Circulation. 2011;124(4):e54–130.

11. Ederle J, Dobson J, Featherstone RL, et al. Carotid artery stenting compared with endarterectomy in patients with symptomatic carotid stenosis (International Carotid Stenting Study): an interim analysis of a randomised controlled trial. Lancet. 2010;375(9719):985–97.
12. Bonati LH, Dobson J, Featherstone RL, et al. Long-term outcomes after stenting versus endarterectomy for treatment of symptomatic carotid stenosis: the International Carotid Stenting Study (ICSS) randomised trial. Lancet. 2015;385(9967):529–38.
13. Mas JL, Chatellier G, Beyssen B, et al. Endarterectomy versus stenting in patients with symptomatic severe carotid stenosis. N Engl J Med. 2006;355(16):1660–71.
14. Mas JL, Trinquart L, Leys D, et al. Endarterectomy versus angioplasty in patients with symptomatic severe carotid stenosis (EVA-3S) trial: results up to 4 years from a randomised, multicentre trial. Lancet Neurol. 2008;7(10):885–92.
15. Eckstein HH, Ringleb P, Allenberg JR, et al. Results of the Stent-Protected Angioplasty versus Carotid Endarterectomy (SPACE) study to treat symptomatic stenoses at 2 years: a multinational, prospective, randomised trial. Lancet Neurol. 2008;7(10):893–902.
16. Ringleb PA, Allenberg J, Bruckmann H, et al. 30 day results from the SPACE trial of stent-protected angioplasty versus carotid endarterectomy in symptomatic patients: a randomised non-inferiority trial. Lancet. 2006;368(9543):1239–47.
17. Yadav JS, Wholey MH, Kuntz RE, et al. Protected carotid-artery stenting versus endarterectomy in high-risk patients. N Engl J Med. 2004;351(15):1493–501.
18. Gurm HS, Yadav JS, Fayad P, et al. Long-term results of carotid stenting versus endarterectomy in high-risk patients. N Engl J Med. 2008;358(15):1572–9.
19. Brott TG, Hobson 2nd RW, Howard G, et al. Stenting versus endarterectomy for treatment of carotid-artery stenosis. N Engl J Med. 2010;363(1):11–23.
20. Bonati LH, Lyrer P, Ederle J, Featherstone R, Brown MM. Percutaneous transluminal balloon angioplasty and stenting for carotid artery stenosis. Cochrane Database Syst Rev. 2012;9:Cd000515.
21. Economopoulos KP, Sergentanis TN, Tsivgoulis G, Mariolis AD, Stefanadis C. Carotid artery stenting versus carotid endarterectomy: a comprehensive meta-analysis of short-term and long-term outcomes. Stroke; J Cereb Circ. 2011;42(3):687–92.
22. Bangalore S, Bhatt DL, Rother J, et al. Late outcomes after carotid artery stenting versus carotid endarterectomy: insights from a propensity-matched analysis of the Reduction of Atherothrombosis for Continued Health (REACH) Registry. Circulation. 2010;122(11):1091–100.
23. Lal BK, Beach KW, Roubin GS, et al. Restenosis after carotid artery stenting and endarterectomy: a secondary analysis of CREST, a randomised controlled trial. Lancet Neurol. 2012;11(9):755–63.
24. Arquizan C, Trinquart L, Touboul PJ, et al. Restenosis is more frequent after carotid stenting than after endarterectomy: the EVA-3S study. Stroke; J Cereb Circ. 2011;42(4):1015–20.
25. Bonati LH, Ederle J, McCabe DJ, et al. Long-term risk of carotid restenosis in patients randomly assigned to endovascular treatment or endarterectomy in the Carotid and Vertebral Artery Transluminal Angioplasty Study (CAVATAS): long-term follow-up of a randomised trial. Lancet Neurol. 2009;8(10):908–17.
26. Cohen DJ, Stolker JM, Wang K, et al. Health-related quality of life after carotid stenting versus carotid endarterectomy: results from CREST (Carotid Revascularization Endarterectomy Versus Stenting Trial). J Am Coll Cardiol. 2011;58(15):1557–65.
27. Mahoney EM, Greenberg D, Lavelle TA, et al. Costs and cost-effectiveness of carotid stenting versus endarterectomy for patients at increased surgical risk: results from the SAPPHIRE trial. Cathet Cardiovasc Interv: Off J Soc Card Angiography Interv. 2011;77(4):463–72.

28. Vilain KR, Magnuson EA, Li H, et al. Costs and cost-effectiveness of carotid stenting versus endarterectomy for patients at standard surgical risk: results from the Carotid Revascularization Endarterectomy Versus Stenting Trial (CREST). Stroke; J Cereb Circ. 2012;43(9):2408–16.
29. Crawley F, Stygall J, Lunn S, Harrison M, Brown MM, Newman S. Comparison of microembolism detected by transcranial Doppler and neuropsychological sequelae of carotid surgery and percutaneous transluminal angioplasty. Stroke; J Cereb Circ. 2000;31(6):1329–34.
30. Atkins MD, Bush RL. Embolic protection devices for carotid artery stenting: have they made a significant difference in outcomes? Semin Vasc Surg. 2007;20(4):244–51.
31. Cremonesi A, Manetti R, Setacci F, Setacci C, Castriota F. Protected carotid stenting: clinical advantages and complications of embolic protection devices in 442 consecutive patients. Stroke; J Cereb Circ. 2003;34(8):1936–41.
32. Cosottini M, Michelassi MC, Puglioli M, et al. Silent cerebral ischemia detected with diffusion-weighted imaging in patients treated with protected and unprotected carotid artery stenting. Stroke; J Cereb Circ. 2005;36(11):2389–93.
33. Kastrup A, Groschel K, Krapf H, Brehm BR, Dichgans J, Schulz JB. Early outcome of carotid angioplasty and stenting with and without cerebral protection devices: a systematic review of the literature. Stroke; J Cereb Circ. 2003;34(3):813–9.
34. Gensicke H, Zumbrunn T, Jongen LM, et al. Characteristics of ischemic brain lesions after stenting or endarterectomy for symptomatic carotid artery stenosis: results from the international carotid stenting study-magnetic resonance imaging substudy. Stroke; J Cereb Circ. 2013;44(1):80–6.
35. Macdonald S, Evans DH, Griffiths PD, et al. Filter-protected versus unprotected carotid artery stenting: a randomised trial. Cerebrov Dis (Basel, Switzerland). 2010;29(3):282–9.
36. Barbato JE, Dillavou E, Horowitz MB, et al. A randomized trial of carotid artery stenting with and without cerebral protection. J Vasc Surg. 2008;47(4):760–5.
37. Hernandez-Fernandez F, Parrilla G, Garcia-Villalba B, et al. Comparison between proximal versus distal protection devices in 287 cases of carotid revascularization using angioplasty and stenting: periprocedure complications, morbidity, and mortality. Cardiovasc Intervent Radiol. 2014;37(3):639–45.
38. Mokin M, Dumont TM, Chi JM, et al. Proximal versus distal protection during carotid artery stenting: analysis of the two treatment approaches and associated clinical outcomes. World Neurosurg. 2014;81(3–4):543–8.

Arteriovenous Malformations: How We Changed Our Practice

14

Christoph J. Griessenauer, Parviz Dolati, Ajith Thomas, and Christopher S. Ogilvy

Introduction

Brain arteriovenous malformation (AVM) is a cluster of direct connections of arteries to draining veins without an intervening capillary bed [4]. The three main components of an AVM are one or more feeding arteries, the nidus as the site of the arteriovenous shunt, and the draining venous structures. Arteriovenous malformations are high-flow, low-resistant shunts due to a significant pressure difference between the arterial and venous side. The pressure gradient and resultant high flow trigger remodeling of both arteries and draining veins. Arteries may be dilated and thin walled due to degeneration of the media and elastic lamina or thickened from endothelial proliferation, hypertrophy of the media, and changes in the basal lamina. Remodeling of the venous system is referred to as arterialization and includes thickening of the wall due to cellular proliferation without an organized elastic lamina [4, 10]. The draining veins commonly coalesce and form a major draining vein that eventually drains into a dural venous sinus. The pathogenesis of the AVM has not been fully elucidated. The predominant theory is that AVMs are congenital in nature and result from incomplete or abnormal resolution of a primitive vascular plexus that occurs during early embryogenesis [2]. One explanation for why they are rarely detected in utero or in infants is that they first appear in utero but then continue to grow after birth. There is also growing evidences for postnatal de novo formation of these lesions [7, 17, 21]. Recent studies have identified some of the factors that may be involved in the formation of AVMs. One of them is endothelin-1, found throughout the normal cerebral vasculature, and a potent vasoconstrictor that plays a role in vascular cell growth. Local repression of endothelin-1 within the

C.J. Griessenauer, MD • P. Dolati, MD • A. Thomas, MD • C.S. Ogilvy, MD (✉)
Neurosurgical Service, Beth Israel Deaconess Medical Center, Brain Aneurysm Institute, Harvard Medical School, Boston, MA, USA
e-mail: cogilvy@bidmc.harvard.edu

E. Veznedaroglu (ed.), *Controversies in Vascular Neurosurgery*,
DOI 10.1007/978-3-319-27315-0_14

AVM has been implicated in the pathophysiology underlying AVMs [23]. Endothelial cell-specific tyrosine kinases that are normally found in developing embryonic blood vessels and vascular endothelial growth factor have been shown to be increased in association with AVMs [12].

Anatomic Features

Arteriovenous malformations are equally distributed between both hemispheres and most commonly seen in the frontal and parietal lobes. Typically, AVMs are pyramidal-shaped lesions with the base oriented toward the meninges and the apex pointing to the ventricle or deep into the brain. Three types of feeding arteries have been described and include terminal, pseudoterminal, and indirect, or en passage, feeders [10]. The surrounding parenchyma may be stained from previous hemorrhage, and the overlying meninges tend to have a thickened, fibrotic appearance. While there is usually no functional brain tissue within the AVM, AVM vessels may be separated by the normal brain in diffuse lesions [10]. The brain parenchyma surrounding or within the nidus may show evidence of edema, necrosis, and gliosis as a result of ischemic injury related to vascular steal and venous hypertension.

Epidemiology and Natural History

Estimates of the prevalence of AVMs range from 0.005 to 0.6 % in the general population and are believed to be about one-tenth as common as intracranial aneurysms [10]. The incidence of first ever AVM hemorrhage is 0.51 per 100,000 person-years. Arteriovenous malformations are slightly more common in males and diagnosed at a mean age of 31.2 years [10]. Up to 9 % of patients have multiple AVMs, and most of these patients have an associated vascular syndrome such as hereditary hemorrhagic telangiectasia, Wyburn-Mason syndrome, or Sturge-Weber syndrome. While the majority of AVMs are sporadic, familial intracranial AVMs have also been reported [10].

Hemorrhage was the most common manifestation prior to noninvasive imaging. In recent decades, the detection rates of unruptured AVMs have doubled due to availability and advances in imaging [1, 27]. Early retrospective data including previously ruptured AVMs estimated the annual rupture rate at approximately 4 % [20]. A more recent prospective study estimated rupture rates as low as 0.9 % per year for unruptured AVMs [28]. On the other hand, annual rupture rates may be as high as 34.4 % for AVMs that have ruptured previously and are located deep in the brain with deep venous drainage [28]. A meta-analysis estimated the overall annual rupture rate at 3 % with a rate of rupture of 2.2 % and 4.5 % for unruptured and previously ruptured AVMs, respectively [8]. The risk of re-rupture is greatest in the first year after the initial hemorrhage at about 7 % [9].

Features that pose increase risk of rupture include previous hemorrhage, particularly within 1 year, deep location, deep venous drainage, associated aneurysms along the feeding vessels or within the nidus, location in the posterior fossa or intra- and periventricular, and venous outflow obstruction [6, 8, 13, 28]. The effects of AVM size on hemorrhage risks are controversial [10]. Overall, an annual rupture risk of 2–4 % is frequently cited for unruptured AVMs [10].

Clinical Presentation

The most common presentation for an AVM is hemorrhage located in the brain parenchyma often with intraventricular extension. Isolated intraventricular hemorrhage and subarachnoid hemorrhage may also occur [16]. Cortically based AVMs are more likely to cause subarachnoid hemorrhage [22]. The initial hemorrhage or hemorrhage during follow-up appears to carry a lower morbidity than intracranial hemorrhage from other causes [5, 29]. After hemorrhage, seizures are the second most common-presenting symptom in about 20–25 % of patients [10]. In a series of patients with unruptured AVMs, specific angioarchitectural characteristics such as location, fistulous component in the nidus, venous outflow stenosis, and the presence of a long pial course of the draining vein were identified as the strongest predictors of seizures [25]. Lastly, headaches, focal neurological deficits, and developmental learning disorders have been reported [10].

Management

Management options for patients with an AVM include expectant management, surgery, radiosurgery, endovascular embolization, or a combination [10, 11, 29]. Surgery and radiosurgery comprise the mainstay of treatment with embolization as a useful preparatory step for either of the two treatment options. Expectant management is indicated for large lesions that are difficult to treat and associated with significant morbidity and mortality.

Surgery

Surgical resection is the gold standard for small, accessible AVMs, and the decision-making process begins with stratification according to the Spetzler-Martin grading system. Surgery accomplishes obliteration rates of 94–100 % for Spetzler-Martin grade I–III AVMs, which account for approximately 60–80 % of all AVMs. There is a paucity of data on obliteration rates for surgery on Spetzler-Martin IV and V AVMs alone as most of these lesions are subject to multimodality treatment. There is a good correlation of increasing morbidity and mortality with higher Spetzler-Martin grades [10, 26].

Radiosurgery

Radiosurgery involves the administration of multiple beams of radiation that meet at one target or isocenter. The radiation primarily damages the endothelial cells within the AVM which leads to progressive occlusion of the vessel due to proliferation of smooth muscle cells and myofibroblasts and an accumulation of an extracellular collagen. Chronic inflammation induces the formation of the granulation tissue in proximity to the AVM [10]. Radiosurgery is minimally invasive and relatively low risk and can be used for surgically inaccessible lesions. Obliteration is delayed by approximately 2–3 years from initial treatment and most effective for AVMs that are smaller in size. While at 2–5 years of follow-up, 70–95 % of AVMs with a nidus diameter of <3 cm are obliterated that rate drops to <70 % of AVMs >3 cm. The risk of hemorrhage during the latency period is somewhat controversial but may be reduced compared to the pre-radiation risk [15]. An unsecured aneurysm proximal to the nidus increases the risk of rupture, and even after complete angiographic AVM obliteration, there may be a low risk of rupture of 0.3 % [10]. Seizures are effectively treated with radiosurgery with seizure-free rates ranging from 51 to 80 % [10]. There is a good dose-response correlation for treatment with up to 25 Gy with minimal additional benefit in regard to obliteration rates and substantial increase in side effects above that dose [10].

Embolization

Embolization as the sole treatment for a cure of an AVM is uncommon and accomplished in only 5–10 % of cases as most AVMs have multiple feeders, and not all of them can be safely catheterized. Embolization is currently applied mostly presurgical or pre-radiosurgical and used to occlude deep feeders. Preoperative embolization decreases the morbidity associated with surgery for higher Spetzler-Martin grades to the level of lower-grade lesions that are not embolized preoperatively [14]. Some argue that at least 50 % of the AVM nidus has to be obliterated with embolization to accomplish a definitive gain during surgical resection [31]. Permanent morbidity related to presurgical embolization varied from 4 to 8.9 % [3]. The main goal of pre-radiosurgery embolization is to decrease the size of the nidus, thus reducing the radiation dose necessary [10].

Medical Management With or Without Interventional Therapy for Unruptured Brain Arteriovenous Malformations (ARUBA) Trial

The ARUBA trial was a prospective, non-blinded, randomized trial that enrolled 223 adult patients with unruptured AVMs at 39 clinical sites in nine countries and compared interventions (using any treatment modality alone or in combination) to medical management. The trial was stopped prematurely after the primary endpoint of stroke or death was reached and found to be significantly higher in the interventional compared to the observational arm (hazard ratio 0·27, 95% CI 0·14–0·54) [18]. The ARUBA trial, or the "elephant in the room of AVM management" as it has been referred to [30], has sparked animated discussions among all disciplines involved in the care of patients with AVMs. The enrolled cohort had a heterogenous group of unruptured AVMs with >10% of lesions Spetzler-Martin grade IV, and >25% were grade III AVMs, namely, those known to carry higher risks with treatment [2]. Any comparison of an intervention with expectant management is initially in favor of the expectant management as any intervention comes with an up-front risk that may be offset over time due to the natural history of the disease. This is of particular importance for a lifelong disease such as an untreated AVM. Furthermore, there was a high rate of embolization as the sole treatment (32% of patients), a treatment modality known to be associated with a low rate of obliteration. Only 5% of patients were treated with surgery, the only imminent cure for AVMs, despite two-thirds of patients harboring Spetzler-Martin grade I and II AVMs, which were amendable to surgical treatment. Neither accurately reflects current AVM management in the United States. Likewise, some well-known and recognized clinical centers have published their experience with ARUBA-eligible patients and found excellent outcomes with surgery in patients with AVMs of Spetzler-Martin grades I and II [19]. One of the studies concluded that the results in ARUBA-eligible patients managed outside the trial led to an entirely different conclusion about AVM intervention, due to the primary role of surgery, judicious surgical selection with established outcome predictors, and technical expertise developed at high-volume AVM centers [24]. Lastly, clinical equipoise is a necessary element in ensuring unbiased enrollment of patients into any trials. Concerns for lack of equipoise and resultant selective enrollment were the primary objection to participation in the trial and explanations for the low number of clinical sites in the United States involved [2].

The Treating Physicians

Given the complexity of decision-making in the management of brain AVMs, it is often of benefit to have a multidisciplinary team for the detailed discussions of risks and benefits of treatment of each modality and of projected combined treatment. In addition, the patient's age and overall medical condition are extremely important in balancing the risks of observation with no treatment compared to the risks of treatment. A team should consist of the surgeon experienced in the removal of brain AVMs, endovascular experts who routinely treat AVMs, and individuals who perform radiosurgery on a regular basis. The ARUBA data presented earlier is not significantly changed or management strategies for patients with brain AVMs. Young patients with low-grade lesions are often treated with surgical excision or embolization followed by surgical excision (Fig. 14.1). Older patients with higher Spencer Martin grade lesions are typically followed clinically without intervention.

One major advantage in the treatment of brain AVMs is to have individuals who perform endovascular treatments and open surgical resections. There is a

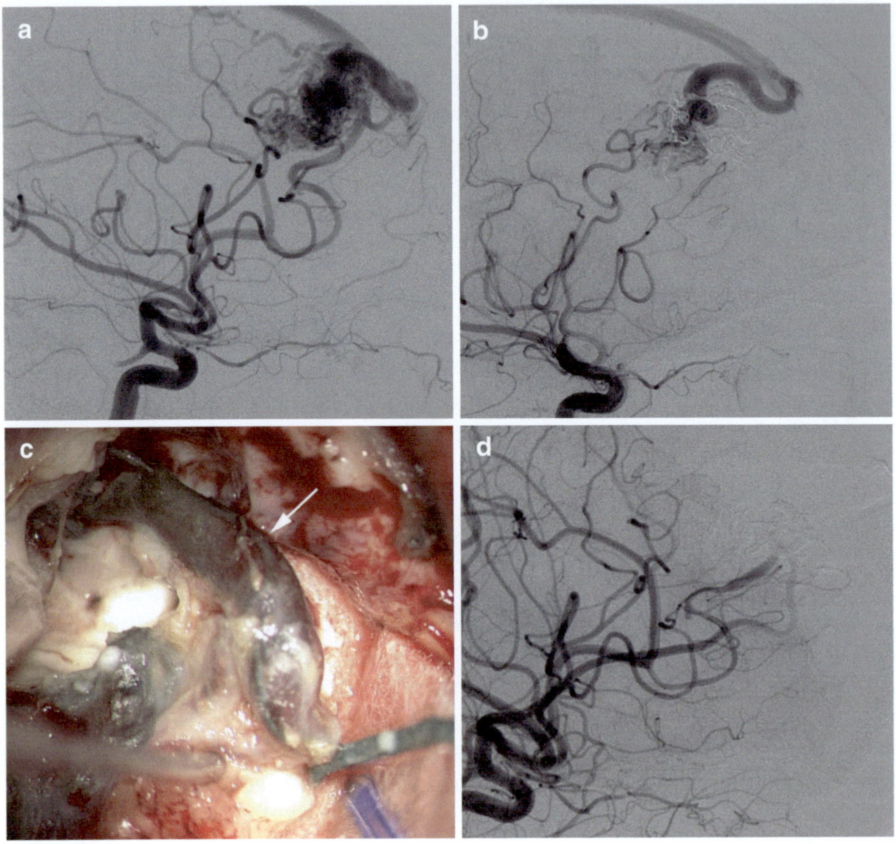

Fig. 14.1 A 32-year-old female presenting with headaches found to have left medial frontal Spetzler-Martin grade II AVM. The patient favored treatment and was preoperatively embolized with Onyx® (Covidien, Mansfield, MA) and subsequently underwent a craniotomy for AVM resection. Neurologically, she did well throughout the course of her treatment. Panels (**a, b**) show the Spetzler-Martin grade II AVM on a lateral injection of the left internal carotid artery before and after embolization, respectively. Intraoperatively, the detachable Apollo™ Detachable Tip microcatheter tip (Covidien, Mansfield, MA) (*white arrow*) used for Onyx injection was visualized in the main feeding artery (Panel **c**). Postoperative lateral angiogram of the left common carotid artery showed complete resection of the AVM (Panel **d**)

greater appreciation for the detailed angioarchitecture acquired during embolization procedures. Armed with this information, the surgeon has a much better sense of the anatomy and physiology of the AVM on the day of surgical excision. By having been the individual who treated the patient with embolization on anywhere from one to three previous treatments, the surgeon had time to digest the remaining details of the AVM for surgical excision. While it is difficult to prove how this helps statistically, individuals who perform embolization and then the surgery can attest to the increased safety and efficacy of this type of approach.

If indeed the person performing embolization is a different individual of the one performing surgical resection, there has to be an excellent and detailed communication between the two individuals regarding the anatomy and physiology of the AVM. Review session should be undertaken to salute all parties involved in understanding the different components of the AVM, where embolization has been performed, and what remains for subsequent surgical or radiosurgical obliteration. Working in a center that manages a high volume of AVM patients facilitates an increased understanding of the pathophysiology and management of brain AVMs.

References

1. Al-Shahi R, Bhattacharya JJ, Currie DG, Papanastassiou V, Ritchie V, Roberts RC, et al. Scottish Intracranial Vascular Malformation Study Collaborators: prospective, population-based detection of intracranial vascular malformations in adults: the Scottish Intracranial Vascular Malformation Study (SIVMS). Stroke J Cereb Circ. 2003;34:1163–9.
2. Amin-Hanjani S. ARUBA results are not applicable to all patients with arteriovenous malformation. Stroke J Cereb Circ. 2014;45:1539–40.
3. Castel JP, Kantor G. Postoperative morbidity and mortality after microsurgical exclusion of cerebral arteriovenous malformations. Current data and analysis of recent literature. Neurochirurgie. 2001;47:369–83.
4. Challa VR, Moody DM, Brown WR. Vascular malformations of the central nervous system. J Neuropathol Exp Neurol. 1995;54:609–21.
5. Choi BS, Park JW, Kim JL, Kim SY, Park YS, Kwon H-J, et al. Treatment strategy based on multimodal management outcome of Cavernous Sinus Dural Arteriovenous Fistula (CSDAVF). Neurointervention. 2011;6:6–12.
6. Da Costa L, Wallace MC, Ter Brugge KG, O'Kelly C, Willinsky RA, Tymianski M. The natural history and predictive features of hemorrhage from brain arteriovenous malformations. Stroke J Cereb Circ. 2009;40:100–5.
7. Fujimura M, Kimura N, Ezura M, Niizuma K, Uenohara H, Tominaga T. Development of a de novo arteriovenous malformation after bilateral revascularization surgery in a child with moyamoya disease. J Neurosurg Pediatr. 2014;13:647–9.
8. Gross BA, Du R. Natural history of cerebral arteriovenous malformations: a meta-analysis. J Neurosurg. 2013;118:437–43.
9. Halim AX, Johnston SC, Singh V, McCulloch CE, Bennett JP, Achrol AS, et al. Longitudinal risk of intracranial hemorrhage in patients with arteriovenous malformation of the brain within a defined population. Stroke J Cereb Circ. 2004;35:1697–702.
10. Harrigan M, Deveikis J. Arteriovenous malformations. In: Handbook of cerebrovascular disease and neurointerventional technique. New York: Humana Press, Springer; 2009. p. 511–27.
11. Hartmann A, Mast H, Mohr JP, Pile-Spellman J, Connolly ES, Sciacca RR, et al. Determinants of staged endovascular and surgical treatment outcome of brain arteriovenous malformations. Stroke J Cereb Circ. 2005;36:2431–5.
12. Hatva E, Jääskeläinen J, Hirvonen H, Alitalo K, Haltia M. Tie endothelial cell-specific receptor tyrosine kinase is upregulated in the vasculature of arteriovenous malformations. J Neuropathol Exp Neurol. 1996;55:1124–33.
13. Hernesniemi JA, Dashti R, Juvela S, Väärt K, Niemelä M, Laakso A. Natural history of brain arteriovenous malformations: a long-term follow-up study of risk of hemorrhage in 238 patients. Neurosurgery. 2008;63:823–9; discussion 829–831.
14. Jafar JJ, Davis AJ, Berenstein A, Choi IS, Kupersmith MJ. The effect of embolization with N-butyl cyanoacrylate prior to surgical resection of cerebral arteriovenous malformations. J Neurosurg. 1993;78:60–9.

15. Karlsson B, Jokura H, Yamamoto M, Söderman M, Lax I. Is repeated radiosurgery an alternative to staged radiosurgery for very large brain arteriovenous malformations? J Neurosurg. 2007;107:740–4.
16. LeBlanc R, Ethier R, Little JR. Computerized tomography findings in arteriovenous malformations of the brain. J Neurosurg. 1979;51:765–72.
17. Miller BA, Bass DI, Chern JJ. Development of a de novo arteriovenous malformation after severe traumatic brain injury. J Neurosurg Pediatr. 2014;14:418–20.
18. Mohr JP, Parides MK, Stapf C, Moquete E, Moy CS, Overbey JR, et al. International ARUBA investigators: medical management with or without interventional therapy for unruptured brain arteriovenous malformations (ARUBA): a multicentre, non-blinded, randomised trial. Lancet. 2014;383:614–21.
19. Nerva JD, Mantovani A, Barber J, Kim LJ, Rockhill JK, Hallam DK, et al. Treatment outcomes of unruptured arteriovenous malformations with a subgroup analysis of ARUBA (A Randomized Trial of Unruptured Brain Arteriovenous Malformations)-eligible patients. Neurosurgery. 2015;76:563–70; discussion570; quiz 570.
20. Ondra SL, Troupp H, George ED, Schwab K. The natural history of symptomatic arteriovenous malformations of the brain: a 24-year follow-up assessment. J Neurosurg. 1990;73: 387–91.
21. O'Shaughnessy BA, Getch CC, Bendok BR, Batjer HH. Microsurgical resection of infratentorial arteriovenous malformations. Neurosurg Focus. 2005;19:E5.
22. Perret G, Nishioka H. Report on the cooperative study of intracranial aneurysms and subarachnoid hemorrhage. Section VI. Arteriovenous malformations. An analysis of 545 cases of cranio-cerebral arteriovenous malformations and fistulae reported to the cooperative study. J Neurosurg. 1966;25:467–90.
23. Rhoten RL, Comair YG, Shedid D, Chyatte D, Simonson MS. Specific repression of the preproendothelin-1 gene in intracranial arteriovenous malformations. J Neurosurg. 1997;86: 101–8.
24. Rutledge WC, Abla AA, Nelson J, Halbach VV, Kim H, Lawton MT. Treatment and outcomes of ARUBA-eligible patients with unruptured brain arteriovenous malformations at a single institution. Neurosurg Focus. 2014;37:E8.
25. Shankar JJS, Menezes RJ, Pohlmann-Eden B, Wallace C, terBrugge K, Krings T. Angioarchitecture of brain AVM determines the presentation with seizures: proposed scoring system. AJNR Am J Neuroradiol. 2013;34:1028–34.
26. Spetzler RF, Martin NA. A proposed grading system for arteriovenous malformations. J Neurosurg. 1986;65:476–83.
27. Stapf C, Mast H, Sciacca RR, Berenstein A, Nelson PK, Gobin YP, et al. New York Islands AVM Study Collaborators: the New York Islands AVM Study: design, study progress, and initial results. Stroke J Cereb Circ. 2003;34:e29–33.
28. Stapf C, Mast H, Sciacca RR, Choi JH, Khaw AV, Connolly ES, et al. Predictors of hemorrhage in patients with untreated brain arteriovenous malformation. Neurology. 2006;66: 1350–5.
29. Van Beijnum J, Lovelock CE, Cordonnier C, Rothwell PM, Klijn CJM, Al-Shahi Salman R. SIVMS Steering Committee and the Oxford Vascular Study: outcome after spontaneous and arteriovenous malformation-related intracerebral haemorrhage: population-based studies. Brain J Neurol. 2009;132:537–43.
30. Van Loveren H. Current treatments of AVM's (66th Southern Neurosurgical Society Annual Meeting). Naples, FL, 2015.
31. Viñuela F, Dion JE, Duckwiler G, Martin NA, Lylyk P, Fox A, et al. Combined endovascular embolization and surgery in the management of cerebral arteriovenous malformations: experience with 101 cases. J Neurosurg. 1991;75:856–64.

Discussion

15

Kenneth M. Liebman, Vikas Y. Rao, and Gerald W. Eckardt

The authors discuss the different treatments available for cerebral arteriovenous malformations (AVMs) and discuss the various studies that may have changed their approach toward AVM management. It is well understood that the main treatment modalities include endovascular embolization, surgical extirpation, and stereotactic radiosurgery. The more likely scenario is using a combination of the above modalities to treat the lesion. Another management option is not to intervene but rather take a conservative approach which entails following the patient radiographically and clinically.

Intracerebral hemorrhage is the most common and devastating presentation of cerebral AVMs. There is little controversy that a hemorrhagic presentation indicates a worse natural history for the lesion and warrants treatment. The main treatment dilemma for neurosurgeons is to determine if intervention is indicated for patients who present with an unruptured AVM. For treatment to be a viable option for all, the risk of treatment and its associated morbidity and mortality must be lower than the natural history of the disease itself, the risk of spontaneous hemorrhage.

As discussed in the chapter, Ondra and Troup's landmark study [1], published in 1990, reported that the risk of bleeding was 2–4 % on an annual basis with a risk of mortality and major morbidity being 2.7 % per year. These statistics were irrespective of presentation – with or without rupture. Since the data from Ondra et al. was acquired, there have been significant advances in the diagnosis and treatment of patients with cerebral AVMs. Although there were many issues with the study that make it not fully applicable to current treatment paradigms, it has often been used to support aggressive treatment of patients with AVMs. Over the last decade, newer studies attempting to better define the natural history of AVMs as well as the risk of AVM treatments have been undertaken. Newer data suggests that those patients who

K.M. Liebman (✉) • V.Y. Rao • G.W. Eckardt
Department of Neurosciences, Drexel University School of Medicine, Philadelphia, PA, USA
e-mail: kliebman@gnineuro.org

E. Veznedaroglu (ed.), *Controversies in Vascular Neurosurgery*,
DOI 10.1007/978-3-319-27315-0_15

present with incidental, unruptured malformations have a lower risk of spontaneous hemorrhage than previously thought [2]. These studies may redirect our approach toward the treatment of cerebral AVM – but then again maybe not.

The chapter authors describe the recently published ARUBA study (A Randomized Trial of Unruptured Brain Arteriovenous Malformations) which compared treatment vs. observation for unruptured brain AVMs [2]. The study concluded that medically managed patients had a significantly lower risk of death, stroke, or worsened functional outcome when compared to the intervention group. So, based on this one study, should all patients who present with unruptured AVMs not undergo an intervention until a hemorrhage occurs?

ARUBA must factor into our treatment algorithm for unruptured AVMs, comparable to the way that the International Study of Unruptured Intracranial Aneurysms (ISUIA) [3] has shaped our understanding and approach to unruptured aneurysms. The treating physicians looking to apply these studies to their patients, however, should understand their limitations.

Some of the key criticisms of the ARUBA study were reviewed including the low number of patients that underwent surgery despite evidence that it is safe and effective especially in the treatment of lower-grade AVMs [4–6], the high rate of embolization being the only modality used for treatment, the short follow-up time of the study, and the better results at particular ARUBA centers for patients not enrolled in ARUBA vs. those that were.

This chapter did not discuss one additional but important issue. The centers involved in this study did not enroll all eligible patients indicating a certain selection bias. Only 226 (13 %) of the 1,740 screened patients were randomized; 323 patients refused to participate, and clinicians selected a treatment outside the randomization process in 177 patients. These centers proceeded with a treatment or observation for the majority of eligible patients based on their clinical necessity – thus they were not randomized.

The authors reference the recent report from the University of California, San Francisco. The paper describes their, experience with ARUBA eligible patients [7]. This study can be utilized as a real-world example from one of the highest volume centers in the USA and illustrates the lack of randomization of eligible patients. Of 87 patients eligible for enrollment during the study period, only 4 (4.6 %) were randomized. The UCSF group presented their treatment and outcomes for a cohort of 74 patients who were eligible but not enrolled in ARUBA. These patients were not enrolled because the authors felt that their pathology necessitated a course of either therapy or observation and deferred randomization for this reason – thus illustrating the selection biases in the ARUBA data.

The ARUBA study, like ISUIA, was touted to be a prospective randomized trial, however harbored a large selection bias. What is very important for the reader to understand is that both studies are also essentially registries. Patients who presented with cerebral AVMs and subsequently underwent therapy were not included in the study, thus were not part of the randomization process. The patients who did not undergo a therapy were indeed randomized to a treatment vs. observation option. Thus, selection bias again is shown to be a significant issue with this study.

Based on the ARUBA trial and taking into account its limitations, it is difficult to truly form conclusions as to whether treatment or observation is more appropriate. Additionally it is even less clear that if treatment is to be performed for an AVM, what the safest and most effective treatment modality. That being said, there is still value in the results of the ARUBA publication. There is clear evidence to support the concept that not all AVMs warrant treatment. We don't disagree with this notion and think it is a valuable conclusion to mature to. Not all patients who present with the diagnosis of an AVM warrant an intervention, but all those patients certainly warrant observation, which includes clinical and radiographic follow up.

At our center, most patients presenting with unruptured AVMs undergo diagnostic cerebral angiography to identify angiographic features that increase the risk of rupture such as intranidal aneurysms, flow-related aneurysms, venous outflow restrictions, and venous varices. If the patients do have these angiographic features and they are identified as low-grade AVMs, surgical extirpation with or without embolization is recommended. This is especially true for the younger population.

This point is well illustrated in Fig. 15.1. This was a 50-year-old female who presented with headaches and was found to have a cerebellar AVM. The patient's Spetzler-Martin grade was 1; however, on diagnostic angiography, she had high-risk features (flow-related aneurysm, an intranidal aneurysm, and a venous varix). The patient underwent embolization followed by surgical extirpation without complication and was discharged 3 days postoperatively. She remains neurologically intact.

We have a propensity to observe patients who have high-grade AVMs (especially those which are >6 cm in size) and present without hemorrhage. One caveat is for those AVMs which are too large to cure but have high-risk features, specifically flow-related or intranidal aneurysms. We may approach these AVMs endovascularly with the goal of improving their natural history by targeting these high-risk features.

The concept of "whittling down" a high-grade AVM to make it more amenable to either radiosurgery or open surgery is often not successful. Embolizations of large AVMs often results in shutting down pedicles of the lesion but not necessarily decreasing the size of the lesion, taking away its deep venous drainage, or removing it from eloquent cortex.

The last decade has also led to advancements in the treatments available for AVMs and likewise potentially more successful and safer treatment algorithms [4–6]. When formulating a treatment plan, the goal of total angiographic obliteration of the disease is vital. While this may seem intuitive, in practice it is often not followed. Situations occur where a treating physician continues to only offer limited modalities of therapy and not graduate to another modality when it could lead to curing the lesion. Continued single modality treatment like this can make treatment of the disease more problematic and may result in the accumulation of the morbidities of each of the treatments. Multimodality approaches to these complex vascular lesions should be planned in such a way that they complement each other and improve the success and decrease the morbidity of subsequent treatments. At our center, all cerebrovascular lesions are treated by comprehensively trained open and endovascular neurosurgeons; thus a treatment algorithm from the onset can be

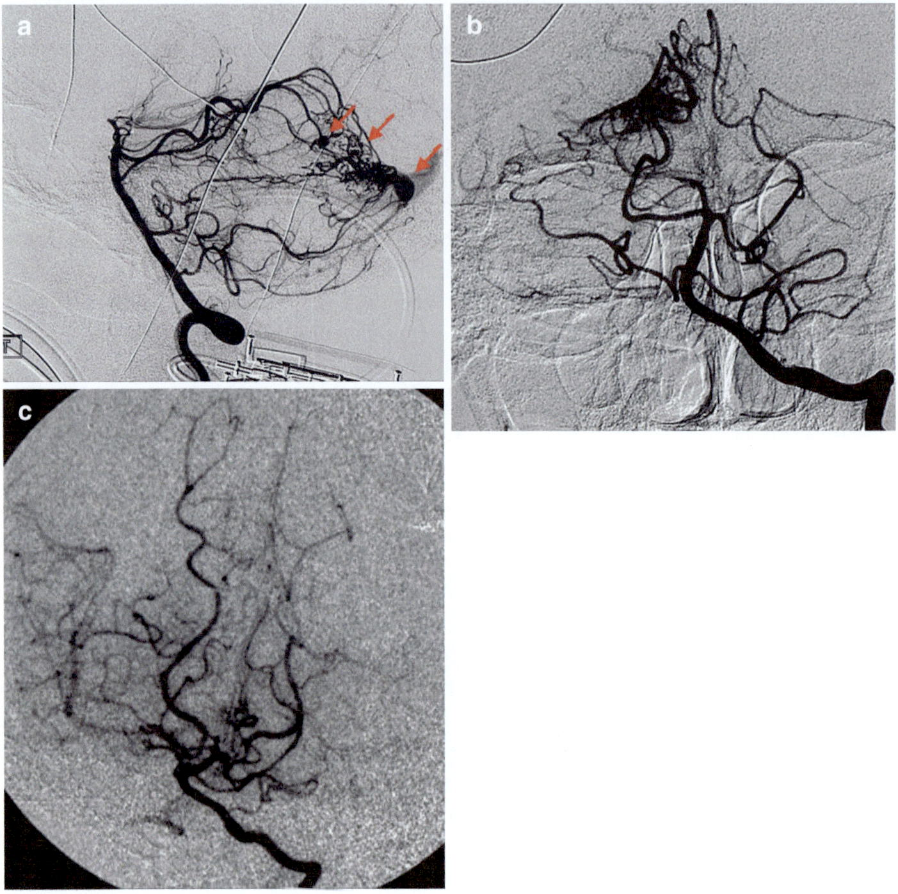

Fig. 15.1 Case example of a 50-year-old female with a Spetzler-Martin grade 1 AVM (**a**, **b**) treated because of high-risk features present on angiography (*arrows* indicating from *left* to *right*: flow-related aneurysm, intranidal aneurysm, and venous varix). The patient underwent embolization followed by surgery and had an excellent angiographic (**c**) and clinical result

directed toward angiographic obliteration without limitation to only open or endovascular techniques.

This point is well illustrated in the case presented in Fig. 15.2. This was a 55-year-old female who underwent multiple embolizations of an occipital AVM at an outside hospital. Her last embolization of this Spetzler-Martin grade 4 AVM left her with a homonymous hemianopsia. Since there was residual filling of this lesion, she was offered yet another embolization at the outside hospital and then came to see the senior author for a second opinion. As the patient already suffered a deficit from the embolization and further embolization was not going to achieve the goal of obliteration, surgery was recommended and subsequently the lesion was easily removed with no additional morbidity (Fig. 15.2c).

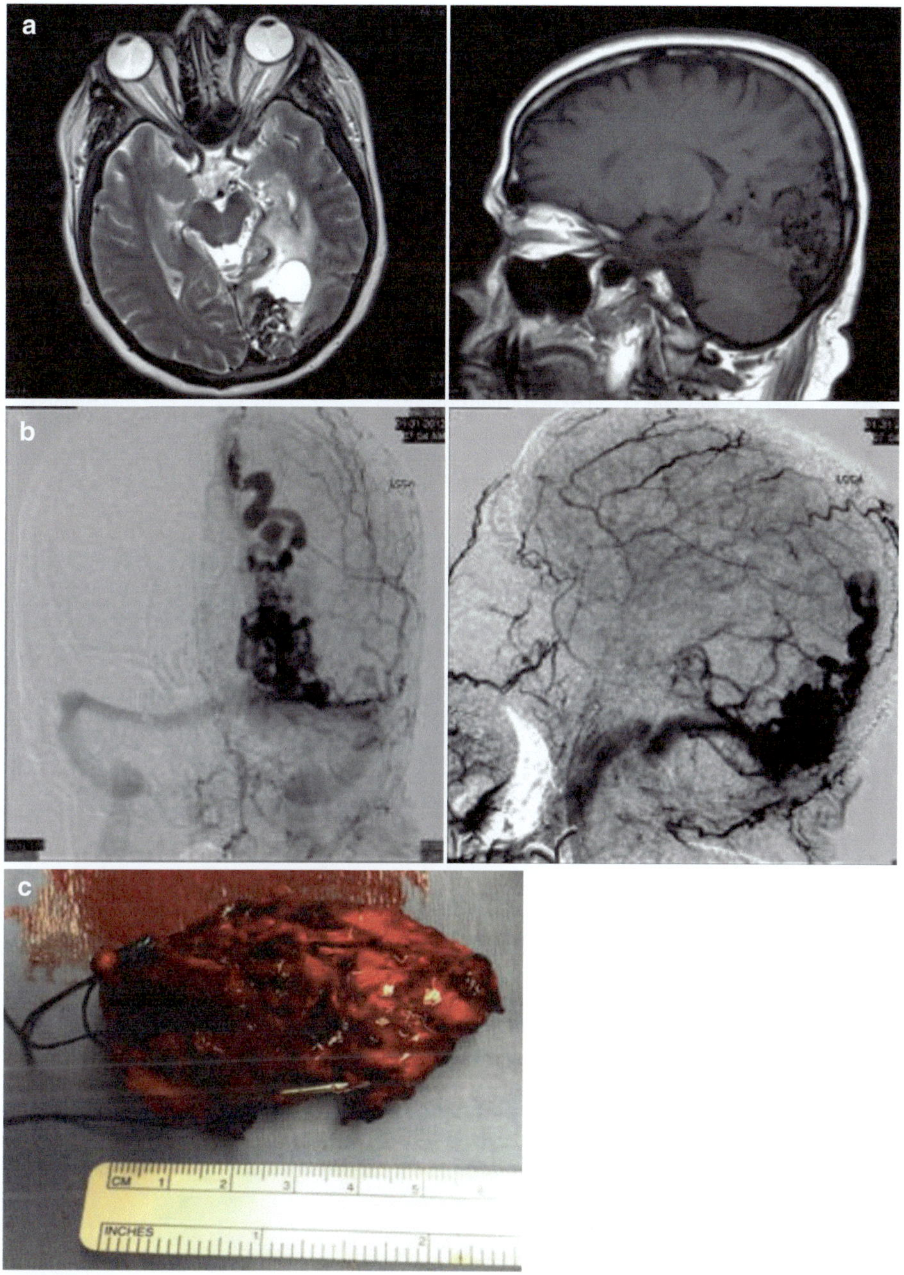

Fig. 15.2 Case example of a 55-year-old female with a Spetzler-Martin grade 4 AVM as seen on MRI (**a**), and angiography (**b**) and was treated with multiple embolizations at an outside institution. The patient eventually suffered homonymous hemianopsia due to the embolization procedures, thus the surgery was able to be performed without additional morbidity

References

1. Ondra SL, Troupp H, George ED, Schwab K. The natural history of symptomatic arteriovenous malformations of the brain: a 24-year follow-up assessment. J Neurosurg. 1990;73:387–91.
2. Mohr JP, Parides MK, Stapf C, Moquete E, Moy CS, Overbey JR, et al. Medical management with or without interventional therapy for unruptured brain arteriovenous malformations (ARUBA): a multicentre, non-blinded, randomised trial. Lancet. 2014;383:614–21.
3. Wiebers DO, Whisnant JP, Huston J, Meissner I, Brown RD, Piepgras DG, et al. Unruptured intracranial aneurysms: natural history, clinical outcome, and risks of surgical and endovascular treatment. Lancet. 2003;362:103–10.
4. van Beijnum J, Lovelock CE, Cordonnier C, Rothwell PM, Klijn CJM, Al-Shahi Salman R, et al. Outcome after spontaneous and arteriovenous malformation-related intracerebral haemorrhage: population-based studies. Brain. 2009;132:537–43.
5. van Beijnum J, van der Worp HB, Buis DR, Al-Shahi Salman R, Kappelle LJ, Rinkel GJE, et al. Treatment of brain arteriovenous malformations: a systematic review and meta-analysis. JAMA. 2011;306:2011–9.
6. Morgan MK, Rochford AM, Tsahtsarlis A, Little N, Faulder KC. Surgical risks associated with the management of grade I and II brain arteriovenous malformations. Neurosurgery. 2007;54:832–7.
7. Rutledge WC, Abla AA, Nelson J, Halbach VV, Kim H, Lawton MT. Treatment and outcomes of ARUBA-eligible patients with unruptured brain arteriovenous malformations at a single institution. Neurosurg Focus. 2014;37:E8.

Intra-arterial Treatment: Who and When

16

Hirad S. Hedayat and Rashid M. Janjua

Stroke causes 9 % of all deaths around the world and is the second most common cause of death after ischemic heart disease [1]. In the United States of America, stroke is the fourth most common cause of death with approximately 795,000 strokes occurring per year at an estimated annual cost of $36.5 billion [2]. Up to 87 % of strokes are ischemic in nature and secondary to embolic or thrombotic etiologies [2] where large vessel occlusions (LVO) fare poorly, with basilar artery, internal carotid artery (ICA), and middle cerebral artery (MCA) occlusions having mortality rates of 50 %, 35 %, and 24 %, respectively [3]. Furthermore, the natural history of acute ischemic stroke (AIS) for patients with a National Institute of Health Stroke Scale (NIHSS) >10 is especially poor, and fewer than 25 % of patients will have a good clinical outcome (modified Rankin score (mRS) ≤2) [4]. As the incidence of stroke continues to increase in combination with greater awareness of the disease in the general population, new treatment options and expanding pathophysiological knowledge have allowed the medical community to delineate which patients benefit most from various treatment options currently available though many questions still remain.

Who to Treat: Age

Advancing age has had a negative correlation with stroke morbidity, mortality, and overall outcome [5–14]. No prospective studies are available in which age has been used to dichotomize treatment, but in one multivariable analysis study, age emerged

H.S. Hedayat, MD
Chief Resident, Department of Neurological Surgery,
Wake Forest University Baptist Medical Center, Winston Salem, NC, USA

R.M. Janjua, MD, MBA (✉)
Director of (Endo)Vascular and Skull Base Surgery,
Novant Healthcare Forsyth Medical Center, Winston Salem, NC, USA
e-mail: rmjanjua@gmail.com

E. Veznedaroglu (ed.), *Controversies in Vascular Neurosurgery*,
DOI 10.1007/978-3-319-27315-0_16

as a significant predictor of outcome independent of stroke severity, etiology, performance of thrombolysis, gender, risk factors, or stroke-related complications [8]. When the age stratum 56–65 years was used as a reference, odds ratios (95 % confidence interval [95 % CI]) of good outcomes were 3.4 (1.9–6.4), 2.2 (1.6–3.2), and 1.5 (1.2–1.9) for patients aged 18–35, 36–45, and 46–55 years and 0.70 (0.60–0.81), 0.32 (0.28–0.37), and 0.18 (0.14–0.22) for those aged 66–75, 76–85, and >85 years ($p<0.001$) respectively. In absolute terms, the regression-adjusted probability of good outcome was highest in the 18–35 years age group and gradually declined by 3.1–4.2 % per decade until age 75 with a steep drop thereafter. Notably, this data applied whether or not patients had received IV thrombolysis.

Given the large aging population nationally, octogenarians are increasingly being treated for stroke. Meta-analysis from four early IA treatment studies suggested a lower likelihood of favorable outcome and higher mortality rate in octogenarians at 1–3 months after their stroke [15], while mortality in octogenarians was more often from extracerebral causes when compared to younger patients [16]. A small meta-analysis of trials with stroke patients treated with IA thrombectomy confirmed the lower likelihood of functional independence, higher mortality, and intracerebral hemorrhage rate in octogenarians [17].

More recent analyses render conflicting data. When evaluating outcomes for IV t-PA alone, a meta-analysis of prospective trials involving a total of 6,756 patients confirmed an improved odds ratio for good outcome in those treated with IV t-PA within 4.5 h without any evidence of lower odds in patients older than 80 years of age [18]. The recently reported MR CLEAN [19] and ESCAPE [20] trials both analyzed data for patients in the <80 and >80 years of age categories and confirmed better outcomes in the endovascular arm of the trials regardless of age. No subgroup analysis was reported on the outcomes between the two age categories.

When to Treat: Time

Currently, the only FDA-approved treatment for AIS is IV t-PA given within 3 h of symptom onset[421]. The National Institute of Neurological Disorders and Stroke (NINDS) rt-PA trial showed good outcomes (mRS <2 at 90 days) in 39 % of those who received IV t-PA versus 26 % of those in the placebo group [21]. Current data supports the expansion of the time window for IV t-PA use up to 4.5 h (albeit with more exclusion criteria than the group presenting in <3 h) from symptom onset [22–24] wherein the data suggests improved outcomes for one in four patients treated within the first 3 h and one in six patients treated between 3 and 4.5 h [23]. No net benefit has been demonstrated beyond 4.5 h [23, 24]. Unfortunately, IV t-PA is only administered in approximately 5.9 % of those arriving within the 3 h time frame and 0.5 % arriving in the expanded 4.5 h window and likely reflects additional contraindications (listed below) introduced in the expanded window along with a smaller number of patients arriving in this time period (3 % versus 22 % in the early time window) [25].

Widespread use of IV t-PA remains limited due to the medical contraindications necessary to mitigate hemorrhagic risks, a constrained time window, and the potential for poor response to IV t-PA seen with LVO. The most common contraindication to IV t-PA administration is delayed presentation to emergency medical facilities after symptom onset with a 2012 study revealing that 75 % of ischemic stroke patients arrive at the ER beyond the indicated treatment window, including the expanded time frame [25]. Medical contraindications include: evidence of intracranial hemorrhage on pretreatment evaluation; clinical presentation suggestive of subarachnoid hemorrhage even with a normal head CT; rapidly improving stroke symptoms; any intracranial or spinal surgery, serious head trauma, or previous stroke within 3 months; history of previous intracranial hemorrhage; uncontrolled hypertension currently (systolic >185 mmHg or diastolic >110 mmHg); active internal bleeding; known bleeding diathesis including but not limited to current/recent use of oral anticoagulants with INR ≥1.7 s, administration of heparin within 48 h preceding onset of stroke and elevated aPTT, and platelet count <100,000/mm; intracranial neoplasm, arteriovenous malformation, or aneurysm; arterial puncture at a noncompressible site in the previous 7 days; blood glucose level <50 mg/dL; and myocardial infarction within the previous 3 months [26]. Relative exclusion criteria include pregnancy, major surgery or serious trauma in the previous 14 days, history of gastrointestinal or urinary tract hemorrhage in the previous 21 days, and seizure at onset with postictal residual neurological impairments [26]. The additional relative exclusion criteria added for IV t-PA given in the 3–4.5 h window include age >80 years, severe stroke (NIHSS >25), taking any oral anticoagulant regardless of INR, and a history of both diabetes and prior ischemic stroke.

The heterogeneity of the patient population afflicted with AIS leads to challenges in treating these patients with a single therapy and, likewise, a high variability in thrombolysis success. In the NINDS [21] and ECASS III [22] studies, the percentage of patients with mRS outcomes of 3–6 ranged from 48 to 57 % [1]. The risk of symptomatic intracranial hemorrhage—seen in 6–7 % of patients who have received IV t-PA [1]—increases with age, hypertension, severe neurological deficits, and hyperglycemia while factors such as LVO, early ischemic changes on CT, and increased time to treatment are found to predict poor outcome with IV t-PA [1].

Proximal LVO is the underlying etiology in 40 % of patients with AIS, and IV t-PA has demonstrated a limited ability to achieve recanalization due to the large thrombus burden which blocks the ability of IV t-PA to penetrate the clot and achieve thrombolysis [27–29]. As a result, these patients often do poorly with a 4.5-fold increased mortality rate and a threefold reduction in odds of a good outcome (mRS ≤2) [30]. Similarly, these patients typically present with a higher NIHSS score (≥10), worse symptoms given that a larger area of the brain is affected and thus resultant greater care and cost requirements overall [1].

There remains lack of strong evidence for the use of acute treatment in the setting of patients who awaken with a stroke, the so-called wake-up stroke with an unknown period of onset. Imaging is critical in the initial evaluation of these patients where MRI evaluates the core infarct with DWI and FLAIR sequence mismatch or a CT perfusion-contrasted study evaluating cerebral blood flow mean transit time versus cerebral blood volume mismatch to elucidate the size of noninfarcted, ischemic salvageable tissue (penumbra) [31]. Thomalla et al. [32] reviewed 543 patients with acute stroke and known time of symptom onset and found DWI-FLAIR mismatch in those patients presenting within 4.5 h of symptom onset with a positive predictive value of 83 % and a negative predictive value of 54 %. This suggested that FLAIR negativity should be weighed somewhat heavily in favor of giving IV lytic agents while FLAIR positivity should be weighted less heavily in favor of withholding IV lytic agents. Multiple prospective trials are underway to evaluate the safety and feasibility of treatment in the "wake-up stroke" population [33–35].

When to Treat: Imaging

The initial imaging evaluation for stroke involves exclusion of an intracerebral hemorrhage or mass. Most commonly, this is performed with a non-contrasted CT (NCT) but can be assessed with a gradient echo (GRE) sequence MRI as well.

While LVO likely increases the risk of deterioration, perfusion imaging can be of great value in identifying ischemic tissue at risk of converting to infarcted tissue (the stroke penumbra) which may benefit from reperfusion therapy. DWI imaging is dynamic in nature and dependent on several factors such as collaterals, blood pressure, and volume status while also identifying the core infarct [36, 37]. Unfortunately, diffusion imaging is more labor and time intensive and requires post-processing, whereas CT perfusion (CTP) can be readily performed, requires less post-processing, and is more rapidly available. CTP allows for evaluation of mean transit time of the contrast in the brain (MTT), cerebral blood volume (CBV), and cerebral blood flow (CBF). Although the CTP cannot identify areas of core infarct as accurately as DWI, this core is well represented by areas with CBV below 2 ml/100 g. The tissue at risk (penumbra) is felt to be defined as that with a relative MTT of >145 % of the contralateral hemisphere [38]. Patients with a relatively large penumbra and small infarct core (perfusion-diffusion mismatch) are thought to benefit most from reperfusion; however, major trials have not unequivocally confirmed this rationale [39].

Desmoteplase in acute ischemic stroke-phase II (DIAS-II) was one of the earlier studies that failed to show the superiority of treatment utilizing perfusion mismatch for penumbral imaging [40], while trials such as DEFUSE, DEFUSE-2, and the Echoplanar Imaging Thrombolysis Evaluation Trial (EPITHET) used a "target mismatch profile" (the ratio of penumbra volume to core infarct) to target a sufficient penumbral tissue volume suitable for endovascular technique. They selected candidates for revascularization beyond 3 h by using DWI and CT perfusion and demonstrated that these patients had better clinical outcomes [41–44]. However, MR RESCUE [45] also used penumbral imaging criteria to select patients but failed to show better clinical outcomes when compared to patients with no selection at all.

The key physiological parameter critical to penumbra survival is cerebral collateral blood supply to the area with cerebral angiography as the gold standard for its assessment. Although it remains the gold standard, it is not a feasible study to perform as an initial evaluation tool for cerebral ischemia given that this information can be obtained through noninvasive perfusion studies, though these may be qualitative at best but without the risks associated with angiography.

Of crucial note is evidence of infarct size >70–100 cc on NCT, DWI, or CTP imaging which should alert the observer to the fact that these patients are more likely to sustain a reperfusion-related hemorrhage and poor outcome [46, 47]. Additionally, patients with ischemic infarct >1/3 of the MCA territory were more likely to suffer from hemorrhagic complications after reperfusion in the ECASS trial [25] and should be carefully evaluated for thrombolytic treatment. The Alberta Stroke Program Early CT (ASPECT) score is a standardized way of discerning the infarct size on a CT angiogram, and a score of <7 has been reliably associated with >1/3 MCA territory infarction [48]. A score of <7 also predicts higher rates of reperfusion-related hemorrhage with IA or IV thrombolytic agents.

Given the heterogeneity of patients presenting with AIS, novel approaches have developed and evolved to meet the crucial need for treatment to improve outcomes. The development of mechanical thrombolysis and mechanical thrombectomy, which occurred secondary to the improved understanding of thrombolytic medications and advances in neuroimaging and angiographic equipment, has advanced patient care significantly. These led to several small case series and pilot studies in the late 1980s and early 1990s and have culminated in our current era of prospective, randomized, endovascular stroke trials.

Mechanical thrombolysis involves the lysing of a clot by IA t-PA delivered at or near the thrombus and/or mechanical manipulation by a guide wire and was the first interventional therapy used to overcome the obstacles posed by IV t-PA [49]. There are significant limitations to this therapy in that the physical disruption of a clot may cause fragments to shower distally causing multiple small infarctions. Moreover, a recent randomized controlled study comparing IV plus IA t-PA versus IV t-PA alone demonstrated similar safety outcomes with no significant difference in functional independence [50].

Mechanical thrombectomy differs significantly from pharmacologic and mechanical thrombolysis in that it utilizes an intra-arterial device to physically remove the clot within 8 h from stroke onset. It is a treatment modality now widely used at comprehensive stroke centers in patients with AIS who are either ineligible for IV t-PA secondary to the aforementioned contraindications or in those in whom IV t-PA failed to cause a response. In the United States, currently approved mechanical thrombectomy devices include the Merci™* Retriever (Stryker/Concentric Medical, Inc.), Penumbra™* System (Penumbra, Inc.), Solitaire FR device (Covidien), and Trevo™* Pro Retrieval System (Stryker/Concentric Medical, Inc.).

There is still much work left to do to elucidate exactly which patients will benefit most from IA treatment and at what point it is best to initiate it. There remains room for much study in this realm as it is a hugely important enterprise which affords life-altering, positive outcomes in the care of our patients.

References

1. Donnan GA, Fisher M, Macleod M, Davis SM. Stroke. Lancet. 2008;371:1612–23.

2. Go AS, et al. Heart disease and stroke statistics – 2013 update: a report from the American Heart Association. Circular. 2013;127:e6–245.
3. Smith WS, et al. Significance of large vessel intracranial occlusion causing acute ischemic stroke and TIA. Stroke. 2009;40:3834–40.
4. Ingall TJ, et al. Findings from the reanalysis of the NINDS tissue plasminogen activator for acute ischemic stroke treatment trial. Stroke. 2004;35:2418–24.
5. Béjot Y, et al. Poststroke disposition and associated factors in a population-based study: the Dijon stroke registry. Stroke. 2012;43:2071–7.
6. Counsell C, Dennis M, McDowall M, Warlow C. Predicting outcome after acute and subacute stroke: development and validation of new prognostic models. Stroke. 2002;33(4):1041–7. doi:10.1161/hs0402.105909.
7. Feigin VL, Parag V, Senior H. Auckland Stroke Outcomes Study. Neurology. 2010;75:1608–16.
8. Knoflach M, et al. Functional recovery after ischemic stroke – a matter of age. Neurology. 2012;78:279.
9. Heuschmann PU, et al. Three-month stroke outcome: the European Registers of Stroke (EROS) investigators. Neurology. 2011;76:159–65.
10. Koennecke H-C, et al. Factors influencing in-hospital mortality and morbidity in patients treated on a stroke unit. Neurology. 2011;77:965–72.
11. König IR, et al. Predicting long-term outcome after acute ischemic stroke: a simple index works in patients from controlled clinical trials. Stroke. 2008;39:1821–6.
12. Weimar C, König IR, Kraywinkel K, Ziegler A, Diener HC. Age and National Institutes of Health Stroke Scale Score within 6 hours after onset are accurate predictors of outcome after cerebral ischemia: development and external validation of prognostic models. Stroke. 2004;35:158–62.
13. Wong KS. Risk factors for early death in acute ischemic stroke and intracerebral hemorrhage: a prospective hospital-based study in Asia. Stroke. 1999;30:2326–30.
14. Andersen KK, Andersen ZJ, Olsen TS. Predictors of early and late case-fatality in a nationwide Danish study of 26 818 patients with first-ever ischemic stroke. Stroke. 2011;42:2806–12.
15. Qureshi AI, Suri MFK, Georgiadis AL, Vazquez G, Janjua NA. Intra-arterial recanalization techniques for patients 80 years or older with acute ischemic stroke: pooled analysis from 4 prospective studies. AJNR Am J Neuroradiol. 2009;30:1184–9.
16. Mono M-L, et al. Intra-arterial thrombolysis for acute ischemic stroke in octogenarians. Cerebrovasc Dis. 2012;33:116–22.
17. Duffis EJ, He W, Prestigiacomo CJ, Gandhi CD. Endovascular treatment for acute ischemic stroke in octogenarians compared with younger patients: a meta-analysis. Int J Stroke. 2014;9:308–12.
18. Emberson J, et al. Effect of treatment delay, age, and stroke severity on the eff ects of intravenous thrombolysis with alteplase for acute ischaemic stroke: a meta-analysis of individual patient data from randomised trials. Lancet. 2014;384:4–10.
19. Berkhemer OA, et al. A randomized trial of intraarterial treatment for acute ischemic stroke. N Engl J Med. 2014;372:11–20.
20. Goyal M, et al. Randomized assessment of rapid endovascular treatment of ischemic stroke. N Engl J Med. 2015;372:1019–30.
21. Troke STS, Roup STG. Tissue plasminogen activator for acute ischemic stroke. The National Institute of Neurological Disorders and Stroke rt-PA Stroke Study Group. N Engl J Med. 1995;333:1581–7.
22. Hacke W, et al. Thrombolysis with alteplase 3 to 4.5 hours after acute ischemic stroke. N Engl J Med. 2008;359(13):1317–29.
23. Lansberg MG, Schrooten M, Bluhmki E, Thijs VN, Saver JL. Treatment time-specific number needed to treat estimates for tissue plasminogen activator therapy in acute stroke based on shifts over the entire range of the modified rankin scale. Stroke. 2009;40:2079–84.
24. Ahmed N, et al. Implementation and outcome of thrombolysis with alteplase 3–4·5 h after an acute stroke: an updated analysis from SITS-ISTR. Lancet Neurol. 2010;9:866–74.

25. De Los Ríos La Rosa F, et al. Eligibility for intravenous recombinant tissue-type plasminogen activator within a population: the effect of the European Cooperative Acute Stroke Study (ECASS) III trial. Stroke. 2012;43:1591–5.
26. Jauch EC, et al. Guidelines for the early management of patients with acute ischemic stroke: a guideline for healthcare professionals from the American Heart Association/American Stroke Association. Stroke. 2013;44:870–947.
27. Saqqur M, et al. Site of arterial occlusion identified by transcranial Doppler predicts the response to intravenous thrombolysis for stroke. Stroke. 2007;38:948–54.
28. De Silva DA, et al. The benefits of intravenous thrombolysis relate to the site of baseline arterial occlusion in the echoplanar imaging thrombolytic evaluation trial (EPITHET). Stroke. 2010;41:295–9.
29. Paciaroni M, et al. Systemic thrombolysis in patients with acute ischemic stroke and Internal Carotid ARtery Occlusion: the ICARO study. Stroke. 2012;43:125–30.
30. Dabus G, Linfante I. The natural history of acute ischemic stroke due to intracranial large-vessel occlusion: what do we know? Tech Vasc Interv Radiol. 2012;15:2–4.
31. Rubin MN, Barrett KM. What to do with wake-up stroke. Neurohospitalist. 2015;5:161–72.
32. Thomalla G, et al. DWI-FLAIR mismatch for the identification of patients with acute ischaemic stroke within 4·5 h of symptom onset (PRE-FLAIR): a multicentre observational study. Lancet Neurol. 2011;10:978–86.
33. Thomalla G, et al. A multicenter, randomized, double-blind, placebo-controlled trial to test efficacy and safety of magnetic resonance imaging-based thrombolysis in wake-up stroke (WAKE-UP). Int J Stroke. 2014;9:829–36.
34. Koga M, et al. THrombolysis for acute wake-up and unclear-onset strokes with alteplase at 0·6 mg/kg (THAWS) trial. Int J Stroke. 2014;9:1117–24.
35. Ma H, et al. A multicentre, randomized, double-blinded, placebo-controlled phase III study to investigate EXtending the time for Thrombolysis in Emergency Neurological Deficits (EXTEND). Int J Stroke. 2012;7:74–80.
36. Kidwell CS, et al. Late secondary ischemic injury in patients receiving intraarterial thrombolysis. Ann Neurol. 2002;52:698–703.
37. Kidwell CS, et al. Thrombolytic reversal of acute human cerebral ischemic injury shown by diffusion/perfusion magnetic resonance imaging. Ann Neurol. 2000;47:462–9.
38. Wintermark M, et al. Perfusion-CT assessment of infarct core and penumbra: receiver operating characteristic curve analysis in 130 patients suspected of acute hemispheric stroke. Stroke. 2006;37:979–85.
39. Butcher KS, et al. Refining the perfusion-diffusion mismatch hypothesis. Stroke. 2005;36:1153–9.
40. Hacke W, et al. NIH public access. Analysis. 2010;8:141–50.
41. Lansberg MG, et al. MRI profile and response to endovascular reperfusion after stroke (DEFUSE 2): a prospective cohort study. Lancet Neurol. 2012;11(10):860–7.
42. Albers GW, et al. Magnetic resonance imaging profiles predict clinical response to early reperfusion: the diffusion and perfusion imaging evaluation for understanding stroke evolution (DEFUSE) study. Ann Neurol. 2006;60:508–17.
43. Davis SM, et al. Effects of alteplase beyond 3 h after stroke in the Echoplanar Imaging Thrombolytic Evaluation Trial (EPITHET): a placebo-controlled randomised trial. Lancet Neurol. 2008;7:299–309.
44. Lansberg MG, et al. RAPID automated patient selection for reperfusion therapy: a pooled analysis of the echoplanar imaging thrombolytic evaluation trial (EPITHET) and the diffusion and perfusion imaging evaluation for understanding stroke evolution (DEFUSE) study. Stroke. 2011;42:1608–14.
45. Kidwell CS, et al. A trial of imaging selection and endovascular treatment for ischemic stroke. N Engl J Med. 2013;368(10):914–23.
46. Edgell RC, Vora NA. Neuroimaging markers of hemorrhagic risk with stroke reperfusion therapy. Neurology. 2012;79(13 Suppl 1):S100–4.
47. Latchaw RE, et al. Recommendations for imaging of acute ischemic stroke: a scientific statement from the american heart association. Stroke. 2009;40:3646–78.

48. Pexman JHW, et al. Use of the Alberta Stroke Program Early CT Score (ASPECTS) for assessing CT scans in patients with acute stroke. Am J Neuroradiol. 2001;22:1534–42.
49. Mortimer AM, Bradley MD, Renowden SA. Endovascular therapy in hyperacute ischaemic stroke: history and current status. Interv Neuroradiol. 2013;19:506–18.
50. Broderick JP, et al. Endovascular therapy after intravenous t-PA versus t-PA alone for stroke. N Engl J Med. 2013;368:893–903.

Acute Ischemic Stroke: Discussion 17

Stephen Jr. Reintjes and Peter Kan

Stroke is the leading cause of disability in adults in North America [1]. In the last 20 years, interest has soared in search of a reperfusion therapy for ischemic stroke caused by vessel occlusion. The revolutionary trial by the National Institute of Neurologic Disorders and Stroke (NINDS) showed that intravenous thrombolysis could be achieved with an intravenous tissue plasminogen activator (tPA). The effectiveness of tPA is time-dependent, and benefit has been shown up to 4.5 h after the onset of stroke. Although tPA can be initiated quickly after a new ischemic stroke is suspected, the short treatment window excludes many patients from therapy. There are also other risks such as development of asymptomatic and symptomatic intracranial hemorrhage (ICH) as well as failure of therapy [2, 3]. These limitations in IV tPA therapy have led to the development of procedural-based interventions such as intra-arterial thrombolytics and mechanical thrombectomy. In 2013, utilization of endovascular therapy was called into question by three randomized controlled trials, showing no benefit of endovascular treatment of stroke compared to standard care or IV tPA [4–6]. These trials used first-generation devices and intra-arterial chemical thrombolysis as the mainstay of treatment. Recruitment was also not limited to patients with a radiographic documentation of proximal large vessel occlusion. Despite different trial methods and designs, none showed benefit of endovascular therapy compared to less invasive measures (although no harm was shown). As these trial results were published, three other multicenter RCTs were enrolling patients to compare endovascular treatment to standard care in managing acute ischemic stroke. The trials ESCAPE, MR CLEAN, and EXTEND-IA all concluded that endovascular treatment of acute vessel occlusion in the anterior circulation was superior to medical management with IV tPA alone [7–9]. These new trials utilized the recent technology of stent retrievers. They also required radiographic evidence of proximal vessel

S. Jr. Reintjes
Neurosurgery, University of South Florida, Tampa, FL, USA

P. Kan (✉)
Neurosurgery, Baylor College of Medicine, Houston, Texas, USA
e-mail: peterkantzeman@yahoo.ca

E. Veznedaroglu (ed.), *Controversies in Vascular Neurosurgery*,
DOI 10.1007/978-3-319-27315-0_17

occlusion and noninvasive imaging to assess tissue viability. Despite their differences in trial design, these recent trials all showed a benefit to patients with acute ischemic stroke caused by proximal vessel occlusion from endovascular therapy. In this chapter, we will give a brief history of endovascular therapy for stroke, including the changes in technology, and discuss the three primary equivocal studies for stroke intervention as compared to the three recent studies, which favor endovascular therapy for the treatment of acute ischemic stroke.

The initial report of endovascular therapy was over 30 years ago. Local IA tPA was delivered for thrombolysis of vertebrobasilar thromboembolic disease [10]. In 1995, the NINDS showed that intravenous thrombolysis with IV tPA is beneficial if given within 3 h of stroke onset. The following year, the FDA approved the use of tPA for the treatment of acute stroke, based on the NINDS study [2]. The time window for IV tPA expanded after the European Cooperative Acute Stroke Study (ECASS) III investigators concluded that benefit of IV tPA can be extended beyond the 3 h time window previously designated [3]. The limitation of IV thrombolysis therapy led to interventional techniques for intra-arterial therapy and was quickly followed by the development of mechanical thrombectomy devices that further enhanced the armamentarium of endovascular specialists in the treatment of stroke.

PROACT-I and PROACT-II tested the safety and recanalization efficacy of intra-arterial delivery of recombinant pro-urokinase in patients with documented proximal middle cerebral artery occlusion within 6 h. PROACT-I showed superior recanalization compared with placebo and PROACT-II showed that intra-arterial pro-urokinase was associated with higher recanalization rates and significantly improved clinical outcome at 90 days [11, 12]. The results of PROACT-II were combined with the Japanese Middle Cerebral Artery Embolism Local Fibrinolytic Intervention Trial (MELT) and meta-analysis and showed that better outcomes were seen with patients treated with IAT than with placebo [13]. Intra-arterial thrombolysis paved the way for mechanical embolectomy in patients with large vessel occlusion in acute stroke.

The first device designed and trialed for intracranial thrombectomy was the Merci retriever (Stryker Neurovascular, Fremont, California, USA). The MERCI trial, reported in 2005, investigated the safety and efficacy of the Merci retriever for occluded large vessels within 8 h of onset of stroke symptoms in patients ineligible for tPA. Recanalization was achieved in 48 % of patients in whom the device was employed. In those whom recanalization was possible with the Merci retriever, good outcomes at 90 days were seen more often than those with unsuccessful recanalization [14]. In the Multi-MERCI trial, recanalization was successful in 54 % of treated vessels and in 69 % of patients after adjunctive therapy with IAT. Symptomatic hemorrhage was 10 % and 90-day mortality was 34 %, lower than the initial MERCI trial [15].

The Penumbra system (Penumbra, Alameda, California, USA) was developed as an alternative approach for mechanical thrombectomy. The penumbra system uses aspiration for thrombus debulking and thrombus removal. Published in 2009, the Penumbra Pivotal Stroke Trial assessed the safety and effectiveness of the Penumbra system in large vessel occlusion resulting in ischemic stroke. This multicenter study enrolled patients within 8 h of stroke symptoms and documented angiographic occlusion. A total of 125 patients were treated with the penumbra system with 82 % being recanalized to Thrombolysis in Myocardial Infarction (TIMI) grade 2–3. There were 28 % of patients who had intracranial hemorrhage at 24 h and all-cause mortality was 33 % at 90 days. Good outcome mRS of 0–2 was reported in 25 % of patients [16].

The newest generation of mechanical thrombectomy devices is designed to retrieve the thrombus within the occluded vessel with the use of retrievable self-expanding stents. The Solitaire FR device (Covidien, Mansfield, Massachusetts, USA) and the TREVO device (Stryker Neurovascular) were designed for this purpose. In 2012, the SWIFT trial compared the safety and efficacy of the Solitaire device with the Merci retriever. Patients were randomized on a 1:1 basis and the primary endpoint was TIMI score of 2 or 3 in all treatable vessels without symptomatic ICH; this was achieved in 61 % with the Solitaire device compared with 24 % for the Merci retrieval device. More patients also had a good outcome at 3 months with the Solitaire (58 %) versus the Merci retrieval device (33 %) and 90-day mortality was lower in the Solitaire group (17 %) versus the Merci group (38 %). The trial was stopped early after reaching a prespecified efficacy-stopping rule [17]. The most recent stent retriever device, the Trevo Retriever, was studied in the TREVO II trial and again compared the efficacy of the Trevo Retriever versus the Merci Retriever. This investigation included patients with angiographic-confirmed large vessel occlusion and National Institutes of Health Stroke Scale (NIHSS) scores of 8–29 within 8 h of stroke symptom onset. Patients were randomly assigned on a 1:1 basis and primary endpoint was thrombolysis in cerebral infarction (TICI) scores of ≥2. In 2011, 178 patients were randomized to Trevo or Merci devices with 86 % of patients in the Trevo group and 60 % in the Merci group reaching a TICI score of ≥2 while safety did not differ between both groups. Good outcome measured by the mRS at 90 days occurred in 40 % of the TREVO cohort compared with 22 % of the MERCI cohort [18].

The Case Against Mechanical Thrombectomy of Acute Ischemic Strokes

In 2013, there were three major trials that were published comparing outcomes of treatment of acute ischemic stroke with IV tPA compared to interventional methods: IMS III, MR RESCUE, and SYNTHESIS. These trials concurrently failed to show the superiority of endovascular therapy compared to IV tPA for the treatment of acute ischemic stroke. There has been much discussion following the publication of these trials. All three trials were criticized for being outdated by the time of publication and failing to have strict enrollment criteria for endovascular treatment.

IMS III began enrollment in 2006 and stopped in 2012 after interim analysis deemed futility of endovascular therapy. This trial was designed as a phase 3 open-label trial with blinded outcome to test patients who had received IV tPA followed by endovascular therapy compared to patients treated with standard IV tPA treatment. The trial did not limit thrombectomy devices and allowed for new devices to be used as the technology developed. There was no imaging requirement and patients had to be eligible to receive IV tPA within 3 h of symptom onset and randomized within 40 min of receiving IV tPA. Endovascular treatment had to begin within 5 h of stroke onset. Primary outcome measure was mRS at 90 days. There were 656 patients randomized and no significant difference was found between endovascular therapy and patients who received IV tPA. Although there was a trend favoring better outcome among patients receiving endovascular treatment, this difference was not statistically significant. Reperfusion rates were higher for those receiving endovascular therapy and there was a trend toward better outcome in patients who had a time interval between initiation of IV tPA and groin puncture less than 90 min. No differences were seen in patient mortality [4].

MR RESCUE was a phase 2b randomized controlled trial which included patients with NIHSS between 6 and 29 with large vessel anterior circulation stroke randomly assigned within 8 h after symptom onset to undergo mechanical embolectomy or standard medical care. Patients were randomized after treatment with IV tPA and persistent vessel occlusion seen on noninvasive angiographic imaging. Perfusion imaging was completed and a favorable penumbral pattern was defined as an infarct core 90 ml or less. All devices available were allowed in mechanical thrombectomy, and IAT was allowed within 6 h of symptom onset. Primary outcome was assessed with the mRS at 90 days. Secondary outcomes were assessed using the TICI scale and parenchyma reperfusion on post-stroke day 7. A total of 118 patients were successfully randomized (64 to embolectomy, 54 for IV tPA alone). No difference in final infarct volume was seen between both arms, nor did mRS score at 90 days (3.9 v 3.9). Patients with a favorable penumbral pattern seemed to perform better regardless of treatment group. There were no significant differences in rates of reperfusion on day 7 imaging [6].

SYNTHESIS was a multicenter open treatment trial with a blinded endpoint, testing whether outcomes were better with endovascular intervention over IV tPA in acute stroke. Patients had to be randomized within 4.5 h of stroke onset and endovascular therapy group did not receive IV tPA. Patients were assessed with the NIHSS at presentation and at 7 days. Long-term outcome was assessed via telephone interview at 90 days and the primary outcome was disability-free survival. Patients were enrolled from 2008 to 2012 and a total of 362 patients were randomized in 1:1 fashion. Patients randomized to endovascular treatment were given IAT at the interventionalist's discretion. Also, the Solitaire retriever was the most frequently used device for thrombectomy (18 patients), followed by the Penumbra device (9 patients), and the Trevo and Merci devices (5 patients each). At 90 days, 30 % of the patients randomized to endovascular treatment survived with mRS 0–1 compared with 34 % of those in the IV tPA group. No difference in safety was detected between the groups [5].

The Case for Mechanical Thrombectomy of Acute Ischemic Strokes

Recently in 2015, there are three randomized trials which all report improved outcomes with endovascular therapy for acute ischemic strokes. These trials all reinforce the efficacy and the safety of endovascular therapy for the treatment of acute stroke in the anterior circulation with an angiographic proven proximal vessel occlusion. ESCAPE and EXTEND-IA were stopped early because predetermined efficacy boundaries were crossed.

MR CLEAN was a phase 3 multicenter trial with blinded endpoint evaluation of endovascular treatment plus usual care compared to usual care alone. To be included in the randomization process, patients had to have a documented proximal vessel occlusion diagnosed by CTA, MRA, or angiography, with NIHSS >2, and endovascular treatment had to be available within 6 h of stroke onset. Interventionalists were allowed to treat with IA tPA at their discretion. Primary outcome was mRS at 90 days. Secondary outcome focused on vessel recanalization at 24 h, final infarct volume, safety, and NIHSS at 24 h, 7 days, and hospital discharge. TICI score was used to quantify vessel recanalization. Five hundred and two patients were randomized between 2010 and 2014. Overwhelmingly, retrievable stents were used in 190/233 patients randomized to endovascular treatment. The primary outcome favored intervention in all mRS scores except death. The absolute difference in treatment effect was 13.5 %. All secondary outcomes favored intervention as well. NIHSS was on average 2.9 points lower in intervention group; infarction volume was smaller in the intervention group (absolute difference of 19 cc on average). Reperfusion was higher in intervention group (TICI score of 2b or 3 achieved in 115 of 196 patients). There was also no difference in safety between intervention group and usual care group; however, 5.6 % of patients in intervention group developed new stroke in different territories within 90 days compared to 0.4 % of control group [7].

The ESCAPE trial was designed to test whether patients with acute ischemic stroke and proximal vessel occlusion diagnosed on CTA would benefit from rapid endovascular treatment. This multicenter randomized trial with blinded outcome enrolled 316 patients up to 12 h after symptom onset. CT angiogram was completed to target patients with small infarct core and occluded proximal artery with moderate to good collateral circulation. The use of retrievable stents was recommended to interventionalists. The control group received the current standard of care and both groups received IV tPA within 4.5 h after symptom onset if they met local guidelines. The target time from CT to groin puncture was 60 min or less and to reperfusion was 90 min. Patients were not enrolled if there were patient limitations or infrastructure factors that prevented a patient meeting target times. Primary outcome was assessed using the mRS at 90 days. Secondary outcomes included recanalization and reperfusion, new intracranial hemorrhage, and angiographic complications. Both primary and secondary outcomes heavily favored intervention therapy. A median mRS of 0–2 at 90 days was 53 % for the intervention group and 29 % for the control group. Mortality was 10 % for the intervention group and 19 % for the control group. Successful reperfusion, TICI score of 2b or 3, was observed in 72 % (113/156) of intervention group compared with successful recanalization, which was measured by CTA, of 31 % (43/138) patients in the control group [9].

EXTEND-IA was also a multicenter randomized trial of patients who received IV tPA within 4.5 h of stroke onset. Between 2012 and 2014, a total of 70 patients were enrolled within 4.5 h after the onset of anterior circulation stroke and documented proximal MCA or ICA occlusion on CTA. CT perfusion imaging was also completed to identify salvageable penumbra and ischemic cores. Patients were included if endovascular therapy was available within 6 h of stroke onset and completed within 8 h. Primary outcome was reperfusion based on the TICI score and neurologic improvement with a reduction of NIHSS of ≥8 points. Secondary outcome was mRS score at 90 days, death, or symptomatic ICH. Stent retrievers were used most often in the endovascular group. Both primary endpoints favored endovascular therapy with a significant improvement. Endovascular therapy led to improved neurologic recovery at 3 days and functional outcomes (assessed with mRS) at 90 days. There was no difference in safety between the two groups, although there were two nonclinically significant parenchymal hemorrhages and two infarcts in new territories in the endovascular group [8].

In 2013, the three trials failed to demonstrate improved outcomes over standard medical therapy and tPA despite the widespread use of endovascular treatment for acute strokes. These trials had several limitations and were heavily criticized for being outdated by the time of study publication. At the time they were published, there was also no standardized endovascular treatment for acute stroke therapy. This was not just for which device used in therapy but the routine use of CTA or MRA to document a proximal large vessel occlusion. As a result of these trial designs, the three new randomized trials published in 2015 utilized the most recent technology and rigorous criteria for study inclusion. These new trials overwhelmingly favor endovascular therapy for suitable lesions in acute stroke. Two trials, ESCAPE and EXTEND-IA, were halted early because preset efficacy boundaries were reached [8, 9].

Limitations of the early negative studies were multifactorial. IMS III was stopped early for treatment futility in the endovascular arm and did not show a benefit of endovascular therapy on 90-day mRS scores. This trial relied heavily on first-generation devices, such as the Merci retriever, which were available when investigators opened recruitment in 2006. Additionally, randomization did not require an angiographic evidence of proximal vessel occlusion or treatable lesion. MR RESCUE also did not show a clinical or radiographic benefit in patients undergoing embolectomy compared to the control group. Patients were stratified based on favorable penumbral pattern. This trial also began enrollment in 2004 and mainly utilized IA thrombolysis and first-generation devices. The average time to groin puncture was over 6 h after symptom onset and randomization occurred 5.5 h after symptom onset. Investigators concluded that patients with a favorable penumbral pattern did not identify those that would have a clinical benefit to endovascular therapy. The third trial, SYNTHESIS, failed to show superiority of endovascular therapy compared to IV tPA, again with patients mostly treated with first-generation devices. Proximal vessel occlusion was, again, not a requirement for randomization into the treatment arm for the SYNTHESIS trial, and 16 patients randomized to this group did not receive any treatment [5].

The trials reported in 2015 all sought to standardize endovascular treatment as well as use imaging-based approaches to identify which patients are optimally suited for endovascular therapy. These three trials each required CTA, MRA, or angiographic evidence of proximal MCA or ICA occlusion for randomization. MR CLEAN was the first trial to show clinical superiority of endovascular treatment over current standards of care or IV tPA. Investigators required that endovascular treatment be initiated within 6 h and have angiographic proof of vessel. This trial also utilized the widespread availability of stent retrievers, which were shown to be superior in vessel recanalization compared to first-generation Merci retriever [17, 18]. This trial highlights the importance of pretreatment imaging to select which patients might benefit from endovascular therapy, unlike IMS III and SYNTHESIS which did not require radiographic evidence of proximal vessel occlusion prior to randomization [7]. ESCAPE and EXTEND-IA confirmed what MR CLEAN had already shown. Both of these trials were stopped early because a predetermined efficacy point had been reached. ESCAPE used rigorous workflow and time criteria for endovascular therapy, which resulted in improved outcome and decreased mortality in the treatment group. Patients were randomized prior to receiving IV tPA. The time criteria were heavily emphasized in order to achieve early reperfusion, much like the model in acute coronary syndrome. CTA was used as a screening tool in a majority of patients and excluded patients with a large infarct core and poor collateral circulation. Only centers that were able to demonstrate efficient utilization of resources were able to participate in this trial [9]. EXTEND-IA was unique in that it used CT perfusion imaging to select patients with the greatest potential benefit from endovascular treatment, much like MR RESCUE investigators. This possibly excluded patients with large ischemic cores without evidence of clinical salvageable ischemic brain (nearly 25 % of patients were excluded because of this).

In the last 10 years, there has been a dramatic improvement in technology and stroke outcomes for patients with acute stroke caused by proximal vessel occlusion. Advances in technology and standardized stroke care have been the main contributors to the increase in outcome. Although early randomized trials did not show increased benefit for endovascular treatment of stroke, they did overall show that endovascular treatment is safe and patients were not harmed by its use. These results cannot be overlooked. Later trials regulated the workflow, improved the presentation to groin puncture time, and better established criteria and protocol for those patients who might benefit from interventional therapy. Together with the use of modern stent-retrievers, they showed benefit from endovascular treatment in the treatment of acute ischemic stroke. Stroke therapy continues to improve and future study will hopefully continue to advance our understanding of therapy in acute ischemic stroke.

References

1. Mozaffarian D, Benjamin EJ, Go AS, et al. Heart disease and stroke statistics – 2015 update: a report from the American Heart Association. Circulation. 2015;131(4):e29–322.
2. The National Institute of Neurological Disorders and Stroke rt-PA Stroke Study Group. Tissue plasminogen activator for acute ischemic stroke. N Engl J Med. 1995;333(24):1581–7.
3. Hacke W, Kaste M, Bluhmki E, et al. Thrombolysis with alteplase 3 to 4.5 hours after acute ischemic stroke. N Engl J Med. 2008;359(13):1317–29.
4. Broderick JP, Palesch YY, Demchuk AM, et al. Endovascular therapy after intravenous t-PA versus t-PA alone for stroke. N Engl J Med. 2013;368(10):893–903.

5. Ciccone A, Valvassori L, Nichelatti M, et al. Endovascular treatment for acute ischemic stroke. N Engl J Med. 2013;368(10):904–13.
6. Kidwell CS, Jahan R, Gornbein J, et al. A trial of imaging selection and endovascular treatment for ischemic stroke. N Engl J Med. 2013;368(10):914–23.
7. Berkhemer OA, Fransen PS, Beumer D, et al. A randomized trial of intraarterial treatment for acute ischemic stroke. N Engl J Med. 2015;372(1):11–20.
8. Campbell BC, Mitchell PJ, Kleinig TJ, et al. Endovascular therapy for ischemic stroke with perfusion-imaging selection. N Engl J Med. 2015;372(11):1009–18.
9. Goyal M, Demchuk AM, Menon BK, et al. Randomized assessment of rapid endovascular treatment of ischemic stroke. N Engl J Med. 2015;372(11):1019–30.
10. Zeumer H, Hacke W, Ringelstein EB. Local intraarterial thrombolysis in vertebrobasilar thromboembolic disease. AJNR Am J Neuroradiol. 1983;4(3):401–4.
11. del Zoppo GJ, Higashida RT, Furlan AJ, Pessin MS, Rowley HA, Gent M. PROACT: a phase II randomized trial of recombinant pro-urokinase by direct arterial delivery in acute middle cerebral artery stroke. PROACT Investigators. Prolyse in Acute Cerebral Thromboembolism. Stroke J Cereb Circ. 1998;29(1):4–11.
12. Furlan A, Higashida R, Wechsler L, et al. Intra-arterial prourokinase for acute ischemic stroke. The PROACT II study: a randomized controlled trial. Prolyse in Acute Cerebral Thromboembolism. JAMA. 1999;282(21):2003–11.
13. Jayaraman MV, Hussain MS, Abruzzo T, et al. Embolectomy for stroke with emergent large vessel occlusion (ELVO): report of the Standards and Guidelines Committee of the Society of NeuroInterventional Surgery. J Neurointerventional Surg. 2015;7(5):316–21.
14. Smith WS, Sung G, Starkman S, et al. Safety and efficacy of mechanical embolectomy in acute ischemic stroke: results of the MERCI trial. Stroke J Cereb Circ. 2005;36(7):1432–8.
15. Smith WS. Safety of mechanical thrombectomy and intravenous tissue plasminogen activator in acute ischemic stroke. Results of the multi Mechanical Embolus Removal in Cerebral Ischemia (MERCI) trial, part I. AJNR Am J Neuroradiol. 2006;27(6):1177–82.
16. Penumbra Pivotal Stroke Trial I. The penumbra pivotal stroke trial: safety and effectiveness of a new generation of mechanical devices for clot removal in intracranial large vessel occlusive disease. Stroke J Cereb Circ. 2009;40(8):2761–8.
17. Saver JL, Jahan R, Levy EI, et al. Solitaire flow restoration device versus the Merci Retriever in patients with acute ischaemic stroke (SWIFT): a randomised, parallel-group, non-inferiority trial. Lancet. 2012;380(9849):1241–9.
18. Nogueira RG, Lutsep HL, Gupta R, et al. Trevo versus Merci retrievers for thrombectomy revascularisation of large vessel occlusions in acute ischaemic stroke (TREVO 2): a randomised trial. Lancet. 2012;380(9849):1231–40.

Arterial Bypass

18

David J. Langer, Mohammed Labib, and
Hussam Abou Al-Shaar

Introduction

When M. Gazi Yaşargil performed the first extracranial-intracranial (EC-IC) bypass in 1967 for a patient with carotid artery occlusion [1], a new field of neurovascular surgery had begun. The interest cerebrovascular bypass surgery as a viable option for flow augmentation grew exponentially in the 1980s. However, the results of EC-IC [2, 3] and the more recent COSS [4] trials, which compared the effects of EC-IC bypass plus best medical therapy to medical therapy alone in patients with ischemic cerebrovascular disease, were very disappointing. Despite the declining indications for cerebral revascularization in the management of ischemia, bypass surgery remains an important tool in the armamentarium of the neurosurgeon treating complex aneurysms, skull base tumors, and moyamoya disease.

D.J. Langer (✉)
Department of Neurosurgery, North Shore LIJ/Hofstra School of Medicine,
Lenox Hill Hospital, New York, NY, USA
e-mail: langerd@mac.com

M. Labib
Department of Neurosurgery, North Shore LIJ/Hofstra School of Medicine,
Hempstead, NY, USA

H. Abou Al-Shaar
College of Medicine, Alfaisal University, Riyadh, Saudi Arabia

E. Veznedaroglu (ed.), *Controversies in Vascular Neurosurgery*,
DOI 10.1007/978-3-319-27315-0_18

Bypass Indications

The current indications for cerebral revascularization include:

1. Intracranial aneurysms
2. Moyamoya disease
3. Cerebral ischemia
4. Skull base tumors

Intracranial Aneurysms

Cerebral revascularization for intracranial aneurysms is employed in the management of giant and complex aneurysms not amenable to endovascular intervention or clipping. Giant aneurysms represent 3–5 % of all intracranial aneurysms and present with a variety of symptoms (related to mass effects or ischemia) such as visual deficits, cranial nerve palsies, hemiparesis, and hydrocephalous. Subarachnoid hemorrhage due to aneurysmal rupture can present in up to 35 % of patients. If managed conservatively, these aneurysms carry a 5-year mortality rate of up to 80 % [5].

There are many factors that classify an aneurysm to be complex including the presence of a very broad neck (dome-to-neck ratio <1.5), fusiform and saccular-fusiform aneurysms, symptomatic dissecting aneurysms, small blister aneurysms, the presence of severe atherosclerosis or calcification of at the neck, the presence of extensive aneurysmal thrombosis, and the origin of critical branches from the aneurysm sac or neck [6].

Bypass surgery for intracranial aneurysms should take into account the age and clinical condition of the patient, location and size of the aneurysm, possible treatment alternatives, and the risks involved with each modality, as well as the surgeon's preference and level of comfort with the different bypass strategies.

Flow replacement to major cerebral territories prior to surgical or endovascular aneurysmal occlusion is the ultimate goal. Specifically, EC-IC bypass is performed during the treatment of a complex intracranial aneurysm when the parent vessel or one of the major branches needs to be sacrificed. Moreover, temporary bypass using vessel graft may be performed during protracted temporary clipping of the parent artery to provide adequate collateral circulation to the brain [6].

Conventional EC-IC bypass procedures for complex aneurysms require harvest of the transplanted conduit, cervical incision for the proximal anastomosis, craniotomy for distal anastomosis, and parent vessel occlusion. In addition, they carry a risk of graft compression and kinking, and in the event of graft complication, only a partial view of the total graft length is visualized [7, 8]. Recently, a new technique has been established to utilize the internal maxillary artery (IMAX) as a potential donor for cerebral revascularization. The IMAX can be easily localized anterior and parallel to a line between the foramen rotundum and the foramen ovale. The advantages of this subcranial-intracranial (SC-IC) bypass procedure over the traditional EC-IC include the avoidance of a long cervical incision, the complete visualization of the graft length, better long-term patency due to the relatively short length of the graft, the avoidance of graft "kinking" and compression in the subcutaneous compartment, and the concentration of the surgeon's focus on one microscopic field instead of translating back and forth between the head and neck. The IMAX-IC bypass can be utilized in cases that require high flow replacement where the use of the cervical carotid is contraindicated (i.e., after neck surgery or in the setting of occlusion of the common carotid artery) [7, 8]. The radial artery, saphenous vein, and brachiocephalic vein can be used as bypass grafts in such cases [7–9].

IC-IC bypass is performed less frequently compared to EC-IC bypass procedures. It is mainly allocated for a few aneurysms of the anterior cerebral artery territory, posterior inferior cerebellar artery, and middle cerebral artery. There are four main surgical techniques utilized during IC-IC bypass procedures. In situ bypass (most commonly used) utilizes a parallel and proximate donor artery that is connected to the recipient artery with a side-to-side anastomosis [10]. Reanastomosis bypass (least commonly utilized) repairs the parent artery directly by reconnecting the afferent and efferent arteries with an end-to-end anastomosis. Reimplantation bypass reattaches the recipient artery to a parent or other donor artery with an end-to-side anastomosis. In cases where the anatomy is unfavorable for any of the IC-IC bypasses described above, an interpositional bypass uses a harvested graft from the radial artery or saphenous vein to connect the donor and recipient arteries with two or more anastomoses [11].

When a vessel graft is needed, the choice should be based on the size of the recipient vessel, availability of a donor vessel, degree of blood flow augmentation required, and availability of graft material [6]. Recently Amin-Hanjani and Charbel described a novel methodology to guide graft selection [12]. Their flow-assisted surgical technique (FAST) uses flow measurements of the vessel to be bypassed to quantify the volume of blood to be replaced. Once this volume is quantified using a microvascular ultrasonic flow probe, the STA "cut flow" is measured similarly to determine whether the STA alone can act as an adequate replacement donor. If the STA is found inadequate, a larger flow donor must be utilized. STA stump or a transplanted conduit graft for the cervical carotid may then be necessary. The superficial temporal artery (STA) and occipital artery are the main vessels utilized in lower flow (<50 mL/m) bypasses, the radial artery can provide intermediate flows (50–150 mL/m) graft, while vein grafts usually provide the highest flows (100–200 mL/m) [5, 6, 9]. The decision for the optimal graft is based on the factors indicated above. The minimum caliber needed for the vessel to be harvested and used in bypass surgery is 1 mm for the STA, 2.4 mm for the radial artery, and 3 mm for the saphenous vein [6].

The radial artery is easier to harvest than the saphenous vein. However, radial artery spasm may develop during or after harvesting the graft. Therefore, the use of pressure distention techniques may aid in the prevention of this undesirable problem [13]. It is essential to perform Allen's test preoperatively where the radial artery is to be harvested and used as a graft. The saphenous or brachiocephalic vein can be utilized as well. Vein grafts have a thin wall and are more prone to kinking or extreme turbulence because of the high flow. They may also arterialize or undergo accelerated atherosclerosis [6, 9, 13]. The patency rate of the radial artery at 3 weeks post-operation was 95 % compared to 86 % at 30 days post-operation for the saphenous vein graft [14, 15]. Vein grafts are somewhat easier to handle and sew to the intracranial recipient due to their thin walls. The decision to use radial artery versus vein is in reality at the discretion of the surgeon and is more often than not based upon personal preference. Harvest of the donor can be performed both conventionally and via endoscopic technique.

The optimal surgical exposure should allow for the visualization of the aneurysm and the donor and recipient vessels in addition to allow proximal and distal control. This might be achieved with one surgical approach or more depending on the location of the aneurysm and the planned bypass [11]. Intraoperative flow measurements using the Transonic Charbel flow probe are critical. Indocyanine green angiography can be helpful to assess patency; however, we utilize intraoperative angiography for all bypasses for aneurysms. We defer any vascular deconstruction until an adequate bypass is demonstrated utilizing conventional angiography. Often with giant aneurysms of the middle cerebral artery or PICA, we defer direct aneurysm deconstruction. We prefer to deconstruct these lesions utilizing interventional technique postoperatively, thus avoiding dissection of critical perforators and cranial nerves that are often associated with these locations. It is of critical importance to stress the bypass prior to continuing on to the INR suite. A bypass without demand is likely to thrombose, and partial deconstruction or vessel sacrifice is usually performed to increase bypass flow demand prior to moving angiography. Hybrid rooms allow this to be done more efficiently and are ideal for these bypass/vascular deconstruction procedures.

Moyamoya Disease

Moyamoya disease was first described in Japan in the 1960s as narrowing of the distal ICAs that gives rise to an oligemic state, which stimulates the formation of collaterals with a typical "puff of smoke" appearance on angiography [16]. The majority of patients present with symptoms related to cerebral hypoperfusion and stroke, with some patients developing cerebral hemorrhage.

To date, different medical interventions have failed to improve the symptomology and prognosis in such patients. Forty to 82 % of symptomatic patients treated medically develop a new stroke within 5 years [17–19]. Moreover, 32 % of those with unilateral disease will progress to bilateral disease in 5 years [20]. Cerebral revascularization represents the only treatment modality to improve the symptoms and prognosis in symptomatic patients. It was reported that 71 % and 87 % of moyamoya patients undergoing cerebral revascularization have symptomatic and functional improvement, respectively [21].

Different modalities have been developed to address the condition and aid in the development of collateral circulation to improve the brain perfusion. These are divided into two major categories, direct and indirect revascularization procedures [22]. Direct revascularization procedures include EC-IC bypass utilizing an

STA-MCA bypass or radial artery bypass grafting. The direct procedures are advocated for adult patients with symptomatic disease. The indirect revascularization procedures include encephaloduroarteriosynangiosis (EDAS), encephalomyosynangiosis (EMS), encephaloduroarteriomyosynangiosis, omental flaps, and multiple burr hole procedure. Those procedures have been advocated in the child population. Both procedures have been proven to be effective among moyamoya patients. Combinations of both direct and indirect procedures have been utilized by some surgeons with promising results [21–24].

The direct revascularization through an STA-MCA bypass is performed by exposing the parietal and frontal branches of the STA. The frontal STA branch is used in the anastomosis with a cortical branch of the MCA, while the parietal branch is made adherent to the cortex by suturing it to the pia with the underlying arachnoid being opened at multiple sites to enhance spontaneous angiogenesis. The bone and muscle flaps should allow the vessels to enter and exit without compression or kinks [23]. The direct bypass enhances the perfusion acutely in the majority of patients [21–25]. This anastomosis will enlarge as much as 50 % with time [25]. The recent report of the JAM trial showed that direct bypass surgery for adult patients with hemorrhagic moyamoya significantly decreased the rate of all adverse events and rebleeding attacks and improved patients' prognosis within 5 years. The authors concluded that these results strongly suggest that the newly established bypass flow can influence the hemodynamic state of the collateral vessels and lessen their overstress [27]. However, there are still some potential disadvantages to direct anastomoses including the development of a stroke from an embolic event, cross-clamping of recipient vessels, hyperperfusion syndrome, hypotension, long operative time, and the technical challenges of anastomoses [21]. In one series of 450 revascularization procedures in children and adults, 91 % of whom were treated with direct anastomoses, symptoms resolved within 1 month of direct bypass. The risk of perioperative or subsequent stroke or hemorrhage was only 5.5 % over 5 years, and 71 % of patients had functional improvement as measured by the modified Rankin scale (mRS) [28]. The technical complications can be avoided by utilizing the microscope for STA exposure, using an adventitial flap around the parietal branch of the STA to avoid iatrogenic injury and vasospasm, extensive cleaning of the distal end of the frontal branch of the STA, and meticulous wound closure to avoid graft compression and kinking [23].

Adults with a small fragile STA or cortical MCA branches of <0.7 mm in diameter and children should undergo indirect revascularization procedure [21, 23]. There are many indirect procedures reported in the literature with EDAS being the most commonly used procedure due to its high success rates (92 %) [29]. In EDAS, the parietal STA branch should be dissected with a cuff of galea and tacked to an avascular section of pia with or without dural inversion. Indirect procedures are generally associated with shorter operative times, fewer technical challenges, and similar outcomes to direct procedures [21, 23]. However, one major disadvantage is the delay of angiogenesis, which may take weeks to months to develop (mean 3–4 months) [26, 30]. The indirect bypass will enhance cerebral perfusion in the long term. Thus, we, as well as other authors, advocate to combine both direct and indirect procedures in symptomatic adult patients in order to enhance the perfusion acutely (direct) and in the long term (indirect) based on the concept that direct and indirect bypass procedures are temporally complementary and inversely related to one another as observed by graft shrinkage over time as a response to reduced demand due to collateral vessel formation [23, 24, 30].

Cerebral Ischemia

Revascularization in cerebral ischemia is still a controversial issue among cerebrovascular neurosurgeons and continues to be under evaluation. The results of the major trials (EC-IC and COSS) [2–4] comparing EC-IC bypass with the best medical therapy to the best medical therapy alone in ischemic cerebrovascular disease have failed to demonstrate the effectiveness of bypass surgery over medical therapy. Despite the high bypass patency rates, stroke and mortality rates were significantly higher in the bypass group compared to the medically treated group.

Therefore, bypass for cerebral ischemia is used as a last resort in a limited number of patients who fail to improve despite receiving maximal medical therapy [31]. In one study by the Barrow Neurological Institute, the authors reported their experience with 28 bypass procedures on 27 patients with cerebral occlusive vascular disease. They found that the bypass patency rate was 100 % in their long-term follow-up. Interestingly, only 55.5 % of patients improved symptomatically with 14.3 % of patients developing morbidities [25].

Skull Base Tumors

With recent advances in radiotherapy and chemotherapy, the rate of bypass surgery for skull base tumors has tremendously decreased. Some authors advocate for bypass as it aids in the resection of skull base tumors and improves both patient and tumor outcomes. Others, however, believe that carotid artery preservation should be always maintained even in the event of iatrogenic laceration.

It is essential to determine if the vessel is invaded or only encased by the tumor. Of similar importance is the evaluation of the presence of collaterals. With the exception of meningiomas, benign tumors, like schwannomas and pituitary adenomas, can generally be dissected away from the vessel [6]. On the other hand, meningiomas tend to invade and narrow the vessel, making vessel sacrifice a must for complete surgical resection [32]. However, many surgeons prefer to leave a residual, which can be tackled by radiosurgery. Chordomas and chondrosarcomas are similar to benign lesions, in which vessel skeletonization could be achieved surgically in the majority of patients. For slow-growing malignant neoplasms such as adenoid cystic carcinomas, vessel sacrifice is needed for optimal and complete tumor removal. In such procedures, vessel sacrifice enables the surgeon to pay extra attention to cranial nerve preservation [6].

References

1. Yaşargil MG. Anastomosis between superficial temporal artery and a branch of the middle cerebral artery. Stuttgart: Georg Thieme Verlag; 1969.
2. The EC/IC Bypass Study Group. Failure of extracranial-intracranial arterial bypass to reduce the risk of ischemic stroke. Results of an international randomized trial. N Engl J Med. 1985;313(19):1191–200.
3. The EC/IC Bypass Study group. The International Cooperative Study of Extracranial/Intracranial Arterial Anastomosis (EC/IC Bypass Study): methodology and entry characteristics. Stroke. 1985;16(3):397–406.
4. Powers WJ, Clarke WR, Grubb Jr RL, Videen TO, Adams Jr HP, Derdeyn CP, COSS Investigators. Extracranial-intracranial bypass surgery for stroke prevention in hemodynamic cerebral ischemia: the Carotid Occlusion Surgery Study randomized trial. JAMA. 2011;306(18):1983–92.
5. Drake CG. Giant intracranial aneurysms: experience with surgical treatment in 174 patients. Clin Neurosurg. 1979;26:12–95.
6. Sekhar LN, Natarajan SK, Ellenbogen RG, Ghodke B. Cerebral revascularization for ischemia, aneurysms, and cranial base tumors. Neurosurgery. 2008;62(6 Suppl 3):1373–408; discussion 1408–10.
7. Nossek E, Costantino PD, Eisenberg M, Dehdashti AR, Setton A, Chalif DJ, Ortiz RA, Langer DJ. Internal maxillary artery-middle cerebral artery bypass: infratemporal approach for subcranial-intracranial (SC-IC) bypass. Neurosurgery. 2014;75(1):87–95.
8. Abdulrauf SI, Sweeney JM, Mohan YS, Palejwala SK. Short segment internal maxillary artery to middle cerebral artery bypass: a novel technique for extracranial-to-intracranial bypass. Neurosurgery. 2011;68(3):804–8; discussion 808–09.
9. Liu JK, Kan P, Karwande SV, Couldwell WT. Conduits for cerebrovascular bypass and lessons learned from the cardiovascular experience. Neurosurg Focus. 2003;14(3):e3.
10. Korja M, Sen C, Langer D. Operative nuances of side to side in situ posterior inferior cerebellar artery to posterior inferior cerebellar artery bypass. Neurosurgery. 2010;67:ons471–7.
11. Abla AA, Lawton MT. Anterior cerebral artery bypass for complex aneurysms: an experience with intracranial-intracranial reconstruction and review of bypass options. J Neurosurg. 2014;120(6):1364–77.
12. Amin Hanjani S, Charbel FT. Flow assisted surgical technique in cerebrovascular surgery. Surg Neurol. 2007;68(S1):S4–11. 1.
13. Sekhar LN, Bucur SD, Bank WO, Wright DC. Venous and arterial bypass grafts for difficult tumors, aneurysms, and occlusive vascular lesions: evolution of surgical treatment and improved graft results. Neurosurgery. 1999;44(6):1207–23; discussion 1223–4.
14. Houkin K, Kamiyama H, Kuroda S, Ishikawa T, Takahashi A, Abe H. Long-term patency of radial artery graft bypass for reconstruction of the internal carotid artery. Technical note. J Neurosurg. 1999;90(4):786–90.
15. Regli L, Piepgras DG, Hansen KK. Late patency of long saphenous vein bypass grafts to the anterior and posterior cerebral circulation. J Neurosurg. 1995;83(5):806–11.
16. Hoffman HJ. Moyamoya disease and syndrome. Clin Neurol Neurosurg. 1997;99 Suppl 2:S39–44.
17. Chiu D, Shedden P, Bratina P, Grotta JC. Clinical features of moyamoya disease in the United States. Stroke. 1998;29(7):1347–51.
18. Hallemeier CL, Rich KM, Grubb Jr RL, Chicoine MR, Moran CJ, Cross 3rd DT, Zipfel GJ, Dacey Jr RG, Derdeyn CP. Clinical features and outcome in North American adults with moyamoya phenomenon. Stroke. 2006;37(6):1490–6.
19. Shirane R, Yoshida Y, Takahashi T, Yoshimoto T. Assessment of encephalo-galeo-myo-synangiosis with dural pedicle insertion in childhood moyamoya disease: characteristics of cerebral blood flow and oxygen metabolism. Clin Neurol Neurosurg. 1997;99 Suppl 2:S79–85.

20. Kelly ME, Bell-Stephens TE, Marks MP, Do HM, Steinberg GK. Progression of unilateral moyamoya disease: a clinical series. Cerebrovasc Dis. 2006;22(2–3):109–15.
21. Abla AA, Gandhoke G, Clark JC, Oppenlander ME, Velat GJ, Zabramski JM, Albuquerque FC, Nakaji P, Spetzler RF, Wanebo JE. Surgical outcomes for moyamoya angiopathy at barrow neurological institute with comparison of adult indirect encephaloduroarteriosynangiosis bypass, adult direct superficial temporal artery-to-middle cerebral artery bypass, and pediatric bypass: 154 revascularization surgeries in 140 affected hemispheres. Neurosurgery. 2013;73(3):430–9.
22. Baaj AA, Agazzi S, Sayed ZA, Toledo M, Spetzler RF, van Loveren H. Surgical management of moyamoya disease: a review. Neurosurg Focus. 2009;26(4):E7.
23. Nossek E, Langer DJ. How I do it: combined direct (STA-MCA) and indirect (EDAS) EC-IC bypass. Acta Neurochir (Wien). 2014;156(11):2079–84.
24. Amin-Hanjani S, Singh A, Rifai H, Thulborn KR, Alaraj A, Aletich V, Charbel FT. Combined direct and indirect bypass for moyamoya: quantitative assessment of direct bypass flow over time. Neurosurgery. 2013;73(6):962–7; discussion 967–8.
25. Kalani MY, Rangel-Castilla L, Ramey W, Nakaji P, Albuquerque FC, McDougall CG, Spetzler RF, Zabramski JM. Indications and results of direct cerebral revascularization in the modern era. World Neurosurg. 2015;83(3):345–50.
26. Veeravagu A, Guzman R, Patil CG, Hou LC, Lee M, Steinberg GK. Moyamoya disease in pediatric patients: outcomes of neurosurgical interventions. Neurosurg Focus. 2008;24(2):E16.
27. Miyamoto S, Yoshimoto T, Hashimoto N, Okada Y, Tsuji I, Tominaga T, Nakagawara J, Takahashi JC, JAM Trial Investigators. Effects of extracranial-intracranial bypass for patients with hemorrhagic moyamoya disease: results of the Japan Adult Moyamoya trial. Stroke. 2014;45(5):1415–21.
28. Guzman R, Lee M, Achrol A, Bell-Stephens T, Kelly M, Do HM, Marks MP, Steinberg GK. Clinical outcome after 450 revascularization procedures for moyamoya disease. Clinical article. J Neurosurg. 2009;111(5):927–35.
29. Isono M, Ishii K, Kamida T, Inoue R, Fujiki M, Kobayashi H. Long-term outcomes of pediatric moyamoya disease treated by encephalo-duro-arterio-synangiosis. Pediatr Neurosurg. 2002;36(1):14–21.
30. Houkin K, Kamiyama H, Takahashi A, Kuroda S, Abe H. Combined revascularization surgery for childhood moyamoya disease: STA-MCA and encephalo-duro-arterio-myo-synangiosis. Childs Nerv Syst. 1997;13(1):24–9.
31. Reynolds MR, Derdeyn CP, Grubb Jr RL, Powers WJ, Zipfel GJ. Extracranial-intracranial bypass for ischemic cerebrovascular disease: what have we learned from the Carotid Occlusion Surgery Study? Neurosurg Focus. 2014;36(1):E9.
32. Kotapka MJ, Kalia KK, Martinez AJ, Sekhar LN. Infiltration of the carotid artery by cavernous sinus meningioma. J Neurosurg. 1994;81(2):252–5.

Cranial Dural AV Fistulas: Making Sense of Who to Treat and How

19

Rami James N. Aoun, Mithun G. Sattur, Andrew R. Pines, Tariq K. Halasa, Youssef J. Hamade, Samer G. Zammar, and Bernard R. Bendok

Introduction

Cranial dural arteriovenous fistulas (DAVFs) are abnormal vascular malformations of the cranial dura that involve direct connections between meningeal arteries draining into veins adjacent to dural venous sinuses. Their etiology remains unknown, though dural fistulas are known to occur after venous sinus thrombosis and trauma. Microsurgical, radiosurgical, and interventional approaches all play critical roles in dural fistula management. These modalities can be used in isolation or in tandem depending on a number of factors including location, anatomy of the fistula, and the feasibility of both arterial and venous access to the nidus and draining vein(s). Observation may be appropriate for select dural fistula when they are low grade and not affecting quality of life. Careful assessment of clinical symptoms, the physical exam, noninvasive imaging, and a thorough cranial angiogram are the bedrock of safe and effective patient management. This chapter is augmented with a compendium of interesting illustrative case examples of DAVFs that have been managed by the senior author and clearly illustrates the concept of a multimodal management strategy.

R.J.N. Aoun, MD, MPH (✉) • M.G. Sattur, MD • A.R. Pines, MA • T.K. Halasa, MD
Y.J. Hamade, MD, MSCI • B.R. Bendok, MD, MSCI
Department of Neurosurgery, Mayo Clinic, Phoenix, AZ, USA
e-mail: aoun.rami@mayo.edu

S.G. Zammar, MD, MPH
Department of General Surgery, Mayo Clinic, Phoenix, AZ, USA

E. Veznedaroglu (ed.), *Controversies in Vascular Neurosurgery*,
DOI 10.1007/978-3-319-27315-0_19

Table 19.1 Location distribution of DAVFs in the brain [3]

DAVF location	Frequency (%)
Transverse and sigmoid sinus	61
Cavernous sinus	10
Middle fossa	7.7
Convexity	6.5
Confluence of sinuses	3.1
Frontobasal	3.1
Tentorium	2.7
Superior sagittal sinus	2.3
Foramen magnum	1.9
Other	1.9

Epidemiology

The rate of detection of dural arteriovenous fistulas has been increasing in parallel to the evolution of imaging modalities [1–4]. Yearly population incidence rates for DAVFs are 0.15 per 100,000 individuals, but have been reported as high as 0.29 per 100,000 (Japan) to 0.51 per 100,000 (Finland) [3, 5, 6]. These lesions have a 1:1 male to female predilection and typically present during the fifth and sixth decades [1, 3]. The anatomic distribution of cranial dural fistulas varies widely as outlined in Table 19.1.

Clinical Presentation

The range and severity of symptoms depends on the location, hemodynamics, and venous drainage patterns of the dural AVFs [7]. Patients may present with a wide variety of symptoms ranging from mild to severe and even fatal [8–11]. Symptoms are known to correlate to location. DAVFs related to the cavernous sinus typically manifest with ocular symptoms such as exophthalmos, visual disturbance, orbital pain or swelling, and ophthalmoplegia (Case 19.5) [1, 12, 13]. DAVFs related to the transverse-sigmoid junction can present with pulsatile tinnitus as they are contiguous to the auditory apparatus [12, 14]. DAVFs draining into the superior sagittal sinus or deep veins may manifest with symptoms of prolonged intracranial hypertension and venous congestion, such as hydrocephalus, seizures, and papilledema [1, 10, 14]. Fistulas involving the brainstem may present with cranial nerve involvement, motor weakness, or paralysis [15]. Rarely, fistulas may present with cognitive dysfunction and memory loss (Cases 19.1 and 19.4).

Diagnostic Approach and Imaging

The history, physical exam, and noninvasive imaging are all important for proper selection of patients for further workup with a diagnostic cerebral angiogram. MRA and CTA in patients who present with brain hemorrhage can show clues that point toward the diagnosis of dural fistula (Case 19.3). Fundamentally a cerebral angiogram remains the gold standard of diagnosis and the most helpful modality for treatment decision-making [3, 16–18]. It is crucial to include both external carotid systems in the angiographic injection, in addition to the internal carotid and vertebral systems.

Grading

The first classification system for dural arteriovenous fistulas was proposed by Djindjian and Merland who analyzed angiographic findings in relation to hemorrhagic risk. Accordingly, they classified dural fistulas into grades I–IV (Table 19.2). Contemporary classification systems currently followed in clinical practice, however, are the Cognard and Borden classification systems [10, 19]. Borden classified DAVFs into three grades

Table 19.2 Merland and Djindjian classification of dural AVFs [19]

Merland and Djindjian type	
I	Dural sinus or meningeal vein
II	Dural sinus with cortical venous reflux
III	Purely into cortical vein
IV	Cortical vein with supra- or infratentorial venous lake

Table 19.3 Borden classification of dural AVFs [19]

Borden classification	Description
1	Venous drainage directly into venous sinus or meningeal veins
2	Venous drainage into dural venous sinus with CVR
3	Venous drainage directly into subarachnoid veins (CVR) only

Table 19.4 Cognard classification of dural AVFs [10]

Grade	Venous drainage	Venous sinus flow	Cortical venous flow	Hemorrhage risk (%)	Description
I	Venous sinus	Antegrade	Antegrade	~0	Venous drainage into dural venous sinus with antegrade flow
IIa	Venous sinus	Retrograde	Antegrade	~0	Venous drainage into dural venous sinus with retrograde flow, no cortical vein involvement
IIb	Venous sinus	Antegrade	Retrograde	20	Venous drainage into dural venous sinus with antegrade flow and cortical vein reflux
IIa+b	Venous sinus	Retrograde	Retrograde	6	Venous drainage into dural venous sinus with retrograde flow and cortical vein reflux
III	Cortical veins	N/A	Retrograde	45	Drains directly into cortical veins
IV	Cortical veins	N/A	Retrograde	60	Drains directly into cortical veins with venous ectasia
V	Spinal medullary veins	N/A	N/A	N/A	Spinal perimedullary venous drainage, associated with progressive myelopathy

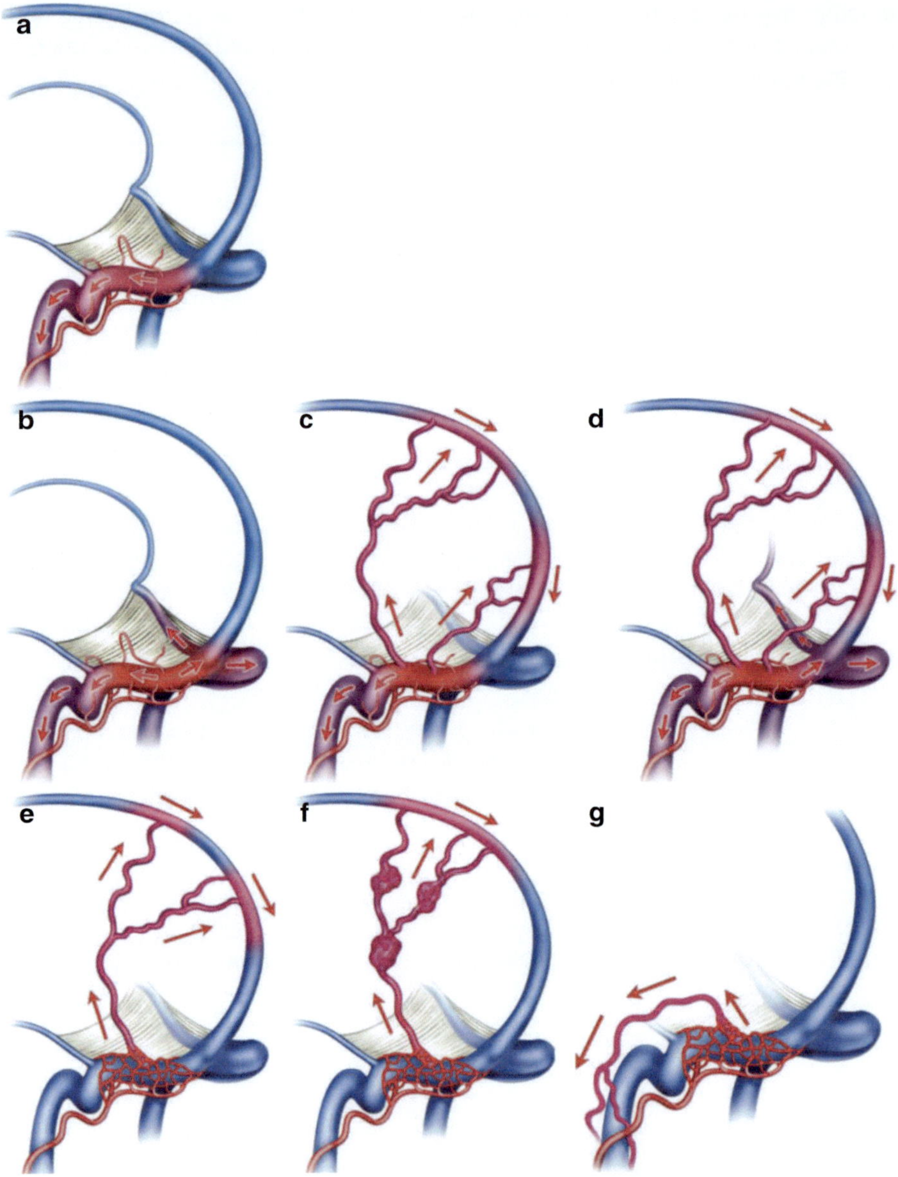

Fig. 19.1 Cognard (C) and Borden (B) DAVF classification. The fistula is located in the wall of the transverse sinus in each example: (**a**) C1, B1, antegrade flow in sinus. (**b**) C2a, B1, retrograde flow in the sinus. (**c**) C2b, B2, retrograde reflux into cortical veins with antegrade flow in sinus. (**d**) C2a+b, B2, retrograde flow in the sinus and reflux into cortical veins. (**e**) C3, B3, direct fistula drainage into cortical veins. (**f**) C4, B3, similar to E but associated with venous ectasia. (**g**) C5, drainage directly into perimedullary spinal veins [20]

Table 19.5 Barrow classification of carotid cavernous fistulas [21]

Grade	Characteristics
A	Direct internal carotid artery (ICA)-cavernous sinus fistula
B	Dural ICA branch-cavernous sinus fistula
C	Dural external carotid artery branch-cavernous sinus fistula
D	ICA/ECA dural branches-cavernous sinus fistula

(I–III) (Table 19.3), while Cognard classified the lesions into five grades (grade I–V) with three subtypes for class II DAVFs (IIa, IIb, and IIa+b) (Table 19.4) (Fig. 19.1). Based on the Cognard classification, the annual risk of hemorrhage from a type I or type IIA arteriovenous fistula is zero. Type II B is associated with an overall risk of 20%, whereas types III and IV are associated with an overall hemorrhage risk of 40% and 65%, respectively. In both classifications, type I and II fistulas drain into the venous sinuses, and type III into cortical veins. Additionally, in Cognard's classification, type IV fistulas drain into cortical veins and are associated with venous ectasia, and type V drain into perimedullary spinal veins (Fig. 19.1).

Carotid cavernous sinus fistulas (CCFs) are classified separately using the Barrow classification system (Table 19.5). The typical "dural" CCFs are types B–D. Type A is a direct carotid to cavernous sinus fistula that typically presents acutely with aggressive symptomatology [21].

Natural History and Clinical Course

In the absence of cortical venous reflux (CVR), DAVFs typically present as incidental findings or with signs and symptoms of increased dural venous drainage (bruit, tinnitus) [1, 12, 13, 22]. In a study of 68 patients with dural arteriovenous fistulas and no cortical venous drainage [23], none of the patients had neurological deficits and only 1 (1%) developed intracranial hemorrhage during a mean follow-up period of 27.9 months. Furthermore, among 50 patients who underwent angiography at follow-up, only 2 (4%) patients developed cortical venous drainage [23]. Studies tend to indicate that dural fistulas without cortical venous drainage typically follow a benign natural history [24, 25].

In the presence of cortical venous reflux, however, patients with DAVFs are at an increased risk for intracranial hemorrhage or nonhemorrhagic neurological deficits. A study by van Dijk et al. [23] included 20 patients with DAVFs and cortical venous drainage who were treated partially or followed conservatively for a mean period of 4.3 years. 16 (80%) patients developed intracranial hemorrhage or neurological deficits. The calculated annual risks for intracranial hemorrhage and neurological deficits were 8.1% and 6.9%, respectively [23]. In a meta-analysis conducted by Awad et al. on 360 tentorial DAVFs, 31 of 32 (96%) patients with cortical venous drainage developed hemorrhagic or nonhemorrhagic neurological sequelae. Other studies have also shown an increased risk of intracranial hemorrhage and neurological deficits for patients who have venous varices and anomalies involving the deep venous system [1, 24, 26, 27].

Treatment

Patient Selection for Treatment

The key decision in DAVF management is to identify patients who need treatment. The presence of cortical venous reflux (Borden types II, III; Cognard types II b, II a+b, III, IV, and V) is a potentially concerning feature and should lead to strong consideration of treatment [28–34]. Careful consideration should be given not to attribute an unrelated hemorrhage or progressive neurological symptoms to a low-grade fistula (Borden and Cognard types I). High-grade fistulas that present with hemorrhage are invariably selected for treatment to obliterate the fistula [30]. The importance of a thorough, unhurried clinical encounter with a patient cannot be overemphasized; unilateral pulsatile tinnitus with a low-grade fistula that is interfering with quality of life is a potential indication for treatment. Observation is a valid strategy for DAVFs that are low grade, but conversion of a low-grade fistula to a high-grade one while on observation can occur at an annual rate of about 1 % [35]. Hence periodic surveillance with MR imaging is warranted in patients who are being observed [36–39].

Formulating a Treatment Strategy

Once a decision is made to treat a DAVF, the goals and methods of treatment should be formulated by careful analysis of all imaging with special emphasis on the angiogram. However, visualizing the fistula is only one component of this analysis. Important questions that should be considered are:

1. The location of the fistula: certain locations favor endovascular therapy while others favor microsurgical treatment.
2. The anatomy of arterial and venous access from both microsurgical and interventional perspectives.
3. The relationship of feeding arteries to cranial nerves and potential extracranial to intracranial collateral.
4. The relationship of normal venous drainage to the arterialized sinus or arterialized cortical veins (drainage can be mixed).
5. What is the safest and easiest way to eliminate CVR?
6. Can the benign anatomic features of the fistula be treated safely and easily?

Endovascular Management

Advances in endovascular surgery and approaches over the past two decades have allowed for an increasing proportion of dural fistulas to be effectively treated with this approach (Case 19.2). Several embolic materials have been used for successful DAVF occlusion: NBCA (n-butyl cyanoacrylate glue) (Codman Neuro, Raynham, MA), Onyx (ethylene vinyl alcohol copolymer) (ev3 Endovascular Inc., Plymouth, MN), and coils. Our preferred agent for most embolizations is Onyx for a number of reasons: First, Onyx possesses cohesive properties, as opposed to the adhesive character of NBCA, which allows for more controlled and prolonged injections [40, 41]. Second, Onyx allows for the possibility of precise, controlled injections, including stopping intermittently for short durations. Careful analysis of the angiogram can define the potential safety and success rate of both transvenous and transarterial approaches. Transarterial approaches can be quite straightforward if access can be achieved close to the nidus via a meningeal artery branch that is not in close proximity to cranial nerves. When cranial nerve proximity or potential extracranial to intracranial collaterals are at stake, then transvenous approaches may be preferable. When considering occlusion of venous structures, however, careful attention should be given to assure lack of normal venous drainage to those structures (mixed drainage). Adjuncts to transarterial Onyx may be required in technically challenging circumstances such as high-flow fistulas, in which the liquid material may quickly gain access and occlude the venous side or cause pulmonary embolism. This may take the form of balloon or coil assistance (flow control techniques) [41, 42]. Balloon- or coil-assisted Onyx embolization can potentially utilize a transarterial or transvenous route for either the balloon or coil and then employ Onyx through either route in various combinations [42, 43]. Novel dural lumen catheters have been used successfully [44, 45].

In some instances, an occluded sinus may be navigated using a microcatheter [41]. The transvenous route is by far most reliably used in management of type B–D CCFs. For non-CCFs, it has been primarily employed for TS-SS DAVFs (because anatomically they tend to have various routes for a transvenous approach) [46]. On the other hand, some DAVFs located at the tentorial incisura or anterior cranial fossa may not have accessible venous routes. Problems with transvenous occlusion include propagating venous thrombosis [47].

Obliteration rates with Onyx embolization are in the 68–92 % range [40, 48–50]. However, DAVFs that show complete obliteration on immediate postprocedure angiography have been demonstrated to occasionally recanalize or regrow on follow-up [50, 51].

Recanalization rates of around 10 % have been reported [52]. This reinforces the necessity of continued follow-up. It has been suggested that a short-term angiographic follow-up may be more predictive of long-term occlusion than relying on the immediate posttreatment angiogram [51].

Complications of cranial nerve paresis include those in the cavernous sinus (3–6) and the posterior fossa cranial nerves 7 and 9–12 with tentorial and TS-SS DAVFs and are described to occur in about 8 % of cases in most contemporary series [41, 53]. Mechanical complications such as catheter adherence and breakage are known to occur but do not necessarily translate into clinically significant problems.

Microsurgical Management

Despite the vast majority of DAVFs being treated with endovascular means, select circumstances in Borden types 2 and 3 (with CVR) lesions mandate open surgical approaches. Such cases include instances where embolization was not performed due to difficult access, critical anastomoses, or the presence of arterial feeders with critical normal supply. An example of the latter is ethmoidal DAVFs with ophthalmic artery supply, which present an increased risk of vision impairment with transarterial embolization (Case 19.4). Microsurgery is also considered when embolization is not possible and angiography shows persistent filling [54]. Based on location, tentorial DAVFs are noted to have multiple tortuous arterial feeders that supply several cranial nerves along with less accessible transvenous routes. These factors make microsurgical management for these treacherous lesions an important option [55].

Current surgical techniques are vastly different from the traditional extensive resections in the pre-embolization/early embolization era [56, 57]. Contemporary surgical strategies may take the form of interruption of the draining vein close to the fistula using image guidance, surgical excision of the involved sinus, or direct sinus packing of a nonfunctional sinus. Hybrid approaches may involve burr hole placement to access an arterialized sinus with catheter-based occlusion then delivered endovascularly [58–60]. As a "hybrid" procedure, direct surgical access of the superior ophthalmic vein, a cortical vein, the vein of Galen, or the middle meningeal artery to deliver embolic material can be employed (Case 19.3) [61–63]. Some authors make a distinction between DAVFs with CVR that drain directly into the leptomeningeal vein (non-sinus type) and ones that occur via drainage into a venous sinus (sinus type) [64]. Non-sinus-type lesions are approached with interruption of the vein close to the dura, by clipping or by coagulation, and then sectioning without tackling the arterial feeders. The sinus-type lesions can be dealt with by sinus occlusion. An important caveat for a surgical approach is recognizing that the initial scalp, bony, and dural openings may be excessively bloody due to extensive external carotid arterial feeders. Preoperative embolization can ameliorate this issue [31]. Various technical adjuncts for surgery include frameless stereotaxy, intraoperative angiography or ICG videoangiography, and intraoperative Doppler ultrasound [39].

Stereotactic Radiosurgery

Stereotactic radiosurgery (SRS) has a delayed obliteration effect on dural fistulas. While this latency period may be tolerated for benign fistulas, the high annual hemorrhage rate for fistulas with CVR makes radiosurgery problematic as a first-line therapy [30, 33, 34]. SRS is, hence, chosen as a modality in situations where the lesion is not amenable to safe endovascular/microsurgical methods of obliteration or in a patient with severe medical comorbidities. Benign residual fistula after treatment can also be targeted with SRS to potentially reduce recurrence risk or eliminate residual pulsatile tinnitus. In case of low-flow/low-risk DAVFs such as CCF types B–D or Borden type 1, SRS may have more applicability, especially to treat a postembolization residual lesion [60]. The most common radiosurgery platform used is the Gamma Knife; however, any platform may be used for treatment delivery. The radiosurgical target is the nidus which typically is located in the wall of the dural venous sinus. The dose depends on the lesion size and location and ranges from 14 to 25 Gy [65]. A recent meta-analysis of SRS for DAVFs reported a complete obliteration rate of 68.2 % over an overall mean follow-up period of 28.9 months [66]. Following SRS, there is an overall risk of hemorrhage that is in the range of 1.2–1.6 % [66, 67] over follow-up periods ranging from 2 to 11.4 years. This risk persists till complete obliteration and is higher in patients with CVR.

Cases

Case 19.1 High-Grade Dural Arteriovenous Fistula Simulating a Bilateral Thalamic Neoplasm

Summary: A 51-year-old male presented with bilateral thalamic lesions causing cognitive dysfunction. MRI demonstrated bilateral enhancing thalamic lesions with minimal mass effect (Fig. 19.2). Angiography revealed a thalamic DAVF supplied by bilateral middle meningeal arteries, marginal tentorial arteries from both ICAs, and a posterior meningeal artery from the left vertebral artery (Fig. 19.3). Transarterial endovascular embolization of the fistula was performed via both middle meningeal arteries using Onyx 18. Post-op angiography revealed complete resolution of the fistula (Fig. 19.4). Patient returned to his cognitive base-line 3 weeks after treatment.

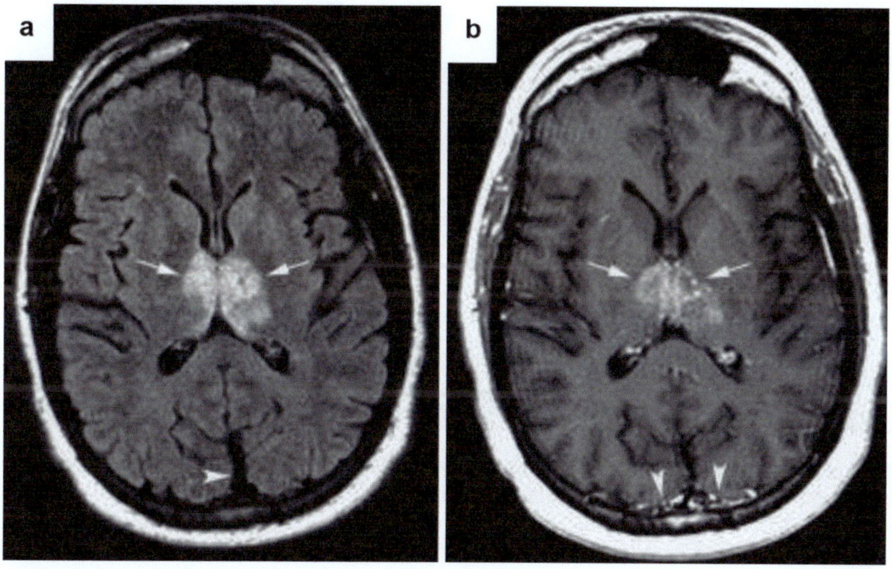

Fig. 19.2 (**a**) Axial FLAIR MRI sequence demonstrating hyperintense bilateral thalamic signal, represented by *arrows*. (**b**) T1 post-gadolinium showing bilateral thalamic enhancement, represented by *arrows*, and increased vascularity near the falcine sinus, represented by *arrowheads*

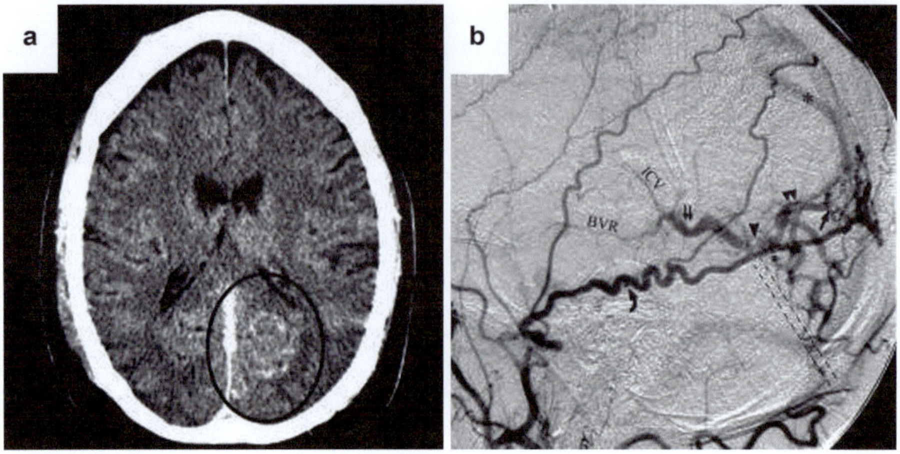

Fig. 19.3 (**a**) "Non-contrast" head axial CT (performed after an abdominal CT study for hematuria of unrelated etiology) shows enhancement of the left occipital cortical veins. (**b**) Right external carotid artery preoperative lateral cranial angiography shows an enlarged middle meningeal artery with a small flow-related aneurysm, represented by curved arrow, and supplying a leash of vessels which converge on a fistula, represented by *arrow*, draining into the posterior falcine sinus, represented by *double arrowheads*

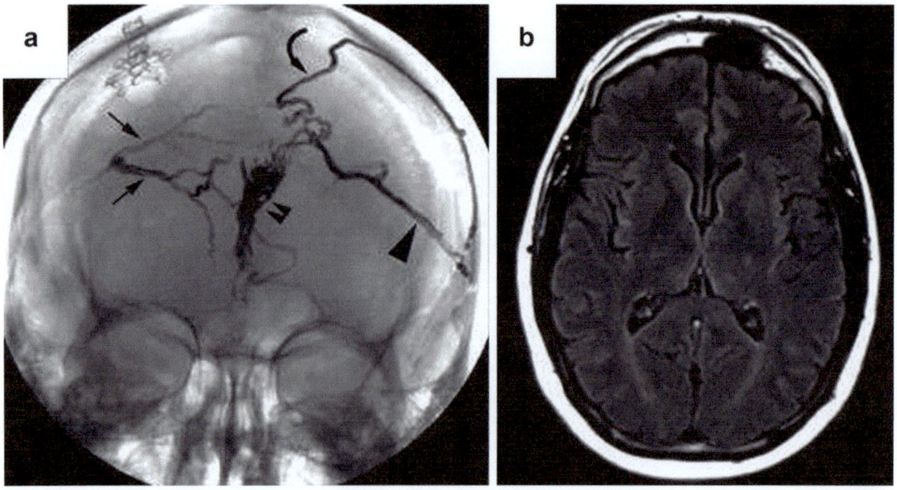

Fig. 19.4 (**a**) Angiogram following embolization of both the right middle meningeal feeders, represented by *arrows*, and left meningeal feeders, represented by *double arrowheads*. These structures were opacified by the injected Onyx. The *curved arrow* pinpoints reflux along a separate dural feeder which occurred during embolization on the *left*. (**b**) Follow-up magnetic resonance imaging (FLAIR) at 3 months interval exhibited resolution of the bithalamic high-signal aberrancy (Source: Sugrue et al. [68])

Case 19.2 Reversal of Diffusion Restriction After Embolization of Dural Arteriovenous Fistula

Summary: A 54-year-old male patient presents with a 5-day history of confusion and mental status changes. Computed tomography (CT) demonstrated gyral swelling and sulcal effacement associated with a small subcortical parenchymal hemorrhage in the left parietal region. MRI that was then performed demonstrated a broad zone of T2/FLAIR hyperintensity and restricted diffusion (Fig. 19.5). Cerebral angiogram revealed a Cognard type III left lateral tentorial DAVF with cortical venous drainage, resulting in significant left parieto-temporo-occipital venous hypertension (Fig. 19.6). The DAVF was treated by occluding the fistulous nidus endovascularly using Onyx 18. Postoperative cerebral angiography demonstrated complete obliteration with normalization of the venous drainage (Fig. 19.7). Follow-up MRI examination performed 4 weeks after the embolization revealed resolution of the previously seen area of restricted diffusion (Fig. 19.8). The patient was neurologically intact and seizure-free upon follow-up.

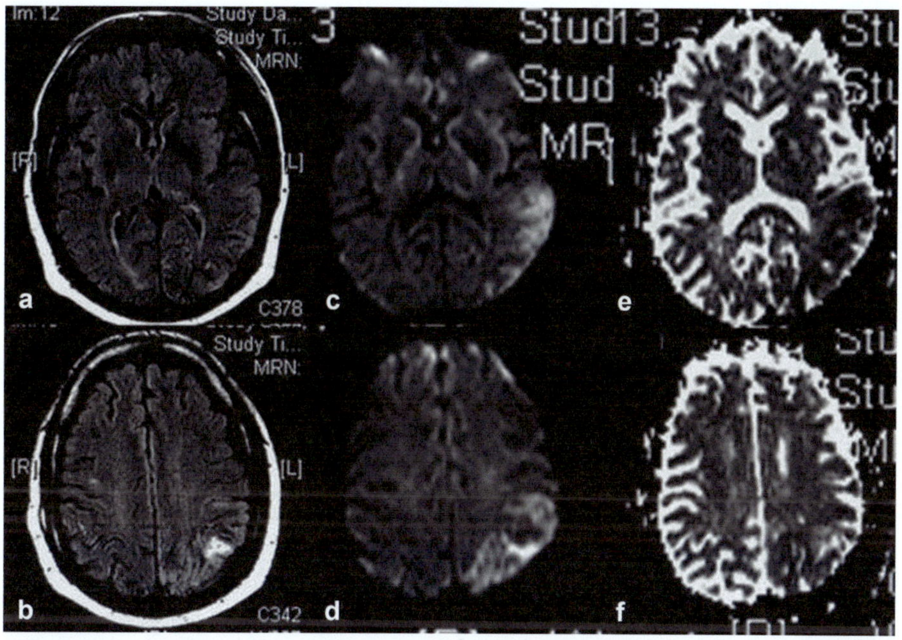

Fig. 19.5 (**a**, **b**) Magnetic resonance imaging (FLAIR sequence) showing a signal increase patient's left parietotemporal region. (**c**, **d**) Diffusion restriction is observed within the same area. (**e**, **f**) ADC map signal reduction is recognized as well

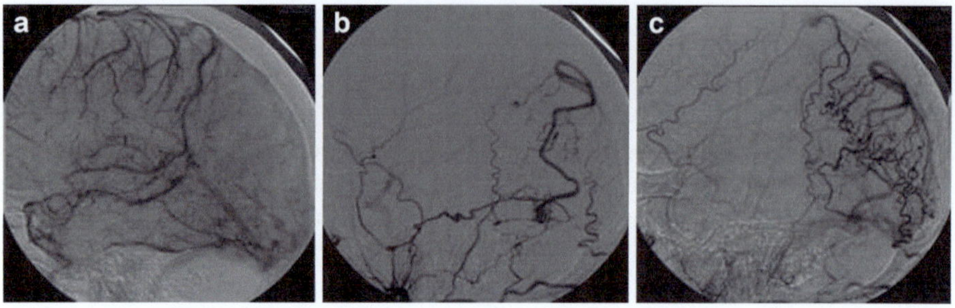

Fig. 19.6 Digital subtraction angiography (DSA) of left parieto-temporo-occipital region showing lack of cortical venous opacification. (**a**) Lateral venous phase of left internal carotid artery injection. (**b**, early phase, and **c**, late phase) Left external carotid artery injection demonstrating a Cognard type III left lateral tentorial DAVF causing considerable left parieto-temporo-occipital venous hypertension

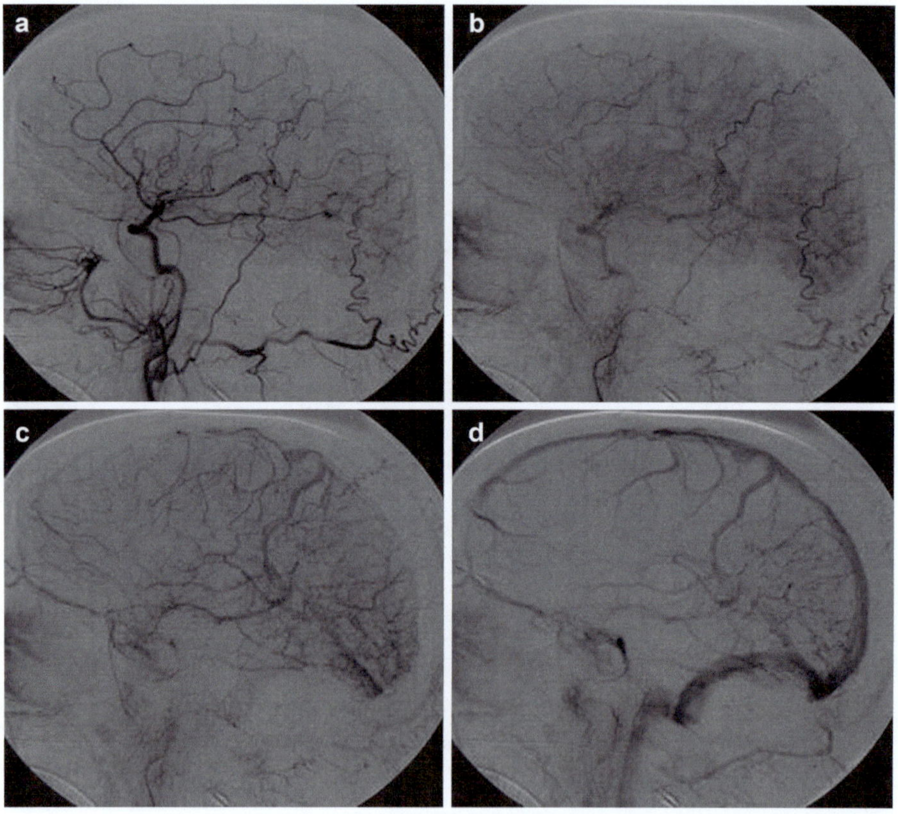

Fig. 19.7 (**a**) Posttreatment cerebral angiography revealing angiographic resolution of the aberrancy. (**b–d**) Restoration of the normal cortical venous drainage in the left parieto-temporo-occipital region

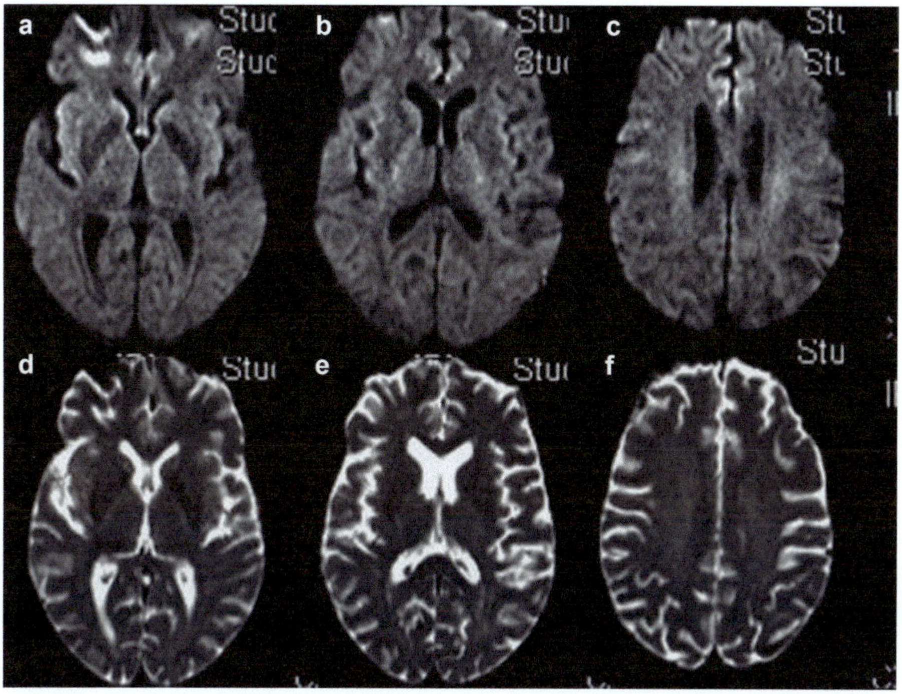

Fig. 19.8 (**a–f**) 4-week posttreatment follow-up magnetic resolution imaging (MRI) scans confirms the complete reversal of the diffusion restriction previously seen (Source: Dabus et al. [69])

Case 19.3 Combined Surgical and Endovascular Access of the Superficial Middle Cerebral Vein to Occlude a High-Grade Cavernous Dural Arteriovenous Fistula

Link: http://links.lww.com/NEU/A393

Summary: A 75-year-old female patient presented with 3-month history of left retro-orbital headaches, 1 week of intermittent vertical and horizontal diplopia, and a few days of worsening slurred speech and RUE weakness. Computed tomography head scan without contrast demonstrated an acute left temporal lobe hemorrhage (Fig. 19.9a). Subsequent, magnetic resonance imaging (MRI) and magnetic resonance angiography (MRA) studies of the head revealed dilated cortical veins in the left sylvian fissure (Fig. 19.9b). Cerebral digital subtraction angiography revealed the presence of a high-grade left CS-DAVF supplied by the bilateral external carotid branches as well as the left ICA feeders (Fig. 19.10a). Drainage from the left CS was solely through the left SMCV into engorged perisylvian cortical veins without involvement of the right CS (Fig. 19.10b). Venous access to the lesion was determined to be challenging. Subsequently, transarterial embolization was attempted and was unsuccessful due to migration of Onyx into the intraorbital left lacrimal artery. Following this, we elected to perform a left orbitozygomatic craniotomy to provide exposure to the anterior left middle cranial fossa for direct access to the SMCV (Fig. 19.11a). The left

SMCV was then punctured with a 21-gauge micropuncture needle (Fig. 19.11b). The microcatheter was navigated over a microguidewire into the CS under fluoroscopic guidance (Figs. 19.12 and 19.13a). 19 detachable coils were then deployed resulting in the complete occlusion of the fistula (Fig. 19.13). Postoperative angiogram 1 week later confirmed complete obliteration of the fistula. At 6 months follow-up, patient had no neurological deficits and no cognitive dysfunction.

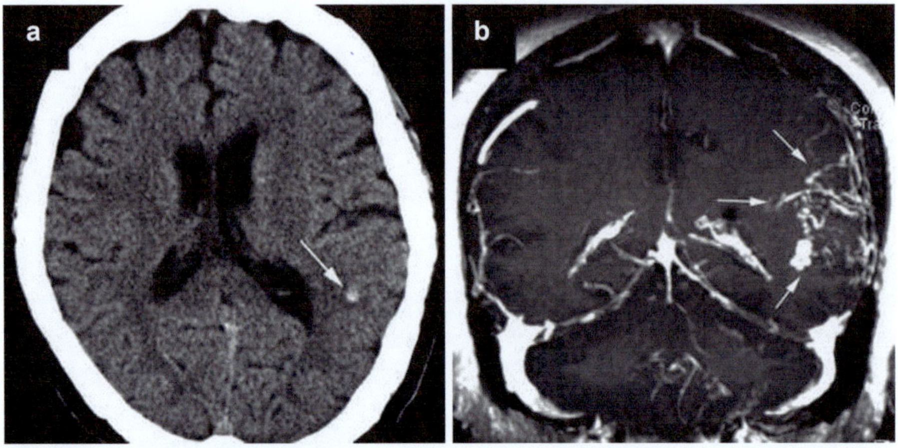

Fig. 19.9 (**a**) Axial head computed tomography without contrast revealing a small left temporoparietal hemorrhage. (**b**) Coronal magnetic resonance imaging (MRI) demonstrating dilated cortical veins in the left perisylvian region

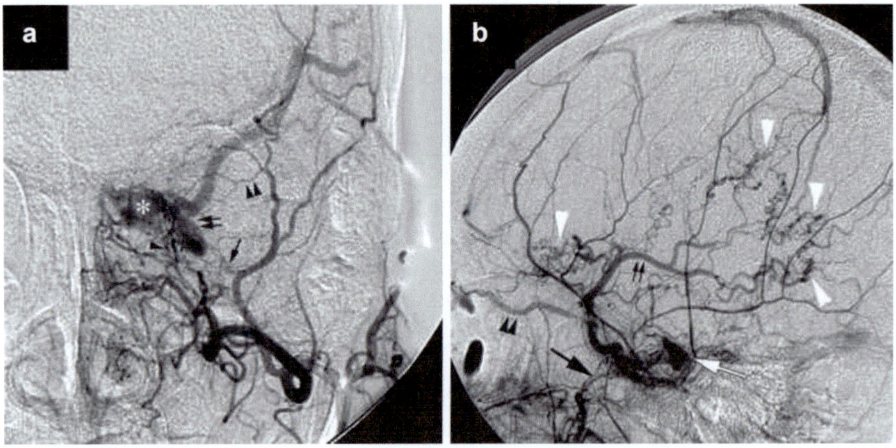

Fig. 19.10 (**a**) AP view of left external carotid digital subtraction angiogram revealing arterial feeders from the middle meningeal cavernous, represented by *arrows*, and recurrent branches, represented by *double arrowheads*, and the artery of the foramen rotundum (FAO), represented by an *arrowhead*, to a fistula centered on the left cavernous sinus (CS), represented by an *asterisk*, draining into the superficial middle cerebral vein (*SMCV*), represented by *double arrows*. (**b**) A lateral view revealing the posterior compartmentalization of the CS fistula, represented by *white arrow*, with FAO feeder, represented by a *black arrow*, and drainage through both the superior ophthalmic vein, represented by *double arrowheads*, and the SMCV, represented by *double arrows*. The *white arrowheads* represent the dilated cortical veins in the perisylvian region

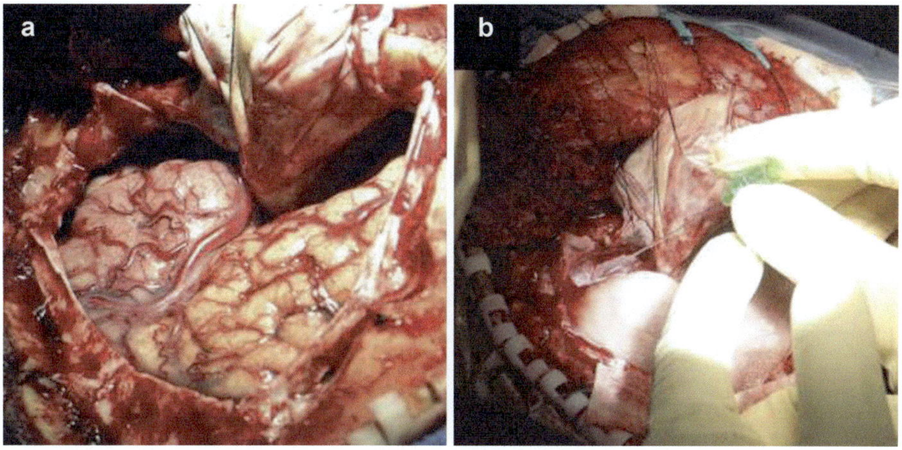

Fig. 19.11 (**a**) Exposure of the arterialized superficial middle cerebral vein (SMCV) and cortical venous tributaries after orbitozygomatic craniotomy. (**b**) Micropuncture of the SMCV

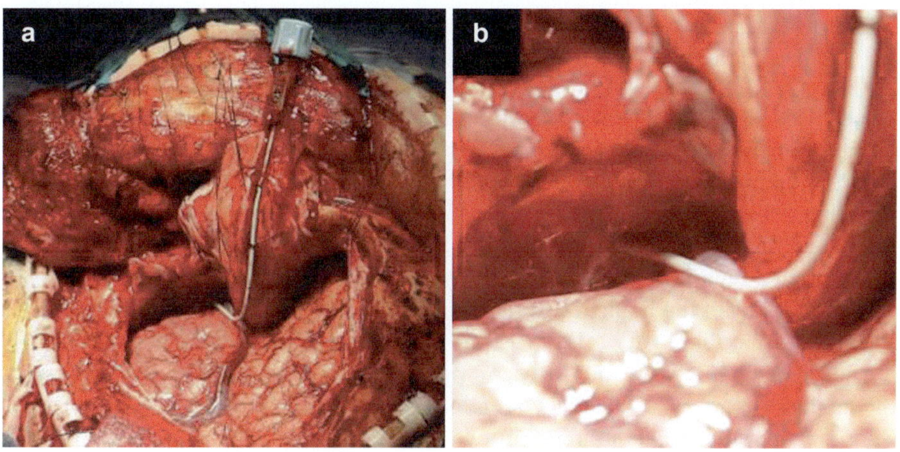

Fig. 19.12 (**a**) 4-French (outer diameter) micropuncture sheath positioned in superficial middle cerebral vein (SMCV). (**b**) Puncture site of sheath into the SMCV

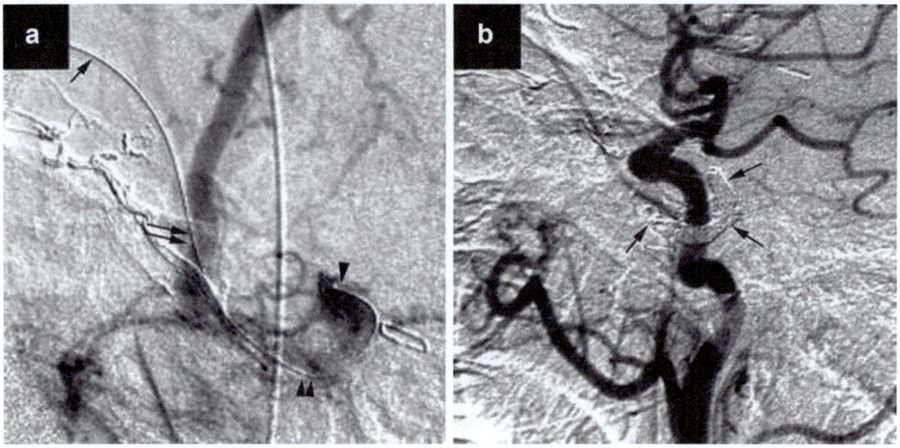

Fig. 19.13 (**a**) Lateral view of intraoperative left external carotid artery DSA showing the microcatheter, represented by an *arrow*, going into the superficial middle cerebral vein (SMCV), represented by *double arrow,* and treading across the floor of the middle cranial fossa, represented by *double arrowhead,* with its tip located in the cavernous compartment, represented by *arrowhead.* (**b**) *Left* carotid angiogram showing the endovascular coils occluding the cavernous sinus (Source: Hurley et al. [70])

Case 19.4 Microsurgical Treatment of an Ethmoidal Dural Fistula: Three-Dimensional Illustration

A 74-year-old male patient presents with memory loss. Magnetic resonance imaging revealed a left high-grade ethmoidal fistula. CTA demonstrated a large vessel emanating from the anterior left skull base with its vein connecting to the superior sagittal vein anteriorly (Fig. 19.14a). Cerebral angiogram revealed the fistula's supply to be from the branches of the ethmoidal artery and meningeal branches of the internal maxillary artery (Fig. 19.14b). The draining on the other hand is through the superior sagittal vein anteriorly. An open procedure was elected due to the risk of ophthalmic artery occlusion via endovascular treatment of ethmoidal fistulas. Subsequently, a bifrontal craniotomy was performed and occlusion of fistula was successfully executed (Fig. 19.15, Video Link 1). Postoperative angiogram revealed complete resolution of the fistula. On 1 month follow-up, patient had no neurological deficits and was able to fully resume his daily activities

Video Link 1: https://www.youtube.com/watch?v=CU5nQfv1BM4

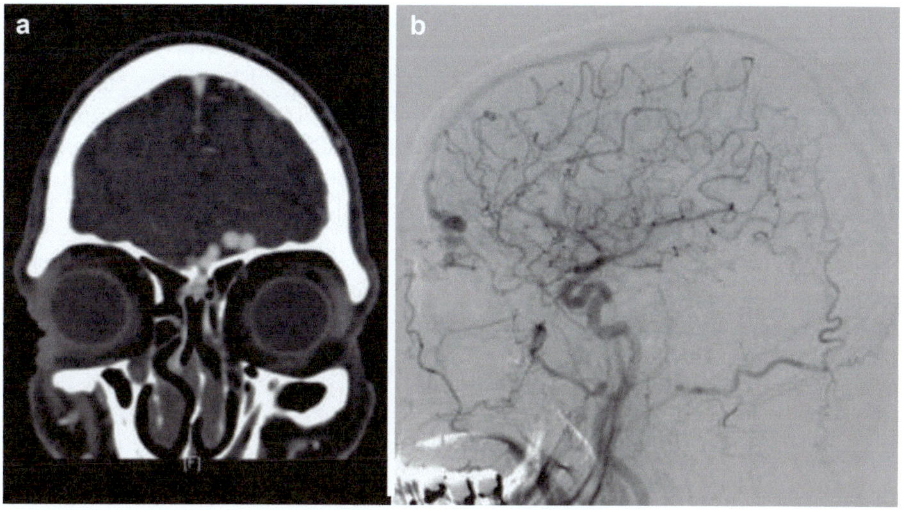

Fig. 19.14 (**a**) Computed tomography angiogram (CTA) and (**b**) digital subtraction angiogram of ethmoidal DAVF showing the large dilated draining vein

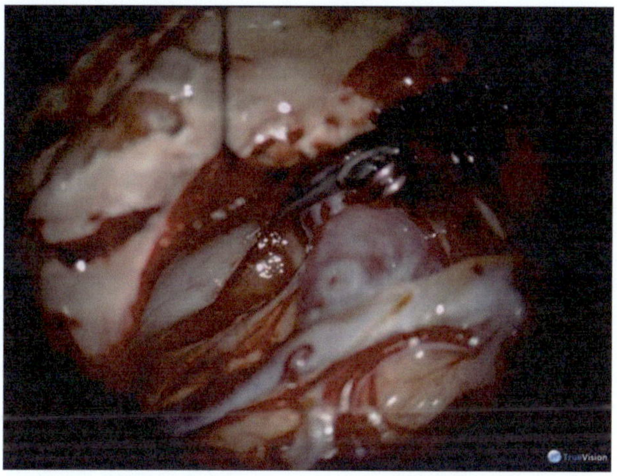

Fig. 19.15 Operative photograph following microsurgical disconnection of DAVF with an aneurysm clip at a site just distal to the exit of the large dilated draining vein just before ablation (Source: Aoun et al. [71])

Case 19.5 *Summary*: A 52-year-old female patient presents with bilateral proptosis and orbital chemosis. Angiography demonstrates bilateral mirror image Barrow type B cavernous sinus fistulas. The fistulas were draining through an ectatic superior ophthalmic vein with focal venous stenosis (Fig. 19.16). A transvenous approach was elected due to the presence of single draining veins from each side accessible through a transvenous approach. Coil-assisted Onyx embolization was carried out on both sides over two procedures with successful obliteration of the fistulas (Figs. 19.17, 19.18, and 19.19). The patient had complete symptom resolution.

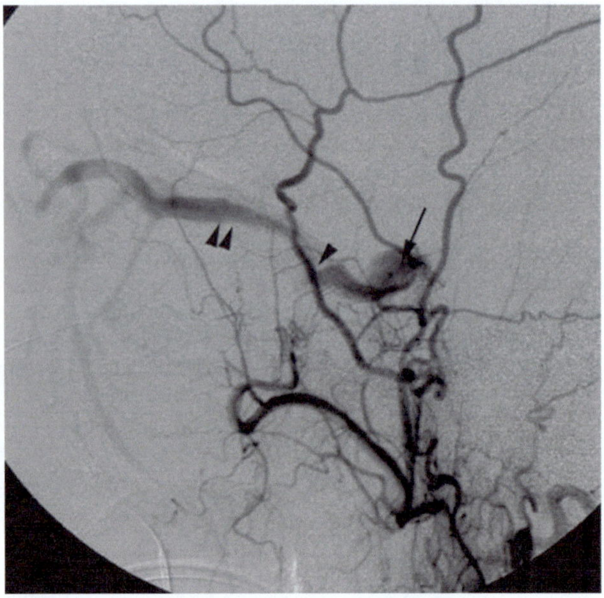

Fig. 19.16 DSA reveals a Barrow type D cavernous sinus fistula, represented by *arrow*, draining through an ectatic superior ophthalmic vein, represented by *double arrowhead*, with a focal venous stenosis, represented by *arrowhead*. Similarly on the contralateral side there was a mirror image fistula of the cavernous sinus (not shown). A transfemoral approach was utilized to navigate the external jugular, angular, and superior ophthalmic veins into the cavernous sinus

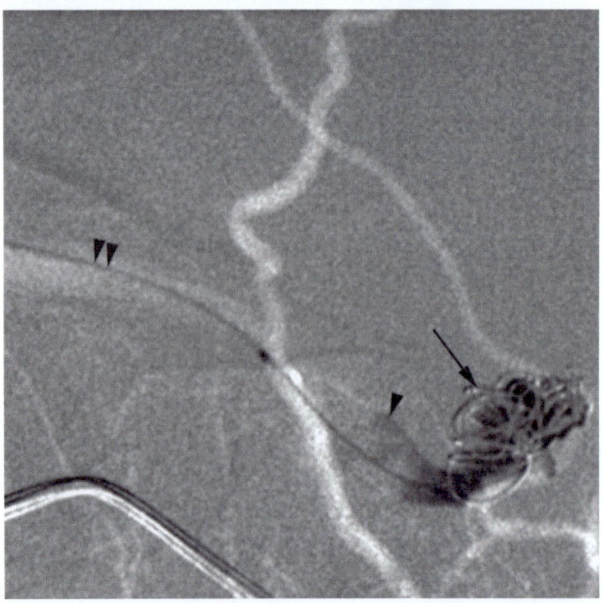

Fig. 19.17 After multiple coils were placed to slow down the flow, 3 cc of Onyx 34 was injected to fill the CS back into the posterior ophthalmic vein

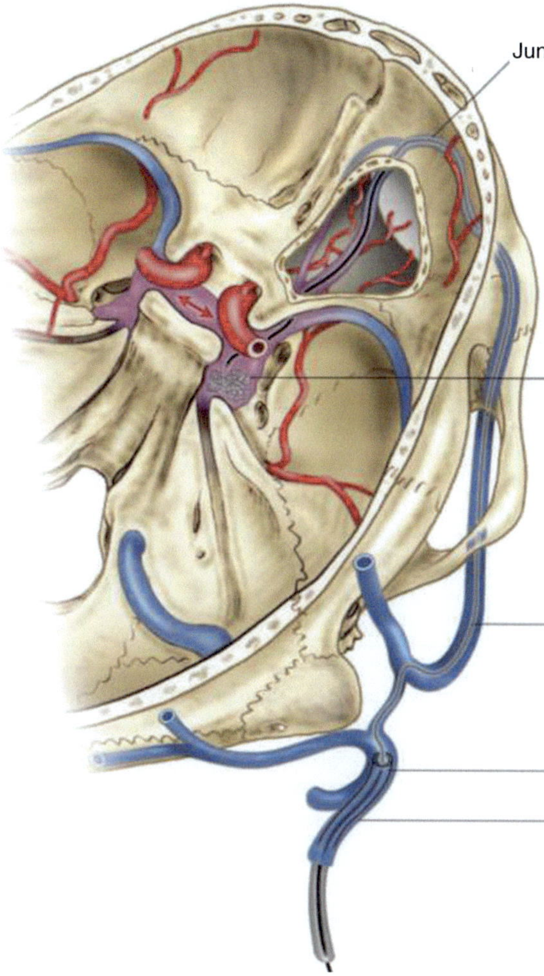

Fig. 19.18 The endovascular technique is rendered above. *CS* cavernous sinus, *EJV* external jugular vein, *SOV* superior ophthalmic vein. Both sides were managed via two elective procedures

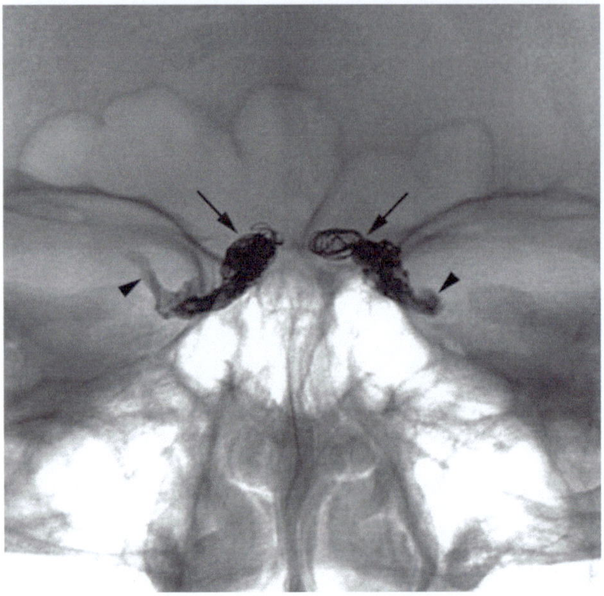

Fig. 19.19 The final appearance of the coils and Onyx is shown above. The *arrowheads* represent the Onyx and the *arrows* represent the coils (Source: Bendok et al. [20])

Conclusions

A comprehensive multidisciplinary evaluation of patients with DAVF is essential to guide best management practices. The decision of whether to observe or treat a fistula should be based on a detailed analysis of clinical and angiographic parameters of the DAVF. These include the presentation, location, and grade of the fistula. Accordingly, if it is decided to pursue treatment, the physician must create and implement an individualized plan based on three types of treatment modalities: endovascular embolization, microsurgery, and stereotactic radiosurgery. Each modality has certain specific strengths and limitations as described in the chapter. It is however fallacious to view the above three options in isolation or mutual exclusion. The ideal approach is an integrative multimodal management strategy that ensures the safety and efficiency of permanent occlusion of cranial dural fistulas.

References

1. Chaichana KL, Coon AL, Tamargo RJ, Huang J. Dural arteriovenous fistulas: epidemiology and clinical presentation. Neurosurg Clin N Am. 2012;23(1):7–13.
2. Newton TH, Cronqvist S. Involvement of dural arteries in intracranial arteriovenous malformations. Radiology. 1969;93(5):1071–8.
3. Piippo A, Niemela M, van Popta J, Kangasniemi M, Rinne J, Jaaskelainen JE, Hernesniemi J. Characteristics and long-term outcome of 251 patients with dural arteriovenous fistulas in a defined population. J Neurosurg. 2013;118(5):923–34.
4. Zipfel GJ, Shah MN, Refai D, Dacey Jr RG, Derdeyn CP. Cranial dural arteriovenous fistulas: modification of angiographic classification scales based on new natural history data. Neurosurg Focus. 2009;26(5):E14.

5. Brown Jr RD, Wiebers DO, Torner JC, O'Fallon WM. Incidence and prevalence of intracranial vascular malformations in Olmsted County, Minnesota, 1965 to 1992. Neurology. 1996;46(4):949–52.
6. Satomi J, Satoh K. Epidemiology and etiology of dural arteriovenous fistula. Brain Nerve. 2008;60(8):883–6.
7. Hacein-Bey L, Konstas AA, Pile-Spellman J. Natural history, current concepts, classification, factors impacting endovascular therapy, and pathophysiology of cerebral and spinal dural arteriovenous fistulas. Clin Neurol Neurosurg. 2014;121:64–75.
8. Awad IA, Little JR, Akrawi WP, Ahl J. Intracranial dural arteriovenous malformations: factors predisposing to an aggressive neurological course. J Neurosurg. 1990;72(6):839–50.
9. Brown R, Wiebers D, Nichols D. Intracranial dural arteriovenous malformations-a clinical, radiologic, and long-term follow-up-study. Stroke, Amer Heart Assoc 7272 Greenville Avenue, Dallas, TX 75231-4596. 1992.
10. Cognard C, Gobin YP, Pierot L, Bailly A-L, Houdart E, Casasco A, Chiras J, Merland J-J. Cerebral dural arteriovenous fistulas: clinical and angiographic correlation with a revised classification of venous drainage. Radiology. 1995;194(3):671–80.
11. Lasjaunias P, Chiu M, Ter Brugge K, Tolia A, Hurth M, Bernstein M. Neurological manifestations of intracranial dural arteriovenous malformations. J Neurosurg. 1986;64(5):724–30.
12. Davies MA, Ter Brugge K, Willinsky R, Wallace MC. The natural history and management of intracranial dural arteriovenous fistulae. Part 2: aggressive lesions. Interv Neuroradiol. 1997;3(4):303–11.
13. Kim MS, Han DH, Kwon OK, Oh CW, Han MH. Clinical characteristics of dural arteriovenous fistula. J Clin Neurosci Off J Neurosurg Soc Australas. 2002;9(2):147–55.
14. Cognard C, Casasco A, Toevi M, Houdart E, Chiras J, Merland JJ. Dural arteriovenous fistulas as a cause of intracranial hypertension due to impairment of cranial venous outflow. J Neurol Neurosurg Psychiatry. 1998;65(3):308–16.
15. Lagares A, Perez-Nunez A, Alday R, Ramos A, Campollo J, Lobato RD. Dural arteriovenous fistula presenting as brainstem ischaemia. Acta Neurochir. 2007;149(9):965–7; discussion 967.
16. Brown RD, Flemming KD, Meyer FB, Cloft HJ, Pollock BE, Link MJ. Natural history, evaluation, and management of intracranial vascular malformations. Mayo Clin Proc. 2005;80:269–81. Elsevier.
17. Houser O, Campbell J, Campbell R, Sundt Jr T. Arteriovenous malformation affecting the transverse dural venous sinus – an acquired lesion. Mayo Clin Proc. 1979;54:651–61.
18. McCormick W. "Pathology of vascular malformations of the brain". Intracranial arteriovenous malformations. Baltimore: Williams & Wilkins; 1984. p. 44–63.
19. Borden JA, Wu JK, Shucart WA. A proposed classification for spinal and cranial dural arteriovenous fistulous malformations and implications for treatment. J Neurosurg. 1995;82(2):166–79.
20. Bendok BR, Naidech AM, Walker MT, Batjer HH. Hemorrhagic and ischemic stroke. New York: Thieme; 2012.
21. Barrow DL, Spector RH, Braun IF, Landman JA, Tindall SC, Tindall GT. Classification and treatment of spontaneous carotid-cavernous sinus fistulas. J Neurosurg. 1985;62(2):248–56.
22. Hashiguchi A, Mimata C, Ichimura H, Morioka M, Kuratsu J. Venous aneurysm development associated with a dural arteriovenous fistula of the anterior cranial fossa with devastating hemorrhage – case report. Neurol Med Chir. 2007;47(2):70–3.
23. van Dijk JM, terBrugge KG, Willinsky RA, Wallace MC. Clinical course of cranial dural arteriovenous fistulas with long-term persistent cortical venous reflux. Stroke J Cereb Circ. 2002;33(5):1233–6.
24. Brown Jr RD, Wiebers DO, Nichols DA. Intracranial dural arteriovenous fistulae: angiographic predictors of intracranial hemorrhage and clinical outcome in nonsurgical patients. J Neurosurg. 1994;81(4):531–8.
25. Satomi J, van Dijk JM, Terbrugge KG, Willinsky RA, Wallace MC. Benign cranial dural arteriovenous fistulas: outcome of conservative management based on the natural history of the lesion. J Neurosurg. 2002;97(4):767–70.

26. Bulters DO, Mathad N, Culliford D, Millar J, Sparrow OC. The natural history of cranial dural arteriovenous fistulae with cortical venous reflux—the significance of venous ectasia. Neurosurgery. 2012;70(2):312–9.
27. Willinsky R, Goyal M, terBrugge K, Montanera W. Tortuous, engorged pial veins in intracranial dural arteriovenous fistulas: correlations with presentation, location, and MR findings in 122 patients. AJNR Am J Neuroradiol. 1999;20(6):1031–6.
28. Davies M, Saleh J, Ter Brugge K, Willinsky R, Wallace M. The natural history and management of intracranial dural arteriovenous fistulae. Part 1: benign lesions. Interv Neuroradiol J Peritherapeutic Neuroradiol Surg Proced Relat Neurosci. 1997;3(4):295–302.
29. Davies MA, TerBrugge K, Willinsky R, Coyne T, Saleh J, Wallace MC. The validity of classification for the clinical presentation of intracranial dural arteriovenous fistulas. J Neurosurg. 1996;85(5):830–7.
30. Gross BA, Du R. The natural history of cerebral dural arteriovenous fistulae. Neurosurgery. 2012;71(3):594–603.
31. Kakarla UK, Deshmukh VR, Zabramski JM, Albuquerque FC, McDougall CG, Spetzler RF. Surgical treatment of high-risk intracranial dural arteriovenous fistulae: clinical outcomes and avoidance of complications. Neurosurgery. 2007;61(3):447–59.
32. Maimon S, Nossek E, Strauss I, Blumenthal D, Frolov V, Ram Z. Transarterial treatment with Onyx of intracranial dural arteriovenous fistula with cortical drainage in 17 patients. Am J Neuroradiol. 2011;32(11):2180–4.
33. Söderman M, Pavic L, Edner G, Holmin S, Andersson T. Natural history of dural arteriovenous shunts. Stroke. 2008;39(6):1735–9.
34. Strom RG, Botros JA, Refai D, Moran CJ, Cross III DT, Chicoine MR, Grubb Jr RL, Rich KM, Dacey Jr RG, Derdeyn CP. Cranial dural arteriovenous fistulae: asymptomatic cortical venous drainage portends less aggressive clinical course. Neurosurgery. 2009;64(2):241–8.
35. Shah MN, Botros JA, Pilgram TK, Moran CJ, Cross 3rd DT, Chicoine MR, Rich KM, Dacey Jr RG, Derdeyn CP, Zipfel GJ. Borden-Shucart type I dural arteriovenous fistulas: clinical course including risk of conversion to higher-grade fistulas. J Neurosurg. 2012;117(3):539–45.
36. Iryo Y, Hirai T, Kai Y, Nakamura M, Shigematsu Y, Kitajima M, Azuma M, Komi M, Morita K, Yamashita Y. Intracranial dural arteriovenous fistulas: evaluation with 3-T four-dimensional MR angiography using arterial spin labeling. Radiology. 2013;271(1):193–9.
37. Jabbour P, Tjoumakaris S, Chalouhi N, Randazzo C, Gonzalez LF, Dumont A, Rosenwasser R. Endovascular treatment of cerebral dural and pial arteriovenous fistulas. Neuroimaging Clin N Am. 2013;23(4):625–36.
38. Jang J, Schmitt P, Kim B-Y, Choi HS, Jung S-L, Ahn K-J, Kim I, Paek M, Kim B-S. Non-contrast-enhanced 4D MR angiography with STAR spin labeling and variable flip angle sampling: a feasibility study for the assessment of Dural Arteriovenous Fistula. Neuroradiology. 2014;56(4):305–14.
39. Youssef PP, Schuette AJ, Cawley CM, Barrow DL. Advances in surgical approaches to dural fistulas. Neurosurgery. 2014;74:S32–41.
40. Hu YC, Newman CB, Dashti SR, Albuquerque FC, McDougall CG. Cranial dural arteriovenous fistula: transarterial Onyx embolization experience and technical nuances. J Neurointerv Surg. 2011;3(1):5–13.
41. VanLandingham M, Fox B, Hoit D, Elijovich L, Arthur AS. Endovascular treatment of intracranial dural arteriovenous fistulas. Neurosurgery. 2014;74:S42–9.
42. Shi Z.-S, Loh Y, Gonzalez N, Tateshima S, Feng L, Jahan R, Duckwiler G, Viñuela F. Flow control techniques for Onyx embolization of intracranial dural arteriovenous fistulae. J Neurointerv Surg Neurintsurg. 2013;5(4):311–6.
43. Huo X, Li Y, Jiang C, Wu Z. Balloon-assisted endovascular treatment of intracranial dural arteriovenous fistulas. Turk Neurosurg. 2014;24(5):658–63.
44. Chiu AHY, Aw G, Wenderoth JD. Double-lumen arterial balloon catheter technique for Onyx embolization of dural arteriovenous fistulas: initial experience. J Neurointerv Surg. 2014;6(5):400–3.

45. Jagadeesan BD, Grigoryan M, Hassan AE, Grande AW, Tummala RP. Endovascular balloon-assisted embolization of intracranial and cervical arteriovenous malformations using dual-lumen coaxial balloon microcatheters and Onyx: initial experience. Neurosurgery. 2013;73:ons238–43.
46. Kirsch M, Liebig T, Kühne D, Henkes H. Endovascular management of dural arteriovenous fistulas of the transverse and sigmoid sinus in 150 patients. Neuroradiology. 2009;51(7):477–83.
47. Gonzalez LF, Chalouhi N, Jabbour P, Teufack S, Albuquerque FC, Spetzler RF. Rapid and progressive venous thrombosis after occlusion of high-flow arteriovenous fistula. World Neurosurg. 2013;80(6):e359–65.
48. Cognard C, Januel A, Silva N, Tall P. Endovascular treatment of intracranial dural arteriovenous fistulas with cortical venous drainage: new management using Onyx. Am J Neuroradiol. 2008;29(2):235–41.
49. Nogueira R, Dabus G, Rabinov J, Eskey C, Ogilvy C, Hirsch J, Pryor J. Preliminary experience with onyx embolization for the treatment of intracranial dural arteriovenous fistulas. Am J Neuroradiol. 2008;29(1):91–7.
50. Rangel-Castilla L, Barber SM, Klucznik R, Diaz O. Mid- and long-term outcomes of dural arteriovenous fistula endovascular management with Onyx. Experience of a single tertiary center. J Neurointerv Surg Neurintsurg. 2014;6(8):607–13.
51. Chandra R, Leslie-Mazwi T, Mehta B, Yoo A, Rabinov J, Pryor J, Hirsch J, Nogueira R. Transarterial Onyx embolization of cranial dural arteriovenous fistulas: long-term follow-up. Am J Neuroradiol. 2014;35(9):1793–7.
52. Adamczyk P, Amar AP, Mack WJ, Larsen DW. Recurrence of "cured" dural arteriovenous fistulas after Onyx embolization. Neurosurg Focus. 2012;32(5):E12.
53. Macdonald JHM, Millar JS, Barker C. Endovascular treatment of cranial dural arteriovenous fistulae: a single-centre, 14-year experience and the impact of Onyx on local practice. Neuroradiology. 2010;52(5):387–95.
54. Gross BA, Du R. Surgical treatment of high grade dural arteriovenous fistulae. J Clin Neurosci. 2013;20(11):1527–32.
55. Lawton MT, Sanchez-Mejia RO, Pham D, Tan J, Halbach VV. Tentorial dural arteriovenous fistulae: operative strategies and microsurgical results for six types. Neurosurgery. 2008;62(3):110–25.
56. Sundt Jr TM, Piepgras DG. The surgical approach to arteriovenous malformations of the lateral and sigmoid dural sinuses. J Neurosurg. 1983;59(1):32–9.
57. Tomak PR, Cloft HJ, Kaga A, Cawley CM, Dion J, Barrow DL. Evolution of the management of tentorial dural arteriovenous malformations. Neurosurgery. 2003;52(4):750–62.
58. Al-Mahfoudh R, Kirollos R, Mitchell P, Lee M, Nahser H, Javadpour M. Surgical disconnection of cortical venous reflux for high grade intracranial dural arteriovenous fistulas. World Neurosurg. 2014;83:652–6.
59. Ghobrial GM, Marchan E, Nair AK, Dumont AS, Tjoumakaris SI, Gonzalez LF, Rosenwasser RH, Jabbour P. Dural arteriovenous fistulas: a review of the literature and a presentation of a single institution's experience. World Neurosurg. 2013;80(1–2):94–102.
60. Natarajan SK, Ghodke B, Kim LJ, Hallam DK, Britz GW, Sekhar LN. Multimodality treatment of intracranial dural arteriovenous fistulas in the Onyx era: a single center experience. World Neurosurg. 2010;73(4):365–79.
61. Chalouhi N, Dumont AS, Tjoumakaris S, Gonzalez LF, Bilyk JR, Randazzo C, Hasan D, Dalyai RT, Rosenwasser R, Jabbour P. The superior ophthalmic vein approach for the treatment of carotid-cavernous fistulas: a novel technique using Onyx. Neurosurg Focus. 2012;32(5):E13.
62. Chaudhary N, Lownie SP, Bussière M, Pelz DM, Nicolle D. Transcortical venous approach for direct embolization of a cavernous sinus dural arteriovenous fistula: technical case report. Neurosurgery. 2012;70:onsE343–8.
63. Houdart E, Saint-Maurice J-P, Chapot R, Ditchfield A, Blanquet A, Lot G, Merland J-J. Transcranial approach for venous embolization of dural arteriovenous fistulas. J Neurosurg. 2002;97(2):280–6.

64. Wachter D, Hans F, Psychogios M-N, Knauth M, Rohde V. Microsurgery can cure most intracranial dural arteriovenous fistulae of the sinus and non-sinus type. Neurosurg Rev. 2011;34(3):337–45.
65. Pan DH, Lee CC, Wu HM, Chung WY, Yang HC, Lin CJ. Gamma knife radiosurgery for the management of intracranial dural arteriovenous fistulas. Acta Neurochir Suppl. 2013;116:113–9.
66. Chen C-J, Lee C-C, Ding D, Starke RM, Chivukula S, Yen C.-P, Moosa S, Xu Z, Pan DH.-C, Sheehan J. P. Stereotactic radiosurgery for intracranial dural arteriovenous fistulas: a systematic review. J Neurosurg. 2015;122(2):353–62.
67. Gross BA, Du R. The natural history of cerebral dural arteriovenous fistulae. Neurosurgery. 2012;71(3):594–602; discussion 602-3.
68. Sugrue PA, Hurley MC, Bendok BR, Surdell DL, Gottardi-Littell N, Futterer SF, Muro K, Batjer HH. High-grade dural arteriovenous fistula simulating a bilateral thalamic neoplasm. Clin Neurol Neurosurg. 2009;111(7):629–32. doi:10.1016/j.clineuro.2009.05.004. Epub 2009 May 31.
69. Dabus G, Bernstein RA, Hurley MC, Shaibani A, Bendok BR, Russell EJ. Reversal of diffusion restriction after embolization of dural arteriovenous fistula: case report. Neurosurgery. 2010;67(4):E1147–51. doi:10.1227/NEU.0b013e3181edadee; discussion E1151.
70. Hurley MC, Rahme RJ, Fishman AJ, Batjer HH, Bendok BR. Combined surgical and endovascular access of the superficial middle cerebral vein to occlude a high-grade cavernous dural arteriovenous fistula: case report. Neurosurgery. 2011;69(2):E475–81. doi:10.1227/NEU.0b013e3182192478; discussion E481–2.
71. Aoun SG, Shafizadeh SF, Bendok BR. Microsurgical treatment of an ethmoidal dural fistula: 3-dimensional illustration. Neurosurgery. 2012;71(1 Suppl Operative):3. doi:10.1227/NEU.0b013e318260518a.

Index

E. Veznedaroglu (ed.), *Controversies in Vascular Neurosurgery*,
DOI 10.1007/978-3-319-27315-0

D

E

MIX
Papier aus verantwortungsvollen Quellen
Paper from responsible sources
FSC® C105338

If you have any concerns about our products,
you can contact us on
ProductSafety@springernature.com

In case Publisher is established outside the EU,
the EU authorized representative is:
Springer Nature Customer Service Center GmbH
Europaplatz 3, 69115 Heidelberg, Germany

Printed by Libri Plureos GmbH
in Hamburg, Germany